Musculoskeletal, Sports, and Occupational Medicine

Rehabilitation Medicine Quick Reference

Ralph M. Buschbacher, MD

Series Editor

Professor, Department of Physical Medicine and Rehabilitation
Indiana University School of Medicine
Indianapolis, Indiana

▨ Spine

Andre N. Panagos

▨ Spinal Cord Injury

Thomas N. Bryce

▨ Traumatic Brain Injury

David X. Cifu and Deborah Caruso

▨ Pediatrics

Maureen R. Nelson

▨ Musculoskeletal, Sports, and Occupational Medicine

William Micheo

Forthcoming Volumes in the Series

Neuromuscular/EMG

Prosthetics

Stroke

Musculoskeletal, Sports, and Occupational Medicine

Rehabilitation Medicine Quick Reference

William Micheo, MD

Professor and Chair
Department of Physical Medicine and Rehabilitation and Sports Medicine
University of Puerto Rico School of Medicine
San Juan, Puerto Rico

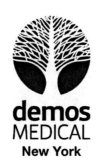

demos
MEDICAL
New York

Acquisitions Editor: Beth Barry
Cover Design: Steven Pisano
Compositor: Newgen Imaging Systems
Printer: Bang Printing
Visit our Web site at www.demosmedpub.com

Medicine is an ever-changing science. Research and clinical experience are continually
expanding our knowledge, in particular our understanding of proper treatment and drug
therapy. The authors, editors, and publisher have made every effort to ensure that all
information in this book is in accordance with the state of knowledge at the time of production
of the book. Nevertheless, the authors, editors, and publisher are not responsible for errors or
omissions or for any consequences from application of the information in this book and make
no warranty, express or implied, with respect to the contents of the publication. Every reader
should examine carefully the package inserts accompanying each drug and should carefully
check whether the dosage schedules mentioned therein or the contraindications stated by the
manufacturer differ from the statements made in this book. Such examination is particularly
important with drugs that are either rarely used or have been newly released on the market.

Library of Congress Cataloging-in-Publication Data

Musculoskeletal, sports, and occupational medicine / [edited by] William Micheo.
        p. ; cm.—(Rehabilitation medicine quick reference)
   Includes bibliographical references and index.
   ISBN 978-1-933864-49-5
   1. Musculoskeletal system—Wounds and injuries—Treatment—Handbooks, manuals, etc.
2. Sports injuries—Treatment—Handbooks, manuals, etc. 3. Musculoskeletal system—
Diseases—Rehabilitation—Handbooks, manuals, etc.
I. Micheo, William. II. Series: Rehabilitation medicine quick reference.
   [DNLM: 1. Musculoskeletal System—injuries—Handbooks. 2. Athletic Injuries—
therapy—Handbooks. 3. Musculoskeletal Diseases—therapy—Handbooks.
4. Occupational Diseases—therapy—Handbooks. WE 39]
   RD732.5.M87 2011
   617.4'7044—dc22   2010033515

Special discounts on bulk quantities of Demos Medical Publishing books are available
to corporations, professional associations, pharmaceutical companies, health care
organizations, and other qualifying groups. For details, please contact:

Special Sales Department
Demos Medical Publishing
11 West 42nd Street, 15th Floor
New York, NY 10036
Phone: 800-532-8663 or 212-683-0072
Fax: 212-941-7842
Email: rsantana@demosmedpub.com

Made in the United States of America

10 11 12 13   5 4 3 2 1

To my wife Vanessa and my children Javier and Francisco,
who encourage me to teach and write, support me in all I do,
and motivate me to continue to improve both as an individual and a professional.

To my parents William and Awilda,
who have always guided me and helped me become who I am today.

To my mentors, who set an example for me to follow.

Contents

Evaluation

Conditions

The Rehabilitation Medicine Quick Reference (RMQR) series is dedicated to the busy clinician. While we all strive to keep up with the latest medical knowledge, there are many times when things come up in our daily practices that we need to look up. Even more importantly…look up quickly.

Those aren't the times to do a complete literature search, or to read a detailed chapter, or review an article. We just need to get a quick grasp of a topic that we may not see routinely, or just to refresh our memory. Sometimes a subject comes up that is outside our usual scope of practice, but that may still impact our care. It is for such moments that this series has been created.

Whether you need to quickly look up what a Tarlov cyst is, or you need to read about a neurorehabilitation complication or treatment, RMQR has you covered.

RMQR is designed to include the most common problems found in a busy practice, but also a lot of the less common ones as well.

I was extremely lucky to have been able to assemble an absolutely fantastic group of editors. They in turn have harnessed an excellent set of authors. So what we have in this series is, I hope and believe, a tremendous reference set to be used often in daily clinical practice. As series editor, I have, of course, been privy to these books before actual publication. I can tell you that I have already started to rely on them in my clinic—often. They have helped me become more efficient in practice.

Each chapter is organized into succinct facts, presented in a bullet point style. The chapters are set up in the same way throughout all of the volumes in the series, so once you get used to the format, it is incredibly easy to look things up.

And while the focus of the RMQR series is, of course, rehabilitation medicine, the clinical applications are much broader.

I hope that each reader grows to appreciate the RMQR series as much as I have. I congratulate a fine group of editors and authors on creating readable and useful texts.

Ralph M. Buschbacher, MD

Preface

The field of physical medicine and rehabilitation continues to evolve, and the knowledge required to deliver quality care continues to expand. Busy practitioners, residents in training, and specialists in related areas of medicine require clinical information that is up-to-date, relevant to their practice, and allows them to provide the best treatment possible for their patients.

This volume of the Rehabilitation Medicine Quick Reference series covers Musculoskeletal, Sports, and Occupational Medicine topics that are commonly seen in our clinical practices. Our goal is to provide the reader with clear, concise, and accurate information that will allow them to better serve their patients. We have contributions from an outstanding set of authors, who have done an excellent job of providing practical clinical knowledge in a format that allows the busy clinician quick access to this information. Each chapter contains specific sections that cover epidemiology, clinical presentation, diagnosis, and patient management including medical treatment, surgery, and rehabilitation of acute and chronic musculoskeletal conditions. The chapters are organized in alphabetical order so that the reader can rapidly find the topic they want to review, making this book a good reference to have in the office or clinic.

Working on a project such as this book can be a challenge (because of the work required to make sure the content is accurate and up-to-date, written in an understandable manner, and relevant to our daily practice), however, one that I am glad we accepted. The end product is one that we are proud of, and one we think will be useful to the clinician caring for athletes, injured workers, and individuals of any age with musculoskeletal injury.

William Micheo, MD

Acknowledgments

Special thanks to Beliza Rohena; without her help this project would not have been completed. In addition, I would like to thank Hilda Camacho, Minerva Abreu, and the University of Puerto Rico, Physical Medicine and Rehabilitation and Division of Sports Medicine staff, for their assistance with this book. Finally, I would like to thank Amarilys Irizarry, our medical illustrator, for her great work.

William Alemany, MD
Department of Gynecology
Hospital HIMA-San Pablo
Bayamon, Puerto Rico

Roxanna Amill, MD
Physical Medicine and Rehabilitation
Residency Training Program
University of Puerto Rico School of Medicine
San Juan, Puerto Rico

Eduardo Amy, MD
Assistant Professor
Department of Physical Medicine and Rehabilitation
   and Sports Medicine
University of Puerto Rico School of Medicine
San Juan, Puerto Rico

Luis Baerga, MD
Assistant Professor
Department of Physical Medicine and Rehabilitation
   and Sports Medicine
University of Puerto Rico School of Medicine
San Juan, Puerto Rico

José A. Báez, MD, FAAPMR
Assistant Professor
Department of Physical Medicine and Rehabilitation and
   Sports Medicine
University of Puerto Rico School of Medicine
San Juan, Puerto Rico

Dave Bagnall, MD
Assistant Professor
Department of Rehabilitation Medicine
State University of New York, Buffalo
Buffalo, New York
Adjunct Clinical Assistant Professor
New York College of Osteopathic Medicine
Glen Head, New York

Zach Beresford, MD
Clinical Instructor
Division of Physical Medicine and Rehabilitation
University of Utah
Salt Lake City, Utah

Jeffrey S. Brault, DO
Assistant Professor
Department of Physical Medicine and Rehabilitation
Mayo Clinic
Rochester, Minnesota

Derek S. Buck, MD, DC
Resident Physician
Department of Physical Medicine and Rehabilitation
University of Arkansas for Medical Sciences
Little Rock, Arkansas

Ralph Buschbacher, MD
Professor of Clinical Physical Medicine/Rehabilitation
Department of Physical Medicine and Rehabilitation
Indiana University School of Medicine
Indianapolis, Indiana

Kevin Carneiro, DO
Assistant Professor
Department of Physical Medicine and Rehabilitation
University of North Carolina
Chapel Hill, North Carolina

David A. Cassius, MD
Physical Medicine and Rehabilitation Clinic
Seattle, Washington

Anne M. Chicorelli, DO, MPH
Orthopedic Pediatric Sports Medicine Fellow
Department of Sports Medicine
Children's Hospital of Boston
Director
Division of Sports Medicine
Children's Hospital of Boston
Clinical Professor of Orthopaedic Surgery
Harvard Medical School
Boston, Massachusetts

Gary P. Chimes, MD, PhD
Assistant Professor
Fellowship Director, Musculoskeletal Sports and
   Spine Fellowship
Department of Physical Medicine and Rehabilitation
University of Pittsburgh Medical Center
Pittsburgh, Pennsylvania

Larry H. Chou, MD
Medical Director
Sports and Spine Rehabilitation Division
Premier Orthopaedic and Sports Medicine
    Associates, LLC
Havertown, Pennsylvania
Clinical Assistant Professor
Department of Physical Medicine and Rehabilitation
University of Pennsylvania School of Medicine
Philadelphia, Pennsylvania

John C. Cianca, MD
Adjunct Associate Professor
Department of Physical Medicine and
    Rehabilitation
Baylor College of Medicine
Houston, Texas

Kenneth Cintrón, MD
Foot and Ankle Specialist
Damas Hospital
Ponce, Puerto Rico

Ana V. Cintrón-Rodríguez, MD, FAAPMR
Assistant Chief, Physical Medicine and Rehabilitation
Residency Program Director
Department of Physical Medicine and Rehabilitation
VA Caribbean Healthcare System
Assistant Professor
Department of Physical Medicine and Rehabilitation and
    Sports Medicine
University of Puerto Rico School of Medicine
San Juan, Puerto Rico

Ricardo E. Colberg, MD
Resident
University of Puerto Rico School of Medicine
San Juan, Puerto Rico

José Correa, MD
Assistant Professor
Department of Physical Medicine and Rehabilitation
    and Sports Medicine
University of Puerto Rico School of Medicine
San Juan, Puerto Rico

Maricarmen Cruz-Jimenez, MD
Associate Chief of Staff for Education
University of Puerto Rico School of Medicine
San Juan, Puerto Rico

Shashank J. Dave, DO
Department of Physical Medicine and Rehabilitation
Indiana University School of Medicine
Indianapolis, Indiana

Efrain Deliz, MD
Attending Physician
Department of Orthopedic Surgery
VA Caribbean Healthcare Center
San Juan, Puerto Rico

Sheila A. Dugan, MD
Department of Physical Medicine and Rehabilitation
Rush University Medical Center
Chicago, Illinois

Ignacio Echenique, MD
Associate Professor Surgery, Ad Hon
University of Puerto Rico School of Medicine
San Juan, Puerto Rico

Sebastian Edtinger, MD
Associate Professor
Department of Physical Medicine and Rehabilitation
Paracelsus Medical University
Salzburg, Austria

Jonathan T. Finnoff, DO
Assistant Professor
Department of Physical Medicine and Rehabilitation
Mayo Clinic
Rochester, Minnesota

Tiffany C.K. Forman, MD
Assistant Professor
Division of Sports Medicine
Department of Family Medicine and Community Health
John A. Burns School of Medicine
Honolulu, Hawaii

Michael Fredericson, MD, FACSM
Professor and Director, Physical Medicine and Rehabilitation
Sports Medicine
Department of Orthopedic Surgery/Physical Medicine
    and Rehabilitation
Stanford University School of Medicine
Stanford, California

Walter R. Frontera, MD, PhD
Dean
University of Puerto Rico School of Medicine
San Juan, Puerto Rico

Michael Furman, MD, MS
Fellowship Program Director
Spine and Sports Medicine Fellowship Program
Orthopedic and Spine Specialists
York, Pennsylvania
Clinical Assistant Professor
Department of Physical Medicine and Rehabilitation
Temple University School of Medicine
Philadelphia, Pennsylvania

Manuel Garcia-Ariz, MD
Chairman and Program Director
Orthopaedic Surgery Training Program
University of Puerto Rico School of Medicine
San Juan, Puerto Rico

Beatriz García-Cardona, MD
Department of Surgery/Orthopaedics
University of Puerto Rico School of Medicine
San Juan, Puerto Rico

Steve Geringer, MD
Professor
Department of Physical Medicine and Rehabilitation
Wayne State University
Detroit, Michigan

Steve Gnatz, MD
Department of Orthopaedics and Rehabilitation
Loyola University Medical Center
Maywood, Illinois

Juan A. González, MD
Director
Emergency Medicine Residency Training Program
University of Puerto Rico School of Medicine
San Juan, Puerto Rico

Ari C. Greis, DO
Clinical Instructor
Department of Physical Medicine and Rehabilitation
The Rothman Institute
Thomas Jefferson University
Philadelphia, Pennsylvania

Michael J. Gruba, MD
Resident
Department of Physical Medicine and Rehabilitation
Mayo Clinic
Rochester, Minnesota

Albert Gunjan Singh, MD
Senior Resident
Department of Physical Medicine and Rehabilitation
University of Indiana
Indianapolis, Indiana

Jonathan S. Halperin, MD
Chief, Physical Medicine and Rehabilitation
Sharp Rees Stealy Medical Group
Voluntary Clinical Faculty
Department of Orthopedics and Rehabilitation
University of California San Diego School of
    Medicine
San Diego, California

Andrew J. Haig, MD
Department of Physical Medicine and Rehabilitation
University of Michigan
Ann Arbor, Michigan

Mark Harrast, MD
Clinical Associate Professor
Department of Rehabilitation Medicine, Orthopaedics, and
    Sports Medicine
University of Washington
Seattle, Washington

Phillip T. Henning, DO
Clinical Instructor
Department of Physical Medicine and Rehabilitation
University of Michigan
Ann Arbor, Michigan

Michael Henrie, DO
Visiting Instructor
Division of Physical Medicine and Rehabilitation
University of Utah
Salt Lake City, Utah

Liza M. Hernández-González, MD
Staff Physician
Department of Physical Medicine and Rehabilitation
VA Caribbean Healthcare System
Associate Professor-Ad Honorem
Department of Physical Medicine and Rehabilitation
    and Sports Medicine
University of Puerto Rico School of Medicine
San Juan, Puerto Rico

Collado Herve, MD
Assistant Professor
Department of Physical Medicine and Rehabilitation
    and Sport Medicine
Public Hospital of Marseille
Marseille University School of Medicine
Phocea Medical Center
Marseille, France

Anne Z. Hoch, DO
Professor
Department of Physical Medicine and Rehabilitation
Women's Sports Medicine Program/Sports Medicine Center
Department of Orthopaedic Surgery
Medical College of Wisconsin
Milwaukee, Wisconsin

Devyani Hunt, MD
Assistant Professor, Physical Medicine and Rehabilitation
Department of Orthopaedic Surgery and Neurology
Washington University School of Medicine
St. Louis, Missouri

Marta Imamura, MD, PhD
Department of Physical Medicine and
   Rehabilitation
University of São Paulo School of Medicine
São Paulo, Brazil

Rui Imamura, MD, PhD
Professor of Otolaryngology
University of São Paulo School of Medicine
São Paulo, Brazil

Satiko Tomikawa Imamura, MD, PhD
Division of Rehabilitation Medicine
Hospital das Clínicas
University of São Paulo School of Medicine
São Paulo, Brazil

Gerald Isenberg, MD, FACS, FACRS
Program Director, President
Colorectal Surgery Residency
Thomas Jefferson University Hospital
Director, Undergraduate Education
Associate Professor of Surgery
Department of Surgery
Jefferson Medical College
Philadelphia, Pennsylvania

Mimi D. Johnson, MD
Clinical Associate Professor
Department of Pediatrics
University of Washington
Seattle, Washington

Rob Johnson, MD
Professor
Family Medicine and Community Health
University of Minnesota
Director
Primary Care Sports Medicine Fellowship Program
Hennepin County Medical Center
Minneapolis, Minnesota

David J. Kennedy, MD
Sports and Spine Fellow
Rehabilitation Institute of Chicago
Chicago, Illinois

Brian J. Krabak, MD, MBA
Program Director, Sports Rehabilitation
   Fellowship
Assistant Professor of Physical Medicine and
   Rehabilitation
Assistant Professor of Orthopaedic Surgery
Johns Hopkins Hospital
Baltimore, Maryland

Christine Lawless, MD, MBA
Associate Professor
President Sports Cardiology Consultants LLC
Department of Cardiology
University of Chicago
Chicago, Illinois

Paul H. Lento, MD
Associate Professor
Department of Physical Medicine and Rehabilitation
Temple University School of Medicine
Philadelphia, Pennsylvania

Carmen E. López-Acevedo, MD
Professor and Associate Director
Department of Physical Medicine and Rehabilitation and
   Sports Medicine
University of Puerto Rico School of Medicine
San Juan, Puerto Rico

Francisco M. López-González, MD, FAAOS
Associate Professor
Department of Orthopedics
University of Puerto Rico School of Medicine
San Juan, Puerto Rico

Stacy L. Lynch, MD
Women's Sports Medicine Fellow
Instructor
Department of Orthopaedic Surgery
Medical College of Wisconsin
Milwaukee, Wisconsin

John MacKnight, MD
Associate Professor, Clinical Internal Medicine and
   Orthopaedic Surgery
Co-Medical Director for Sports Medicine
Primary Care Team Physician
University of Virginia
Charlottesville, Virginia

Eric Magrum, PT
Senior Physical Therapist
University of Virginia-Healthsouth Physical Therapy
Charlottesville, Virginia

Gerald Malanga, MD
Associate Professor
Department of Physical Medicine and Rehabilitation
New Jersey Medical School
Newark, New Jersey

Carmen J. Martínez-Martínez, MD
Emergency Medicine Resident
Emergency Medicine Department
University of Puerto Rico School of Medicine
San Juan, Puerto Rico

Julio A. Martínez-Silvestrini, MD
Medical Director, Outpatient Physical Medicine and
 Rehabilitation Practice
Baystate Physical Medicine and Rehabilitation
Springfield, Massachusetts

Lyle Micheli, MD
Director
Sports Medicine Fellowship Program
Division of Sports Medicine
Department of Orthopaedic Surgery
Children's Hospital
O'Donnell Professor and Clinical Professor
Harvard Medical School
Boston, Massachusetts

William Micheo, MD
Professor and Chair
Department of Physical Medicine and Rehabilitation
 and Sports Medicine
University of Puerto Rico School of Medicine
San Juan, Puerto Rico

Leslie Milne, MD
Emergency Department
Massachusetts General Hospital
Department of Sports Medicine
Children's Hospital Boston
Boston, Massachusetts

Gerardo E. Miranda, MD
Chief Resident
Department of Physical Medicine and Rehabilitation
University of Puerto Rico School of Medicine
San Juan, Puerto Rico

Omar Morales-Abella, MD
Orthopaedic Resident
Department of Orthopaedics
University of Puerto Rico School of Medicine
Trujillo Alto, Puerto Rico

Eduardo Nadal, MD
Resident
Physical Medicine and Rehabilitation Residency Program
VA Caribbean Healthcare System
San Juan, Puerto Rico

Andrew W. Nichols, MD
Professor and Chief, Division of Sports Medicine
Department of Family Medicine and Community Health
John A. Burns School of Medicine
Head Team Physician
Athletics Department
University of Hawaii at Manoa
Honolulu, Hawaii

Maureen Noh, MD
Fellow, Spine and Musculoskeletal Medicine
Department of Orthopaedics and Rehabilitation
University of Florida
Gainesville, Florida

María A. Ocasio-Silva, MD, FAAPMR
Assistant Professor
Pediatric Rehabilitation
Children's Hospital of Wisconsin
Medical College of Wisconsin
Milwaukee, Wisconsin

Antonio Otero-López, MD
Assistant Professor
Department of Orthopaedics
University of Puerto Rico School of Medicine
San Juan, Puerto Rico

Francisco J. Otero-López, MD
Assistant Professor
Department of Orthopaedics
University of Puerto Rico School of Medicine
San Juan, Puerto Rico

Leonardo Pirillo, MD
Resident
Department of Physical Medicine and Rehabilitation
 and Sports Medicine
University of Puerto Rico School of Medicine
San Juan, Puerto Rico

Heidi Prather, DO
Associate Professor, Physical Medicine and Rehabilitation
Department of Orthopaedic Surgery and Neurology
Washington University School of Medicine
St. Louis, Missouri

Joel Press, MD
Reva and David Logan Distinguished Chair of
 Musculoskeletal Rehabilitation
Professor, Physical Medicine and Rehabilitation
Feinberg School of Medicine
Northwestern University
Medical Director, Spine and Sports Rehabilitation Centers
Department of Physical Medicine and Rehabilitation
Rehabilitation Institute of Chicago
Chicago, Illinois

Edwardo Ramos-Cortes, MD
Associate Professor
Department of Physical Medicine and Rehabilition
 and Sports Medicine
University of Puerto Rico School of Medicine
San Juan, Puerto Rico

Per Renstrom, MD, PhD
Professor Emeritus
Karolinska Institute
Stockholm, Sweden

Joshua D. Rittenberg, MD
Department of Physical Medicine and Rehabilitation
Kaiser Permanente East Bay
Oakland, California

Carlos Rivera, MD
Physician
Department of Physical Medicine and Rehabilitation
Campbell Clinic
Collierville, Tennessee

Harry Alverio Rodriguez, MD
Resident
Department of Physical Rehabilitation and Sport Medicine
University of Puerto Rico School of Medicine
Trujillo Alto, Puerto Rico

Rebecca Rodriguez-Negrón, MD, DABFM
Associate Professor and Program Director
Family Medicine Residency Program
Department of Family Medicine
University of Puerto Rico School of Medicine
Loíza, Puerto Rico

Marc Safran, MD
Professor, Orthopaedic Surgery
Associate Director, Sports Medicine
Stanford University
Stanford, California

Thomas Savadove, MD, MPH
Attending Physician
Department of Physical Medicine and Rehabilitation
Abington Memorial Hospital
Abington Rehabilitation Associates
Abington, Pennsylvania

Jay Smith, MD
Professor of Physical Medicine and Rehabilitation
Departments of Physical Medicine and Rehabilitation, and
  Radiology
Mayo Clinic
Rochester, Minnesota

Joanne Snow, MD
Fellow
Department of Pediatric Rehabilitation
Medical College of Wisconsin
Children's Hospital of Wisconsin
Milwaukee, Wisconsin

Antonio Soler, MD
Associate Professor
Department of Orthopedics
University of Puerto Rico School of Medicine
San Juan, Puerto Rico

David A. Soto-Quijano, MD, FAAPMR
Staff Physician
Department of Physical Medicine and Rehabilitation Service
VA Caribbean Healthcare System
Associate Professor-Ad Honorem
Department of Physical Medicine and Rehabilitation
  and Sports Medicine
University of Puerto Rico School of Medicine
San Juan, Puerto Rico

Channarayapatna R. Sridhara, MD
Director
Moss Rehabilitation Electrodiagnostic Center
Elkins Park, Pennsylvania
Clinical Professor
Department of Rehabilitation Medicine
Jefferson Medical College
Philadelphia, Pennsylvania

Christopher J. Standaert, MD
Clinical Associate Professor
Departments of Rehabilitation Medicine, Orthopaedics and
  Sports Medicine, and Neurological Surgery
University of Washington
Seattle, Washington

William Sullivan, MD
Department of Physical Medicine and Rehabilitation
University of Colorado Denver School of Medicine
Denver, Colorado

Jayson Takata, MD
Pacific Physical Medicine Associates
Honolulu, Hawaii

Joshua A. Thomas, DO, MBA
Premier Orthopedics and Sports Medicine
One Medical Center Boulevard
Chester, Pennsylvania

Matthew C. Thompson, MD
Primary Care Sports Medicine Fellow
Department of Orthopedic Surgery
Medical College of Wisconsin
Milwaukee, Wisconsin

Trevin Thurman, MD
Attending Physician
Argires, Becker, & Westphal
Lancaster, Pennsylvania

Margarita Tolentino, MD
Staff Physician
From Pain to Wellness, LLC
Oakbrook Terrace, Illinois
Faculty
Department of Physical Medicine and Rehabilitation
Rush University Medical Center
Chicago, Illinois

George Tsao, DO, MPH
Fellow, Pain Medicine
Baystate Medical Center
Tufts University Medical Center
Springfield, Massachusetts

Irma Valentín, MD
Resident
Physical Medicine and Rehabilitation Residency Program
VA Caribbean Healthcare System
San Juan, Puerto Rico

Enrique Vázquez, MD, MBA
Chief Quality and Informatics Officer
Damas Hospital
Ponce, Puerto Rico
Regional Vice President
Medical Strategies and Management Services
Cayey, Puerto Rico

Manuel Velez, MD
Senior Resident
Department of Physical Medicine and Rehabilitation
University of Puerto Rico
San Juan, Puerto Rico

Christopher J. Visco, MD
Assistant Professor
Department of Rehabilitation and Regenerative Medicine
Columbia University College of Physicians and Surgeons
New York Presbyterian Hospital
New York, New York

Joseph A. Volpe, MD, MEd
Department of Physical Medicine
The Austin Diagnostic Clinic
Austin, Texas

Alison C. Welch, MD
Attending Physician
Department of Physical Medicine and Rehabilitation
Good Samaritan Hospital
Attending Physician
Rainier Rehabilitation Associates, PLLC
Puyallup, Washington

Anton Wicker, MD, PhD
Professor
Department of Physical Medicine and Rehabilitation
Department of Paracelsus Medical University
Salzburg, Austria

Robert P. Wilder, MD, FASCM
Associate Professor
Department of Physical Medicine and Rehabilitation
Medical Director
The Center for Endurance Sport
Team Physician
University of Virginia Athletics
The University of Virginia
Charlottesville, Virginia

Stuart Willick, MD
Associate Professor
Division of Physical Medicine and Rehabilitation
University of Utah
Salt Lake City, Utah

Gregory M. Worsowicz, MD, MBA
Professor of Clinical Physical Medicine and Rehabilitation
Chairman
Department of Physical Medicine and Rehabilitation
University of Missouri, Columbia
Columbia, Missouri

Fernando L. Zayas, MD
Assistant Professor
Department of Physical Medicine, Rehabilitation,
 and Sports Medicine
University of Puerto Rico School of Medicine
San Juan, Puerto Rico

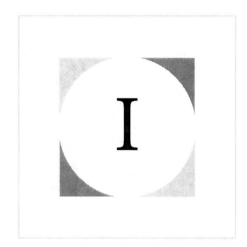

Evaluation

Evaluation of the Individual With Musculoskeletal Injury

Gerardo E. Miranda MD ■ Walter R. Frontera MD PhD

Description

Musculoskeletal injuries are very common and include sports-related injuries and occupational injuries. Sports-related injuries can occur in individuals who exercise for health benefits and in those who participate in recreational and competitive sports. Injuries that occur at the work place are classified as occupational musculoskeletal injuries. An interdisciplinary team approach should be used for adequate evaluation, assessment, diagnosis, treatment, and rehabilitation of these injuries. The majority of musculoskeletal injuries require conservative rather than surgical management. Rehabilitation goals for athletic injuries include the return of the individual to regular activity or competition at the highest level possible and for individuals with occupational musculoskeletal injuries the return to the work place.

Etiology/Types

- Traumatic—sports- or work-related acute trauma
- Overuse due to repetitive overload of anatomic structures, specific sport training errors, poor ergonomics, inappropriate equipment, individual or intrinsic factors, occupational microtrauma, or cumulative trauma disorder

Epidemiology

- The incidence and prevalence of sports-related injuries are influenced by several factors
- The location of the injury may be specific to the type of sport. For example, overhead sports such as baseball, volleyball, and tennis are associated with shoulder and elbow injuries; gymnastics and diving may result in trunk and spine injuries; and running and jumping sports predispose to knee and ankle injuries. Also, the specific diagnosis is influenced by sports-specific activity
- Overhead sports—rotator cuff tendinopathy, shoulder instability
- Trunk twisting and flexion—spondylolysis, disc disease, facet joint syndrome
- Running and jumping—ankle sprains, patellofemoral pain, anterior cruciate ligament tears

Work-related injuries are also influenced by numerous factors. Additionally, their high incidence represents a major economic burden due to elevated medical expenses and decreased labor productivity. Low back pain is the most common cause of disability in people younger than age 45. The type of injury varies with different biomechanical factors, including the extent of tissue damage caused by repetitive or prolonged labor activities, forceful exertion, awkward or static postures, vibration, localized mechanical stress, and extremes of temperatures.

Risk Factors

- Individual or intrinsic factors
  - Age
  - Ligamentous laxity
  - Poor flexibility
  - Malalignment
- Extrinsic factors
  - Training errors
  - Poor ergonomics
  - Sports or occupational demands

Classification of Injury

From a chronological point of view, sports and occupational injuries can be classified as acute, chronic, or an acute exacerbation of a chronic injury. Furthermore, chronic injuries are divided in two subtypes: chronic overuse and acute over chronic. This distinction is important since an acute exacerbation of a chronic injury is treated as an acute injury. Care for an acute injury is divided into three stages: acute (0–4 days), subacute (4–14 days), and post-acute (>14 days). Subsequently, chronic overuse injuries occur as microtrauma accumulation over a longer period of time beyond 3 months.

Diagnosis

The evaluation of the patient should include the following areas:

- History—age, gender, medical history, type of activity, mechanism of injury, severity of injuries, previous history of injury, previous treatment strategies, growth and development, menstrual history, associated medical problems, associated psychological issues

■ Physical examination—observation for asymmetry, range of motion, tenderness on palpation, muscle strength tests, neurological deficits, provocative maneuvers

■ Diagnostic tests
  - Laboratory tests—blood hemogram, blood chemistries, urine analysis, coagulation profile, muscle enzymes, electrocardiogram
  - Imaging studies—conventional x-rays, computed tomography (CT), diagnostic ultrasound, technetium bone scan, magnetic resonance imaging (MRI), CT/MRI arthrography
  - Electrodiagnostic studies—nerve conduction studies and electromyography

Management

■ The majority of musculoskeletal and sports injuries are treated nonsurgically with modification of activity, medications, rehabilitation, and orthotics. If patients fail conservative treatment, have unstable lesions including fractures as well as ligament injuries, or participate in high-level sports, then surgical treatment may be considered

■ Nonsurgical management/rehabilitation is divided into three distinct stages: acute, recovery, and functional phases, each one with specific goals and treatment interventions

■ Acute phase consists of symptomatic treatment by reducing inflammation and pain, and anatomic injury protection by maintenance of pain-free range of motion, muscular atrophy prevention, and cardiovascular fitness
  - Correlates with the inflammatory stage of injury
  - Interventions used in this stage include active rest, analgesics, nonsteroidal anti-inflammatory drugs, cryotherapy, electrical stimulation, protected motion, static and closed chain exercises, and general conditioning

■ Recovery phase consists of correction of deficits in physiological and biomechanical capabilities such as flexibility, muscle strength, cardiovascular endurance, balance, and proprioception
  - Correlates with the fibroblastic repair stage of injury
  - Therapeutic strategies include modalities (superficial heat, ultrasound, electrical stimulation), static and dynamic flexibility exercises, dynamic strengthening exercises, neuromuscular proprioceptive retraining, and initial sports-specific training

■ Functional phase involves more sports-specific training to increase power and endurance, neuromuscular control, and return to training and competition
  - Correlates with the maturation and remodeling stage of tissue healing at injured site
  - The ultimate goal is to prevent future injuries
  - Approaches include plyometrics exercises, increased multiplane neuromuscular control, flexibility, power, and endurance exercises, sports-specific progression, and return to competition

■ Surgery should be considered for patients who fail conservative treatment or in those injuries nonsurgical treatment has been found ineffective
  - Surgical interventions for sports and musculoskeletal injury include tendon repairs, ligament reconstruction, open reduction and internal fixation of fractures, and nerve decompression or transposition. These may be performed open or via arthroscopic surgery. Consultations may be required with orthopedic, spine, and hand surgeons as well as neurosurgeons

Suggested Readings

Micheo WF. Concepts in sports medicine. In: Braddom RL, ed. *Physical Medicine and Rehabilitation*, 3rd ed. London: Elsevier; 2007:1021–1045.

Panagos A, Sable AW, Zuhosky JP, Irwin RW, Sullivan WJ, Foye PM. Industrial medicine and acute musculoskeletal rehabilitation. 1. Diagnostic testing in industrial and acute musculoskeletal injuries. *Arch Phys Med Rehabil.* 2007; 88(3 suppl 1):S3-S9.

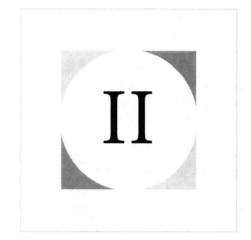

II Conditions

Achilles Tendinopathy

David J. Kennedy MD ■ Joel Press MD

Description
Overuse injury of the Achilles tendon associated with pain, swelling, and impaired performance characterized by chronic degenerative changes of tendinosis rather than the acute inflammatory changes of tendinitis.

Etiology/Types
- Traditionally, tendinosis is thought to occur with overuse and repetitive strain, causing microtrauma resulting in mechanical breakdown of the tendon and scar tissue formation
- Exact etiology remains unclear, although it is likely multifactorial including a combination of overtraining with inherent or acquired biomechanical deficits

Epidemiology
- May occur without sports participation, but incidence dramatically increased in runners and in those in other sports such as tennis, volleyball, and soccer
- Incidence of 7% to 9% in top-level runners and 7% to 18% in club runners, with incidence increasing with advanced age

Pathogenesis
- Functional biomechanical deficits lead to excessive repetitive overload of the Achilles tendon
- Strenuous exercise can subject the tendon to forces up to 12.5 times body weight
- Achilles tendons have naturally decreased blood supply 2- to 6-cm proximal to the calcaneal insertion
- Those with tendinosis have been shown to have higher resting blood flow rates in the tendon
- Tendon may show mucoid degeneration with increased interfibrillar glycosaminoglycans disrupting collagen fiber structure
- Paratendon may show edema, fibrin exudates, and adhesions

Risk Factors
- Runners have a 10-fold increase in incidence
- Excessive mileage or sudden increases in running
- Change of running surface, poor footwear, and toe running
- Functional biomechanical deficits including foot over pronation, gastrocnemius/soleus insufficiency, hindfoot varus, decreased ankle dorsiflexion, limited subtalar joint mobility, weak hip muscles resulting in internal rotation of the femur and tibia
- Increasing age, body weight, and height
- History of contralateral Achilles rupture
- Fluoroquinolone or steroid exposure
- Male sex

Clinical Features
- Posterior heel pain, over the Achilles tendon insertion, or 4- to 6-cm proximal to the tendon insertion, with severity varying from mild to severe
- Pain worse with stairs and walking on tiptoes
- Initially, pain may be experienced only at the beginning and end of a training session; however, as the pathologic process progresses, pain may be felt throughout exercise
- Eventually, pain may adversely affect functional mobility

Natural History
- Worsens with continued training, symptoms temporarily resolve with rest
- Without correction of underlying biomechanical abnormalities, symptoms may be recurrent or chronic in nature

Diagnosis

Differential diagnosis
- Retrocalcaneal bursitis
- Retroachilles bursitis
- Medial calf strain (tennis leg)
- Haglund deformity (enlarged posterior calcaneous)
- Achilles tendon rupture
- Calcaneal fracture
- Referred pain from proximal pathology (i.e., radiculopathy)
- Bone tumor

History
- Gradual onset of pain and dysfunction due to changes in training, running surface, and footwear
- Uncommonly, patients can present with the acute onset of symptoms due to partial or complete tears of the Achilles tendon

Exam

- Physical examination shows tenderness over the muscle-tendon junction proximal to its insertion, with associated swelling, crepitus, and nodules
- Pain with active plantar flexion and passive dorsiflexion
- Squeeze test for Achilles tendon tear

Testing

- Usually none indicated if history classic and patient responsive to conservative treatment
- Plain x-rays are not useful in the diagnosis, although they may reveal associated or incidental bony abnormalities and soft tissue calcifications
- Magnetic resonance imaging (MRI) and ultrasound are sensitive in detecting abnormalities, but findings must be correlated with symptoms
- MRI demonstrates areas of increased signal and ultrasound shows regions of hypoechogenicity
- Ultrasound has potential advantages over MRI, including dynamic nature, decreased cost, and safety for patients with contraindications to MRI. Ultrasound can also be interactive with transducer compression reproducing symptoms leading to improved focus on the abnormal area

Pitfalls

- Failure to correctly identify and treat underlying biomechanical deficiency that predisposes to injury
- Over interpretation of imaging findings

Red flags

- Inability to plantar-flex foot
- Acute onset with significant swelling/bruising

Treatment

Medical

- Relative rest
- Nonsteroidal anti-inflammatory medications may be considered for pain control; however, their role is unclear in the treatment of tendinosis
- Footwear modification, support shoe
- Heel lift, 12 to 15 mm to reduce tensile loading

Exercises

- Mainstay of treatment
- Focus on eccentric training of the gastrocnemius-soleus complex and correction of the underlying biomechanical abnormalities identified
- Core of exercise program is the heel drop, an eccentric exercise in which the heel is lowered from a bench or step until discomfort is felt over the Achilles tendon,

performed with the knee flexed (to strengthen the soleus) and extended (to strengthen the gastrocnemius)
- Manual mobilization to improve foot and ankle range of motion, including subtalar and midtarsal mobilization, stretching of the Achilles tendon
- Functional rehabilitation should progress to multiplanar exercises, single-leg stance to promote normal motor patterns of the lower extremity, and gluteal strengthening
- Jogging should be re-introduced gradually

Modalities

- Cryotherapy can be effective in decreasing pain
- The heel lift should be eliminated after calf flexibility improves and should be used bilaterally

Injections

- Insufficient published data to determine the comparative risks and benefits of corticosteroid injections; controversial due to potential risk of tendon rupture and lack of tendon inflammation in chronic tendinopathy

Surgical

- If 6 months of conservative medical treatment with rehabilitation has failed, and significant pain or decreased function persists, surgery may be considered

Consults

- Physical medicine and rehabilitation
- Orthopedics
- Physical therapy

Complications/side effects

- Tendon rupture
- Pain may cause functional limitations in ankle dorsiflexion and weakness of plantar flexors leading to decreased foot and ankle mobility
- Maladaptive movement patterns including increased flexion at hip and knee

Prognosis

- Overall good but can have protracted course

Helpful Hints

- The key to prevent recurrence is the correct identification and treatment of any underlying biomechanical deficits that may predispose to injury
- Eccentric training indicated for tendinopathy 4 to 6 cm above insertion, not clearly helpful for insertional tendinopathy

Suggested Reading

Sorosky B, Press J, Plastaras C, et al. The practical management of Achilles tendinopathy. *Clin J Sport Med.* 2004;14:40–44.

Achilles Tendon Tear

Per Renstrom MD PhD

Description
Achilles tendon tear is a typical sports injury, mostly in middle-aged men. There is no consensus regarding the optimal treatment for Achilles tendon tears. The question whether surgical or nonsurgical treatment is the treatment of choice is still under debate.

Etiology/Types
- Acute
- Chronic (undiagnosed) longstanding ruptures
- Partial
- Complete
- Injury mechanism
  - Fifty-three percent of the tears occur during weight bearing when the forefoot is pushing off with the knee in extension as seen in sprint starts and in jumping
  - Seventeen percent of the tears follow sudden unexpected dorsiflexion of the ankle, for example, slipping into a hole, and 10% by violent dorsiflexion of a plantarflexed foot, for example, falling from a height

Epidemiology
- The incidence of Achilles tendon tear in developed countries has been determined by the increase over the past two decades
- Most Achilles tendon tears (44%–83%) occur during sporting activities
- Achilles tendon rupture is more common in males, in their third or fourth decade, playing sport occasionally (weekend warriors)
- Increasing incidence in women

Pathogenesis
- The collagen fibers (95% Type I collagen) are tightly packed in parallel bundles containing blood, lymphatic vessels, and nerves
- Achilles tendon tear has been attributed to poor tendon vascularity, degeneration, a suboptimally conditioned musculotendinous unit, age, gender, changes in training pattern, poor technique, previous injuries, and poor footwear
- Degenerative changes are common in tendons of people older than 35 years

- The predominant site of tendon tear is 2- to 6-cm proximal to the tendon insertion
- If the tendon is lengthened more than 3% to 4% of its normal length, it starts to disrupt. At strain levels more than 8%, a macroscopic tear will occur

Risk Factors
- Intrinsic structural, biochemical, and biomechanical changes related to aging may play a significant role
- Training errors and biomechanical factors such as hyperpronation of the foot on heel strike predispose to Achilles tendon tear
- Intratendinous or peritendinous injection of corticosteroids may precipitate a tear

Clinical Features
- Acute swelling, pain, and limited ankle motion following sprint starts jumping, or landing
- Audible pop or tearing sensation
- Difficulty in ambulation
- Inability to rise from a chair or climb stairs
- Although the diagnosis is clinical and straightforward, 20% to 25% of Achilles tendon ruptures are missed by the first examining doctor

Natural History
- Untreated Achilles tendon tears result in ankle/foot muscle weakness and functional disability
- Some patients are able to plantarflex the ankle despite complete tear

Diagnosis
Differential diagnosis
- Ankle sprain
- Gastrocnemius tear (tennis leg)
- Chronic Achilles tendinopathy

History
- Patients report an audible snap following acute event
- They are often unable to bear weight

Exam
- Swelling and a palpable gap in the Achilles tendon approximately 4 to 6 cm above the insertion in the calcaneus

- Calf squeeze test (Thompson's test): patients are placed prone with the feet extended over the end of the table. The gastrocnemius-soleus muscle complex is squeezed by the examiner. It is normal when passive plantarflexion of the ankle occurs (sensitivity 96%, specificity 93%)
- If patient cannot do a single-leg heel rise, this supports the diagnosis

Testing
- X-rays are usually normal but may reveal tendon calcification
- Ultrasonography may show the defect in the tendon, but is operator-dependent
- Tendon stump separation during healing can be identified by ultrasonography
- Magnetic resonance imaging (MRI) is usually not needed but can confirm the diagnosis in doubtful cases
- MRI shows in greater detail the extent of tendon degeneration

Pitfalls
- Missed diagnosis because patient is able to actively plantarflex the ankle

Red Flags
- Persistent weakness and inability to perform heel rise

Treatment

Medical
- Nonoperative management
  - Conservative treatment can be effective in all age groups
  - Although function following nonoperative treatment with immobilization with a cast or an orthosis is generally good, the high re-rupture risk should be considered
  - The lack of tension on the immobilized musculotendinous unit is a major factor in the development of calf atrophy
  - Dynamic mobilization during the second month with an orthosis is now possible
  - Elderly patients, older than 65 to 70 years, can be treated with physiotherapy alone or plaster cast immobilization for a period of 6 to 10 weeks

Exercises
- Gradual range of motion of ankle with the knee in flexion
- Static ankle exercises with the knee in flexion

- Progressive stretching as the tendon heals following immobilization with cast, brace, or surgery
- Dynamic strengthening initial exercises with knee in flexion, progress to knee extension and ankle dorsiflexion gradually
- Aquatic exercises

Modalities
- Cryotherapy following acute injury or surgery to reduce pain/inflammation
- Superficial heat prior to exercise
- Ultrasound in the postimmobilization period or following surgery in patients with restricted ankle motion and tendon contracture
- Electrical stimulation to facilitate gastrocnemious-soleus muscle recruitment

Injection
- Not indicated

Surgery
- Acute tendon tear
  - Surgical treatment is reserved for high-demand patients, whereas sedentary patients are treated conservatively
  - Surgeons favor direct open tendon repair
  - The repair should be put under as much tension as possible as early as possible
  - Surgical repair decreases re-rupture rate from 13% to 20% to 1% to 4%, increases tendon strength, and causes less calf muscle atrophy
  - Higher number of athletes returns to preinjury physical activities
  - Percutaneous repair provides approximately 50% of the initial strength afforded by open repair, and places the sural nerve at risk for injury
  - This technique results in less thick tendons, better cosmesis but demonstrates a higher re-rupture rate as compared with open operative repair
- Chronic tendon tear
  - The tendon should be reconstructed to a functional length
  - The stumps cannot be approximated without undue tension
  - Augmentation with plantaris tendon is recommended
  - A more conservative postoperative management of these patients is recommended, keeping them in plaster for 8 weeks instead of 6 weeks
  - The limitation of dorsiflexion is continued until the sixth week

Consults
- Orthopedic/foot-ankle surgery
- Physical medicine and rehabilitation

Complications/side effects
- Major complications include re-rupture, tendon lengthening, infection, chronic fistula
- Moderate complications include sural nerve injury and wound problems
- Conservative management leads to extensive scarring, lengthening of the tendon, and subsequently suboptimal push-off strength
- The incidence of asymptomatic and symptomatic deep venous thrombosis is high
- Inability to return to competitive sports

Prognosis
- The prognosis for tendon healing after a treated tear is very good

- Return to sport depends on the desired level and character of the sport. Most sports can be resumed within 5 to 6 months

Helpful Hints
- Management of Achilles tendon ruptures should be individualized
- If optimal performance is required, operative management is probably the treatment of choice
- Open operative repair probably produces better functional results than nonoperative treatment, but may lead to higher rate of complications

Suggested Readings
Jozsa L, Kannus P, Jozsa L, Kannus P, eds. *Human Tendon: Anatomy, Physiology and Pathology*. Champaign: Human Kinetics; 1997.

Maffulli N. Rupture of the Achilles tendon. *J Bone Joint Surg Am.* 1999;81(7):1019–1036.

Acromioclavicular Injuries

Rob Johnson MD

Description

The acromioclavicular (AC) joint, a diarthrodial joint that serves as the articulation between the acromion and clavicle, is commonly injured in sports activities. It serves as a pivot point for the clavicle and scapula permitting the scapula to retract and protract around that point. Static stabilizers of the AC joint, which are commonly injured, include the AC ligament and coracoclavicular (CC) ligaments (trapezoid and conoid), with the AC ligament providing anterior-posterior stability and the CC ligaments providing vertical stability.

Etiology/Types

- Traumatic: usually associated with a fall on the shoulder
- Six types of injury to the AC joint have been described based on the degree of displacement of the clavicle (Figure 1):
  - Type I: AC ligaments sprained but no tear; no clavicular displacement from acromion
  - Type II: AC ligaments torn; slight clavicular displacement with anterior-posterior instability
  - Type III: AC and CC ligaments torn with up to 100% displacement of clavicle from acromion; vertical and horizontal instability
  - Type IV: AC and CC ligaments torn with associated tear of deltotrapezius fascia resulting in a fixed posterior displacement
  - Type V: AC and CC ligaments torn with associated tear of deltotrapezius fascia and 100% to 300% vertical displacement of clavicle from the acromion
  - Type VI: AC and CC ligaments torn with a fixed inferior dislocation of the clavicle
- Overuse: may be associated with heavy weight lifting
- Degenerative: seen in older individuals with osteoarthritis who participate in overhead activities

Epidemiology

- AC injuries account for about 9% of all injuries to the shoulder
- Slightly less than one half (43.5%) of AC injuries occur in adults in their 20s
- Frequency is five times greater in men than that in women

Pathogenesis

- The typical mechanism of injury is a direct blow to the shoulder from a fall or collision
- The acromion is driven away from the clavicle injuring the AC and/or CC ligaments

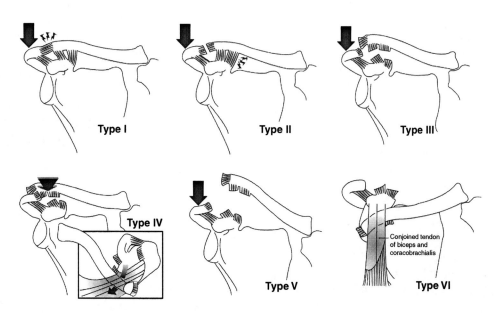

Figure 1. Classification of acromioclavicular injury.

- A fall on an outstretched hand may also injure the AC joint by an indirect force directed along the axis of the radius and humerus forcing the acromion away from the clavicle
- Repeated loading of the joint may lead to injury; damage to the distal clavicle may result in osteolysis

Risk Factors
- Participation in contact sports
- Repetitive overhead activity

Clinical Features
- Pain localized to the AC joint
- Deformity of the AC joint
- Pain with overhead motion

Natural History
- Types I and II injuries improve with conservative treatment
- Type III injuries may improve with conservative treatment but overhead athletes may have persistent symptoms
- AC joint deformity may persist
- Osteoarthritis may develop

Diagnosis

Differential diagnosis
- Distal clavicle fracture
- Scapular fracture
- Rotator cuff tear
- Shoulder (glenohumeral) dislocation
- Osteoarthritis of the shoulder

History
- Shoulder pain following a fall on the tip of the shoulder or direct trauma
- Limited active shoulder motion
- Visible deformity of the AC joint
- Pain and swelling associated with heavy weight lifting

Exam
- Tenderness to palpation of AC joint
- Joint crepitus
- Limited active motion, particularly abduction, adduction, and forward flexion
- Shoulder muscle weakness including deltoid, supraspinatus, and infraspinatus (may be secondary to pain inhibition, or associated rotator cuff injury)
- Scapular dysfunction/winging (weak scapular stabilizers fail to stabilize the scapula, lead to persistent pain)

- Pain with a crossed adduction test (injured shoulder flexed to 90°, reaching across the body to the opposite shoulder)
- Types II to VI injury, visible deformity at the AC joint

Testing
- Standard radiographs can be helpful in determining the severity of traumatic injury. The most helpful views are anteroposterior, 10° to 15° cephalad (Zanca view), and axillary views. In addition, x-rays may show distal clavicle reabsorption in osteolysis, and degenerative changes of arthritis
- Ultrasound may be used to evaluate associated rotator cuff tears
- Magnetic resonance imaging may show rotator cuff or labral tears

Pitfalls
- Missing associated pathology
- Not addressing scapular dysfunction

Red Flags
- Severe AC joint deformity
- Continued pain in older patients may be a symptom of associated rotator cuff tear

Treatment

Medical
- Early immobilization with sling for comfort
- Anti-inflammatory/analgesic medications
- AC separations Types I and II are typically treated symptomatically and with appropriate rehabilitation of the rotator cuff and scapular stabilizers
- Return to play is based on functional testing for pain-free (or minimal discomfort) range of motion (ROM) and strength that is symmetric with the uninvolved limb
- Though there is controversy surrounding the Type III AC separation, most experts agree that nonoperative treatment similar to that employed for Types I and II is appropriate

Exercises
- Active assistive/active range of motion exercises, initially in pain-free range
- Static/closed kinetic chain exercises for scapular stabilizers and the rotator cuff
- Dynamic strengthening (concentric-eccentric) when pain is controlled, start with low rows for the lower trapezius, rotator cuff exercises to 90°, and with the

arm at side, progress to combined motion exercises in sports-specific range of motion
- Core muscle and lower extremity strengthening

Modalities
- Cryotherapy
- Superficial heat
- Electrical stimulation

Injection
- Lidocaine injections for patients during the season of competition may allow participation
- Steroid injections may be used for symptom relief in overuse injury, and osteoarthritis
- Twenty milligrams of triamcinolone or 3 mg of betamethasone, combined with 0.5 mL of xylocaine, can be injected using anterior or superior approaches

Surgical
- Types IV to VI require orthopedic consultation and surgical intervention
- The surgical procedure usually performed is anatomic CC reconstruction
- Distal clavicle resection can be considered in individuals with chronic symptoms

Consults
- Orthopedic surgery
- Sports medicine
- Physical medicine and rehabilitation

Complications/side effects
- Chronic pain and deformity
- Inability to return to same level of performance in overhead sports
- Osteoarthritis

Prognosis
- Good for Types I and II injuries
- Type III injuries appear to respond well to conservative treatment, with results similar to surgical treatment
- Variable results with surgical treatment of Types IV to VI injuries
- Some individuals will persist with obvious deformity, cosmetic defect

Helpful Hints
- Start early rehabilitation in athletes
- Work on scapular muscles to reduce scapular dysfunction

Suggested Readings

Bradley JP, Elkousy H. Decision making: operative versus non-operative treatment of acromioclavicular joint injuries. *Clin Sports Med.* 2003;22(2):277–290.

MacDonald PB, Lapointe P. Acromioclavicular and sternoclavicular joint injuries. *Orthop Clin North Am.* 2008;39:535–545.

Mazzocca AD, Arciero RA, Bicos J. Evaluation and treatment of acromioclavicular joint injuries. *Am J Sports Med.* 2007;35(2):316–329.

Acute Calcific Tendinitis of the Shoulder

Christopher J. Visco MD ▓ Paul H. Lento MD

Description
The acute shoulder may be associated with calcification of a rotator cuff tendon. The calcification may be present for years without symptoms before the pain begins, associated with resorption of calcium. This process can affect shoulder range of motion and quality of life; however, the natural course is usually of spontaneous recovery. Calcific tendinitis may less commonly be found in other tendons, including the hand, forearm, and lower limbs.

Etiology/Types
- Calcifications are composed of hydroxyapatite crystals
- The acutely calcified tendon occurs with insidious onset leading to a sequence of events including severe pain, limited motion, and eventual resolution
- Pathological studies show that tendon aging and degeneration are not precursor to calcification (calcifications in degenerative tendinopathy are different from those in radiographically visible calcific tendinitis)

Epidemiology
- Incidence is unknown; may be 39% to 62% of acutely painful shoulders in large medical center clinics
- Asymptomatic calcification is common
- Affects 30- to 60-year-olds more commonly

Pathogenesis
- The exact pathogenesis of calcifying tendons is unclear and various classification systems have been proposed
- One proposed natural course is divided into precalcific, formative, resorptive, and postcalcific phases
- Precalcific phase is characterized by fibrocartilage ingrowth into the midsubstance of the tendon and is generally asymptomatic
- Formative phase begins with the formation of hydroxyapatite crystals in the substance of fibrocartilage
- During the formative phase, there may be pain with movement, possibly along with a catching sensation
- Resorptive phase is characterized by severe pain and restriction of movement lasting weeks

- Calcium release during the resorptive phase will lead to extravasation of the semisolid substance
- Hydroxyapatite crystals are released into the soft tissues and subacromial bursa, which leads to irritation and inflammation, resulting in pain
- Healing and repair of the rotator cuff occur during the postcalcific phase
- Some pain may last for months, affecting function
- Calcification will most commonly affect the supraspinatus tendon followed by the infraspinatus, teres minor, and subscapularis tendons

Risk Factors
- Insidious onset
- Repetitive loading

Clinical Features
- Clicking or catching sensation
- Constant severe pain
- Limited range of motion
- Low-grade fever, malaise

Natural History
- Spontaneous resolution
- Improvement of pain and range of motion
- Ten percent of patients will have persistent pain that may require arthroscopy and removal of residual calcium

Diagnosis

Differential diagnosis
- Impingement syndrome
- Rotator cuff tear
- Adhesive capsulitis
- Os acromiale
- Labral tear
- Neoplasm

History
- Shoulder pain associated with mechanical symptoms of catching or clicking
- Constant severe pain
- Sharp in nature
- Malaise

Exam
- Tenderness at the affected tendon of the rotator cuff
- Restricted range of motion
- Pain-limited weakness of the affected rotator cuff tendon

Testing
- X-rays, anteroposterior with internal and external rotation, axillary and outlet views show calcification (underpenetrated films may show subtle calcification)
- Sharp contours on radiograph indicates a dense deposit that has not undergone resorption
- Very early or diffuse calcifications may be missed on radiograph
- Musculoskeletal ultrasound is a sensitive test for identifying intrasubstance calcifications, which may not be seen on x-ray or with magnetic resonance imaging (MRI)
- Normal blood chemistries and urine studies

Pitfalls
- Failure to consider acute calcific tendonitis in the differential of shoulder pain

Red Flags
- Fever
- Severe pain not improving with treatment
- Constitutional symptoms
- Neurological dysfunction

Treatment

Medical
- Nonsteroidal anti-inflammatory medications
- Analgesics

Exercises
- Brief period of rest as needed
- Range of motion, Codman and wall-climbing exercises
- Scapular stabilization and correction of underlying muscular imbalance

Modalities
- Heat
- Cryotherapy
- Therapeutic ultrasound
- Extracorporeal shock wave therapy
- Iontophoresis

Injection
- Diagnostic anesthetic injection
- Local steroid injection to the subacromial bursa

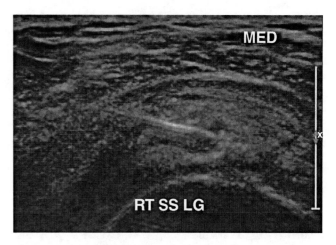

Figure 1. An ultrasound-guided needle lavage of the calcification within the supraspinatus tendon may give dramatic pain relief.

- Lavage and barbotage of calcification with ultrasound guidance (see Figure 1)

Surgical
- Reserved for recalcitrant cases
- Resection of calcification

Consults
- Orthopedic-shoulder surgery for chronic pain despite conservative treatment

Complications/side effects
- Adhesive capsulitis

Prognosis
- Very good for a complete recovery

Helpful Hints
- Modalities may help temporarily; however, they do not change the course of the disease, which is usually self-limiting to full resolution
- Needle lavage and barbotage are effective at giving rapid relief to symptoms. A concomitant bursal steroid injection may also help reduce postprocedure inflammation

Suggested Readings
Uhthoff HK, Loehr JS. Calcific tendinopathy of the rotator cuff: pathogenesis, diagnosis, and management. *J Am Acad Orthop Surg.* 1997;5:183–191.

Wainner RS, Hasz M. Management of acute calcific tendinitis of the shoulder. *J Orthop Sports Phys Ther.* 1998;27(3):231–237.

Adhesive Capsulitis of the Shoulder

Kevin Carneiro DO ■ Paul H. Lento MD

Description
Adhesive capsulitis or "frozen shoulder" is commonly seen but poorly understood. It usually starts spontaneously as shoulder pain and progresses to restricted active and passive range of motion.

Etiology/Types
- Primary or idiopathic
- Secondary causes include intrinsic (rotator cuff tears, tendonitis, bursitis), extrinsic (trauma), and postsurgical causes

Epidemiology
- Prevalence of 2% in the general population
- Cumulative incidence in the general population is 2.4/1000/year
- Women are more affected than men with a ratio of 58:42
- More common in the fifth and sixth decade of life
- Eleven percent prevalence rate in diabetics

Pathogenesis
- Generally thought to be an inflammatory and fibrotic process
- Clinical stages
- During the "freezing stage," there is an insidious onset of pain with active and passive range of motion. Pathology has shown early inflammatory changes with hypervascular synovitis. Duration of this stage 2 to 9 months
- The "frozen stage" is characterized by restricted range of motion and/or a reduction in pain. Pathology has shown a decrease in hypervascularity and synovitis. Arthoscopy shows capsular contraction and thickening. Usually lasts for 4 to 12 months
- The thawing stage is characterized by minimal pain and improved range of motion. Pathology has shown a decrease in capsular thickness and no synovitis. Generally thought to last for 5 to 24 months

Risk Factors
- Diabetes or prediabetes
- Rotator cuff disorders
- Shoulder trauma
- Surgery

Clinical Features
- Insidious onset of pain
- Restricted active and passive range of motion in all directions, including forward flexion, abduction, external, and internal rotation

Natural History
- Is usually self-limiting and improves over an 18- to 24-month period

Diagnosis

Differential diagnosis
- Arthritis
- Rotator cuff tears
- Occult fractures
- Labral tears
- Osteitis
- Infection
- Pancoast tumor

History
- Most patients with primary frozen shoulder have no history of trauma
- Careful history of trauma, cervical radiculopathy, brachial plexus injury, and cardiac ischemia
- Insidious onset of pain followed by a loss of motion
- Pain usually radiates to the deltoid insertion

Exam
- Early in the disease process, the only physical examination finding might be pain produced at the end range of the shoulder motion
- As the disease progresses, there is a loss of both passive and active range of motion, especially in elevation and external rotation (useful in differentiating this condition from rotator cuff tears)
- Weak shoulder girdle muscles
- Normal neurological examination
- Scapular dysfunction

Testing

- Laboratory data are usually normal except in patients with other medical issues, where thyroid-stimulating hormone (TSH), lipids, and fasting blood glucose may be elevated
- X-rays are usually normal
- Arthrography shows decreased shoulder volume
- Arthroscopy, looking for signs of inflammation or fibrosis, is the gold standard
- Ultrasound can demonstrate hypoechoic echotexture and increased vascularity within the rotator cuff interval and/or increased thickness of the coracohumeral ligament
- Magnetic resonance imaging (MRI) imaging to identify acromioclavicular osteoarthritis, rotator cuff tendinopathy, or tears

Pitfalls

- Physical therapy that is too aggressive is thought to delay the normal recovery process

Red Flags

- Worsening pain despite treatment
- Fever/infection
- Neoplasm
- Fracture

Treatment

Medical

- Nonsteroidal anti-inflammatory medications
- Acetaminophen
- Short course of oral steroids
- Benign neglect has been used successfully

Exercises

- Pendulum, active assistive, and active exercises in the pain-free range
- Four-direction shoulder-stretching program that includes passive forward elevation, passive external rotation, passive internal rotation, and passive horizontal adduction
- Mobilization techniques
- Scapular muscle strengthening
- Rotator cuff strengthening

Modalities

- Heat
- Cryotherapy
- Ultrasound
- Transcutaneous electrical nerve stimulation

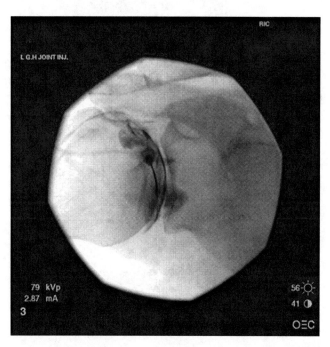

Figure 1. A fluoroscopically guided glenohumeral steroid injection may help improve symptoms.

Injection

- Intra-articular steroid injections with or without arthrographic distention of the glenohumeral joint (hydrodilation) helps to improve symptoms and range of motion. An example of a fluoroscopically guided glenohumeral joint injection is shown in Figure 1.
- Interventional lysis of adhesion (microadhesiolysis)

Surgical

- Manipulation under anesthesia in patients who are symptomatic for more than 6 months
- Arthroscopic capsular release is the main operative treatment
- Open capsular release is not common due to a high complication rate

Consults

- Orthopedic/surgery
- Physical medicine and rehabilitation
- Primary physician to evaluate for prediabetes or diabetes

Complications/side effects

- Osteopenia in the affected humerus
- Residual limitation of motion
- Surgical complications

Prognosis

- Ten percent to 15% of patients suffer from continued pain and limited range of motion
- Recurrence of adhesive capsulitis is extremely rare
- Dominant arm involvement has been shown to have a good prognosis
- Intrinsic pathology and Type 1 diabetes mellitus are poor prognostic indicators

Helpful Hints

- Early intervention with corticosteroids and range of motion therapy has proven to be beneficial.

Would also screen patient for prediabetes or diabetes as there appears to be a significant association

Suggested Readings

Sheridan MA, Hannafin JA. Upper extremity: emphasis on frozen shoulder. *Orthop Clin North Am.* 2006;37: 531–539.

Tasto JP, Elias DW. Adhesive capsulitis. *Sports Med Arthrosc Rev.* 2007;15:216–221.

Ankle Sprain

Ana V. Cintrón-Rodríguez MD FAAPMR

Description
Lateral ankle sprains typically occur when a person falls on a plantar-flexed foot that inverts over the supporting ligaments. This type of injury is commonly related to sports; however, it is prevalent in the general population.

Etiology/Types
- Lateral ankle sprains are common in sports, which require explosive jumping or running such as basketball, volleyball, soccer, and football
- Medial ankle sprains involving the deltoid ligament are less common
- Recurrent ankle sprains are caused by mechanical and functional instability
  - Mechanical instability: failure to achieve stabilization due to ligamentous laxity
  - Functional instability: neuromuscular deficits that contribute to impaired balance

Epidemiology
- One per 10,000 in general population sustains ankle injury every day
- Seven percent to 10% of emergency room daily visits are linked to ankle sprains
- Four percent of people in Western countries suffer ankle sprains
- Forty percent of sports-related injuries are ankle sprains
- Twenty-one percent of people sustaining ankle sprains are absent from school or work
- Recurrence rate of ankle sprains in athletes is approximately 80%
- Thirty percent of patients with ankle sprains develop functional instability

Pathogenesis
- The ankle undergoes forceful plantarflexion and inversion
- The anterior talofibular ligament (ATFL) is the weakest and first ligament injured, followed by the calcaneofibular (CFL) and posterior talofibular ligament (see Figure 1)
- Peroneal muscles are primarily responsible for eversion of the foot against inversion forces when walking on irregular ground

- Peroneal nerve damage has been found in severe injuries
- Lateral ankle sprains are classified as:
  - Grade I: stretching of ATFL, no tear, pain
  - Grade II: tearing of ATFL, sparing CFL
  - Grade III: tearing of both ATFL and CFL, pain is severe, unable to bear Weight

Risk Factors
- Sports activity
- Previous ankle injury
- Absent or incomplete rehabilitation

Clinical Features
- Inability to bear weight on injured ankle
- May be associated with audible "pop"
- Edema in lateral aspect of ankle
- Presence of hematoma
- Tenderness over anterior, lateral, and posterolateral aspects of ankle

Natural History
- Failure to rehabilitate is associated with increased risk of recurrence
- Approximately 10% to 40% will develop chronic instability regardless of initial management

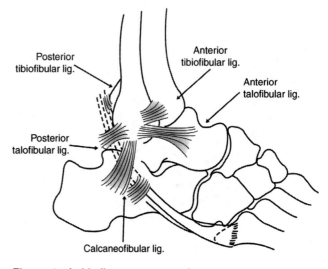

Figure 1. Ankle ligaments complex.

Diagnosis

Differential diagnosis
- Ankle syndesmotic injury
- Fracture at base of fifth metatarsal
- Osteochondral talar dome fracture

History
- Ability to perform weight bearing after injury
- Inversion mechanism of injury
- Previous history of injury
- Neurological symptoms: tingling, numbness, weakness

Exam
- Inspection: hematoma, edema, deformity
- Palpation: tenderness anterior to distal tibia, fibula, and fifth metatarsal base
- Range of motion (ROM): eversion and inversion may be limited due to pain
- Strength: eversion and dorsiflexion weakness but there may be pain inhibition
- Special maneuvers:
  - Anterior drawer sign: assess status of ATFL: if ankle slides anteroposterior more than 5 mm is positive (see Figure 2)
  - Talar tilt test: assess status of CFL. A side-to-side difference is 10° or more is a positive test (see Figure 3)

Testing
- Ankle x-rays: anteroposterior, lateral, and mortise views
- Ankle magnetic resonance imaging (MRI) should be considered if syndesmosis fracture is suspected
- Ottawa ankle rules: obtain ankle x-ray if:
  - Tenderness in posterior or distal aspect of either malleolus
  - Tenderness in navicular bone
  - Tenderness at base of fifth metatarsal
  - Inability to bear weight for four steps
- Ottawa ankle rules: 100% sensitive and 10% to 79% specific for ankle fracture

Pitfalls
- Patients with delay in treatment, severe swelling, and pain may develop complex, regional pain syndrome

Red Flags
- If patient does not improve, suspect occult osteochondral injury
- Injury to deltoid ligament in medial ankle should raise suspicion of proximal fibular fracture (Maisonneuve fracture)
- Inability to bear weight

Treatment

Medical
- Nonsteroidal anti-inflammatory medications use may be considered, although controversial due to effects on tissue repair
- Acetaminophen for pain management, consider weak opioid agonists if pain is severe
- Acute: first 48 to 72 hours. Protection, relative rest, compression, and elevation
- Bracing during functional rehabilitation may prevent recurrent injury. Lace up supports have shown to be

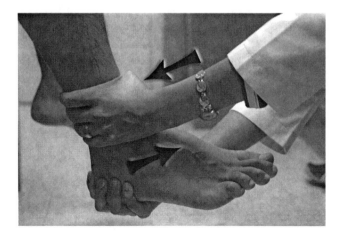

Figure 2. Anterior drawer test.

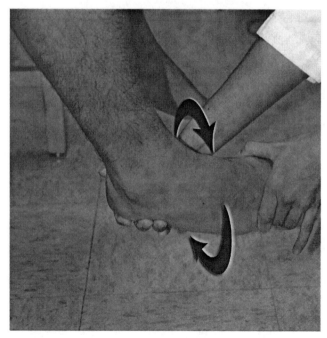

Figure 3. Talar tilt test.

superior to elastic bandages, semirigid supports, and tape in some studies

Exercises
- Functional rehabilitation has been found to be superior to immobilization in all types of ankle injuries
- Rehabilitation of contralateral ankle may improve recovery of injured ankle
- Early phase: restore active ROM (AROM), strength, and begin proprioception training, emphasis on peroneal muscle strengthening
- Late: high-level balance exercises, advanced proprioception exercises, endurance training
- Sports-specific functional rehabilitation

Modalities
- Cryotherapy
- Electrical stimulation
- Ultrasound may be considered although beneficial effect is yet to be proven
- Transcutaneous electrical nerve stimulator (TENS) for pain control

Injection
- Prolotherapy could be considered for lower-grade sprains although scientific evidence is still limited

Surgical
- May be considered for chronic mechanical instability with lateral complex ligamentous laxity
- Surgery vs conservative therapy long-term results have been found to be similar

Consults
- Orthopedics
- Physical medicine and rehabilitation

Complications
- Chronic instability
- Inability to return to high-level sports

Prognosis
- Highly variable
- Literature review has shown that ligament healing may take from 6 weeks to 3 months; however, mechanical laxity and subjective instability may persist for more than a year

Helpful Hints
- Combine bracing with early protected rehabilitation
- Functional bracing continued for 3 to 6 months following injury

Suggested Readings
Hubbard T, Hicks-Little C. Ankle ligament healing after an acute ankle sprain: an evidence-based approach. *J Athletic Train.* 2008;43(5):523–529.

Simmons SM, Zimmerman J. Ankle injuries. In: Frontera WR, Herring SA, Micheli LJ, et al., eds. *Clinical Sports Medicine: Medical Management and Rehabilitation.* Philadelphia: Saunders Elsevier; 2007:459–472.

Stiell IG, Greenberg GH, McKnight RD, et al. Decision rules for the use of radiography in acute ankle injuries: refinement and prospective validation. *JAMA.* 1993;269:1127–1132.

Ankle Syndesmotic Injury

Ana V. Cintrón-Rodríguez MD FAAPMR

Description
Syndesmotic ankle sprains are "high ankle sprains" involving the stabilizing ligaments of the ankle mortise. They are less common, are more severe than lateral ankle sprains, and require a longer recovery.

Etiology/Types
- Ankle external rotation and extreme dorsiflexion are most common mechanisms
- Also reported with severe ankle inversion and eversion injuries
- High or repetitive mechanical loading

Epidemiology
- One percent to 15% of the estimated 25,000 daily ankle injuries
- Incidence of 10% to 20% of all ankle sprains in the general athletic population
- More common in collision sports such as American football and hockey, as well as in skiing
- Isolated syndesmotic ruptures without ankle fractures occur in 20% of patients with lateral ankle sprain

Pathogenesis
- Injury to one or more of the syndesmotic ligaments, including the anterior inferior tibiofibular ligament (AITFL), the posterior inferior tibiofibular ligament (PITFL), the posterior transverse ligament, and interosseous ligament (Figure 1)
- Extreme external rotation and/or hyperdorsiflexion (closed pack position) causes widening of the ankle mortise, causing tension progressively with tearing of the AITFL, the interosseous membrane, and PITFL
- Subsequent talar instability may result
- May have associated deltoid ligament tear and fibular fracture (Maisonneuve fracture)
- Gerber's West Point Ankle Grading System:
  - Grade I: microscopic ligament tearing; no functional loss or instability
  - Grade II: partial tearing, swelling, ecchymosis; moderate functional loss and ankle instability; unable to perform weight bearing
  - Grade III: complete rupture with immediate swelling, ecchymosis; unable to bear weight with associated unstable joint

Risk Factors
- Athletes at risk are football linemen, downhill slalom skiers, soccer, and hockey players

Clinical Features
- Very difficult injury to evaluate, symptoms similar to lateral ankle sprain
- Pain, edema, and tenderness located over the anterolateral tibiofibular joint
- Pain with ambulation at push-off phase, and passive dorsiflexion
- Inability to squat with feet flat

Natural History
- Patients may report a variety of injury mechanisms
- Injury severity is variable, leading to wide variability in recovery and time lost from sport
- Associated injuries include anterior talofibular ligament injury, bone bruises, and talar dome osteochondral lesions
- Heterotopic calcification of the syndesmosis may occur in time

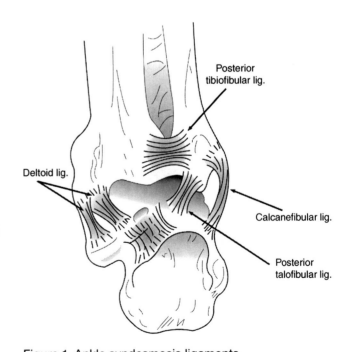

Figure 1. Ankle syndesmosis ligaments.

Diagnosis

Differential diagnosis
- Lateral ankle sprain
- Medial ankle sprain
- Navicular fracture
- Talar dome osteochondral injury
- Achilles tendon rupture

History
- Prolonged recovery of ankle sprain
- Previous history of ankle injury
- Presence of immediate or delayed pain, swelling at the ankle joint, and inability to bear weight after injury

Exam
- Edema, ecchymosis at the ankle joint
- Tenderness at the distal inferior tibiofibular syndesmosis and over the deltoid ligament
- External rotation ankle test—positive with painful motion while ankle in dosiflexion (Figure 2)
- Squeeze test—positive when pain elicited with compression of tibia and fibula distally (Figure 3)
- Crossed leg test—positive with pain at the syndesmosis when midtibia of affected leg is placed over the sound knee
- Squat test—positive with painful dorsiflexion and lateral rotation during squat position

Testing
- Standard anteroposterior, lateral, and mortise views to evaluate for fractures and syndesmosis diastasis
- Stress weight-bearing external rotation and dorsiflexion views may aid in diagnosis of diastasis

- Magnetic resonance imaging (MRI) helps define zone of soft tissue injury including anterior and/or posterior inferior tibiofibular ligaments, talar bone bruise

Pitfalls
- Plain films often negative
- Failure to suspect and diagnose
- Failure to obtain appropriate diagnostic imaging

Red Flags
- Recurrent ankle sprains
- Recurrent pain and swelling
- Mechanical symptoms suggestive of ankle instability

Treatment

Medical
- Acute phase treat with protection, relative rest, compression, and elevation
- Nonsteroidal anti-inflammatory medication use may be considered; controversy exists of its effect on tissue repair
- Immobilization with ankle brace, stirrup, or taping considered in early phase, with use of crutches until gait normal on uneven surfaces

Exercises
- Grades I and II subacute phase goal is to restore mobility, strength, and function with painless ambulation
- Functional training with progressive strengthening, neuromuscular and proprioceptive conditioning, followed by sports-specific training
- Cycle ergometer for early mobilization
- Strengthening exercises to include ankle dorsi/plantarflexors, peroneal muscles

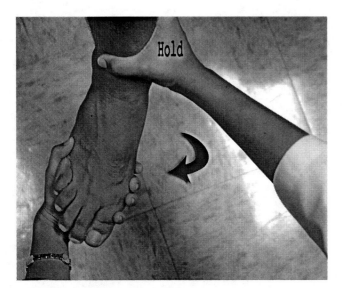

Figure 2. External rotation test.

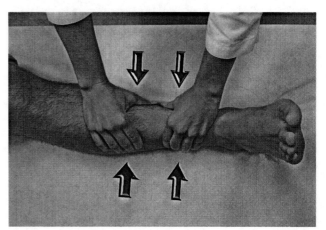

Figure 3. Tibial squeeze test.

- Proprioceptive/balance advanced training as symptoms permit

Modalities
- Heat
- Cryotherapy
- Transcutaneous electrical nerve stimulation
- Ultrasound
- Antiedema massage
- Joint mobilization

Injection
- Generally not indicated

Surgical
- Some Grade II and all Grade III require surgical stabilization of syndesmosis
- In chronic ankle instability related to associated talofibular ligaments when conservative treatment has failed
- Syndesmosis fixation with screws, staples, and suture bottom
- Postoperative management includes a 6-week immobilization period followed by functional rehabilitation

Consults
- Orthopedics
- Physical medicine and rehabilitation
- Sports medicine

Complications/side effects
- Recurrent functional and mechanical instability occurs in approximately 20% to 40% cases
- Recurrent or chronic pain, swelling, and stiffness
- Calcification of syndesmosis (synostosis)
- Posttraumatic arthritis

Prognosis
- Long recovery time common
- Unpredictable return to sports participation

Helpful Hints
- "Tenderness length" or the distance that pain extends proximally over tibiofibular joint has been found to correlate with degree of injury, and recovery time

Suggested Readings
Jackson W. Update on the treatment of chronic ankle instability and syndesmotic injuries. *Curr Opin Orthop.* 2006;17(2):97–102.

Simmons SM, Zimmerman J. Ankle injuries. In: Frontera WR, Herring SA, Micheli LJ, et al. *Clinical Sports Medicine: Medical Management and Rehabilitation.* Philadelphia: Saunders Elsevier; 2007:459–472.

Williams GN. Syndesmotic ankle sprains in athletes. *Am J Sports Med.* 2007;35:1197–1207.

Anterior Cruciate Ligament Tear

Eduardo Amy MD ■ William Micheo MD

Description
A traumatic disruption of the fibers of the anterior cruciate ligament (ACL). Commonly seen in contact and noncontact sports.

Etiology/Type
- Noncontact injury resulting from deceleration, change of direction, or landing from a jump
- Contact injury associated with trauma with valgus stress as a common mechanism
- Isolated injury
- Combined lesion involving the ACL, medial meniscus, and medial collateral ligament (unhappy triad)

Epidemiology
- The incidence of diagnosed and undiagnosed ACL tears is unknown
- More than 100,000 ACL reconstructions are performed in the United States each year
- Women have a higher incidence of injury
- Females with smaller femoral notch, corrected for bone width (low notch width index), have a higher incidence of injury in noncontact sports
- Common in sports such as football, basketball, and soccer

Pathogenesis
- The ACL is a multifilament collagen structure arranged in two bundles: the anteromedial and the posterolateral bundles
- The ligament is made mainly of Types 1 and 3 collagen fibers, which fail in tension and shear stress
- Blood supply is through the middle geniculate arteries
- Nerve supply is through the Ruffini receptors
- Primary function is to control anterior tibial displacement
- Secondary function is to control anterolateral tibial rotation
- Stressed during deceleration in running, cutting, and jumping in noncontact sports

- Placed under stress with valgus forces in contact sports
- Females injured when landing with the knee in valgus and hyperextension (position of no return)

Risk Factors
- Low notch width index (femoral notch size/bone width, <.2) approximately 60 times greater chance
- Contact sports
- Noncontact deceleration, cutting, and jumping sports

Clinical Features
- Acute knee swelling associated with hemarthrosis
- If not diagnosed initially, recurrent knee instability when individual returns to high-risk sports

Natural History
- Progressive laxity of the knee, with frequent giving way on high-demand sports, less so on recreational sports
- Patients with sedentary lifestyle or those who participate in low-demand sports tend to do well with occasional instability
- In continued participation in high-demand sports, patients will have risk of recurrent injury, meniscal tears, chondral lesions, and progressive arthritis

Diagnosis

Differential diagnosis
- Patellar dislocation
- Intra-articular fracture
- Posterior cruciate ligament tear
- Peripheral meniscal tear (vascular zone)

History
- Sudden pop while cutting, jumping, or landing from a jump
- Severe knee pain following traumatic injury, common valgus, and rotation mechanism
- Immediate effusion
- Inability to continue to play

Exam
- Large effusion with pain and loss of motion
- Joint line tenderness associated with lateral femoral, and tibial bone contusion, meniscal tears
- Weak quadriceps muscle
- Positive Lachman's test (evaluates anterior tibial translation with the knee between 15° and 30° of flexion, most important test in acute diagnosis)
- Positive lateral pivot shift test (evaluates and correlates with anterolateral rotatory instability, anterior tibial subluxation on the femur as the knee goes into extension)
- Anterior drawer test (may be false negative in acute injury, secondary stabilizers may reduce anterior tibial displacement with the knee in 90° of flexion)
- Combined injuries, positive valgus stress, and McMurray's tests

Testing
- Magnetic resonance imaging (MRI) is highly sensitive in the acute setting. Findings include large effusion, bone contusion of the lateral femoral condyle, and lateral tibial plateau as well as nonvisualization of the ACL
- X-rays to rule out tibial spine avulsion, and Segond's fracture (lateral capsular sign, associated with avulsion of the capsule)

Pitfalls
- Failure to diagnose acutely may lead to recurrent injury, damage to the meniscus, articular cartilage, and arthritis

Red Flags
- Recurrent symptoms with activities of daily living, work, or sports may indicate need for surgical treatment
- Persistent limited motion may require early surgical intervention (bucket handle meniscal tear)

Treatment

Medical
- Crutch walking partial to full weight bearing
- Analgesics
- Knee immobilizer for comfort

Exercises
- Nonoperative rehabilitation
  - Active range of motion
  - Progress to progressive resisted exercises, in the early postinjury limit resisted terminal extension exercises to protect secondary structures, emphasize hamstrings strengthening
  - Closed chain exercises
  - Functional bracing and progress to jogging 6 to 8 weeks
  - Activity modification
- Postsurgery rehabilitation
  - Accelerated rehabilitation program with early weight bearing
  - Full passive knee extension, active assisted knee flexion
  - Straight leg raising once full extension achieved
  - Avoid isotonic terminal extension resisted exercises for 6 weeks, start with light resisted knee extension from 90° to 30°, and resisted hamstring flexion
  - Closed kinetic chain exercises
  - Stationary bicycle, elliptical trainer, swimming, aquatic exercises
  - Running 3 to 4 months, sports-specific drills 4 to 6 months following injury
  - Return to sports 6 to 8 months following injury

Modalities
- Cryotherapy
- Low-voltage electrical stimulation to the quadriceps muscle (to reduce muscle inhibition, to facilitate muscle recruitment)
- High-voltage galvanic stimulation or transcutaneous electrical stimulation to the knee (reduces pain/arthrogenic muscle inhibition)

Injection
- Aspiration of hemathrosis may be required if slow recovery or inability to participate in rehabilitation

Surgical
- ACL reconstruction using patellar tendon, hamstring tendon, single- or double-bundle techniques results similar in clinical studies
- Autograph or allograft reconstruction techniques produce similar long-term results; slower progression may be required following allograft surgery

Consults
- Orthopedic surgery

Complications/side effects
- Infection 1% to 2%
- Venous thrombosis
- Loss of motion 2% to 3%
- Inability to return to sports
- Re-rupture and graft stretching, reported in up to 8% of cases

- Pain with activity

Prognosis
- Good to excellent results with surgical treatment 85% to 89%
- Return to previous level in sports variable from 70% to 85%
- Early arthritis may occur if not treated appropriately
- A group of "copers" may do well with nonsurgical treatment

Helpful Hints
- Early diagnosis, protection of secondary structures, prevention of recurrent injury with early rehabilitation, or surgery leads to good treatment outcomes

Suggested Readings

Daniel DM, Stone ML, Dobson BR, et al. Fate of the ACL-injured patient: a prospective outcome study. *Am J Sports Med.* 1994;22(5):632–644.

Spindler KP, Wright RW. Clinical practice. Anterior cruciate ligament tear. *N Engl J Med.* 2008;359(20):2135–2142.

Wright RW, Preston E, Fleming BC, et al. A systematic review of anterior cruciate ligament reconstruction rehabilitation. Part I: continuous passive motion, early weight bearing, postoperative bracing, and home-based rehabilitation. *J Knee Surg.* 2008;21(3):217–224.

Wright RW, Preston E, Fleming BC, et al. A systematic review of anterior cruciate ligament reconstruction rehabilitation. Part II: open versus closed kinetic chain exercises, neuromuscular electrical stimulation, accelerated rehabilitation, and miscellaneous topics. *J Knee Surg.* 2008;21(3):225–234.

Anterior Interosseous Neuropathy (Kiloh-Nevin Syndrome)

Ralph Buschbacher MD

Description
Neuropathy of the anterior interosseous nerve (AIN), a branch of the median nerve in the forearm.

Etiology/Types
- Spontaneous
  - Neuralgic amyotrophy type
  - Entrapment from anatomic variants (accessory muscles/vessels, etc.) rare
  - Fascicular constrictions of the nerve itself have been described, often above the branching of the AIN; may be a form of neuralgic amyotrophy
- Traumatic

Epidemiology
- Rare; <1% of compression neuropathies of the upper extremity
- Occasionally bilateral, sometimes recurrent
- Men equal to women, usually 30 to 60 years old, no side preponderance

Pathogenesis
- Largest branch of the median nerve; originates from 5 to 8 cm distal to the level of the lateral epicondyle
- Passes between the deep and superficial heads of the pronator teres and goes under the flexor digitorum superficialis to run on the anterior interosseous membrane
- Runs in an identifiable fascicle of the median nerve as proximal as the brachial plexus
- Carries motor fibers to the flexor digitorum profundus (FDP) of digits 2 (almost always) and 3 (usually), flexor policis longus (FPL), and pronator quadratus (PQ) as well as sensory fibers to the wrist joint; no skin sensory fibers
- Condition may be preceded by a flu-like illness or immunization
- Fascicular constrictions may be due to an inflammatory rather than a mechanical cause

Risk factors
- Unknown

Clinical Features
- With neuralgic amyotrophy type, aching pain in the upper arm/elbow may precede weakness
- Pain may increase with exercise
- Muscle weakness affecting the FPL, PQ, and FDP to digits 2 and 3
- Difficulty with pinch, grip, writing, and picking up objects between the thumb and forefinger
- Normal sensation
- Wrist pain possible
- May affect one muscle more than another

Natural History
- For neuralgic amyotropy type—pain, then weakness
- Spontaneous cases may recover, sometimes slowly—up to a 1- to 2-year period
- Most recover to at least 3 over 5 strength

Diagnosis

Differential diagnosis
- Proximal median neuropathy
- Brachial plexopathy
- Radiculopathy
- Tendon rupture

History
- Pain, then weakness for neuralgic amyotrophy type
- No sensory loss
- Preceding trauma

Exam
- For testing strength of the FPL and FDP, the examiner stabilizes the proximal joints and tests distal flexion
- Testing the PQ is done in elbow flexion to reduce the strength of the pronator teres—not a particularly sensitive test
- Patient is asked to make an "OK sign"—with FPL/FDP weakness, the fingers, not the fingertips, are pushed together (Figure 1)

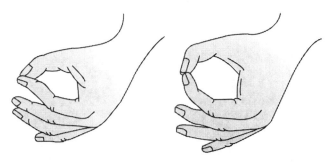

Figure 1. Weakness of the flexor policis longus (FPL)/ flexor digitorum profundus (FDP) leads to inability to flex the distal interphalangeal joint of the index finger and the interphalangeal of the thumb (OK sign).

Testing
- Electromyography (EMG)—sensory studies normal; motor studies to the PQ may show slowing (because of anatomic variability, side to side are comparisons valuable); needle examination reveals denervation; also important to test more .proximal muscles to detect more diffuse neuralgic amyotrophy
- Magnetic resonance imaging (MRI) and ultrasound may reveal obvious causes of compression (if present) and atrophy of affected muscles, but are not usually revealing; cannot visualize the nerve itself

Pitfalls
- Anomalous innervation, especially FDP by the ulnar nerve, flexor digitorum superficialis by the AIN, and FPL directly from the median nerve
- In persons with Martin-Gruber anastomosis, "ulnar-innervated" muscles of hand can be affected, as the anastomosis usually comes off the AIN
- More proximal median neuropathy

Red Flags
- Tendon rupture
- Anatomic derangement that can be reversed

Treatment
Medical
- Rest—avoid aggravating activity (pronation and supination with finger flexion, forceful grip)
- Observe—if no recovery, consider surgical exploration
- Recommend nonoperative care for noncompressive cause (hard to know when this is the case)
- Nonsteroidal anti-inflammatory drugs (NSAIDS)

Exercise
- Not proven

Modalities/bracing
- No evidence of benefit except that bracing may enforce rest or improve function by a stabilizing effect

Injection
- Local block of distal AIN may decrease wrist pain

Surgical
- If suspect a compressive type, with no improvement in 2 months, consider surgery
- If suspect a neuralgic amyotrophy type, surgery results are less predictable
- For neuralgic amyotrophy type, surgery controversial, but if no improvement by 3 months (6 weeks to 1 year have been recommended), consider surgical exploration; this should probably include interfascicular neurolysis, even above the level of the branching of the AIN
- Tendon transfers to improve function if no significant recovery in a year or more

Consults
- Physical medicine and rehabilitation for conservative care
- Orthopedic hand or plastic surgery/neurosurgery
- Neurology or physical medicine and rehabilitation for electrodiagnosis

Complications of treatment
- Surgical risks

Prognosis
- Variable—better if an identifiable cause of compression is released early
- If compression is cause, surgery more likely to help
- For neuralgic amyotrophy type, prognosis variable— generally good, but can take 2 to 3 years

Helpful Hints
- With different forearm lengths, standardized distance measurement for nerve conduction studies is difficult; use obstetric calipers to transfer measure from one side to the other

Suggested Readings
Nagano A. Spontaneous anterior interosseous nerve palsy. *J Bone Joint Surg.* 2003;85B:313–318.
Schollen W, Degreef I, De Smet L. Kiloh-Nevin syndrome: a compression neuropathy or brachial plexus neuritis? *Acta Orthop Belg.* 2007;73:315–318.

Arachnoiditis

Andrew J. Haig MD

Description

Inflammation of the arachnoid covering of the spinal nerves, in most cases asymptomatic, rare, and debated in the medical literature, is related to nerve damage and pain. Radiological and pathological arachnoiditis must be distinguished from symptomatic arachnoiditis.

Etiology/Types

- Trauma: from spine surgery, spine injection, or myelogram
- Infectious: tuberculosis, syphilis, and associated with discitis (rare in developed countries)
- Arachnoiditis ossificans: rare variant

Epidemiology

- Radiologically present in one-third of persons who get myelogram, many surgical patients without consequence
- Historically attributed to various myelogram dyes, but not clearly proven
- Relation with disc degeneration and herniation in nonsurgical cases is debated

Pathogenesis

- Trauma causes inflammation

Risk Factors

- Spinal procedures

Clinical Features

- Unclear. Some claim progressive weakness, paresthesia, and pain

Natural History

- Some believe pain, neurological deficit, and incontinence may progress
- More neurological deficits from surgical attempts to cure than from the disease itself in one study

Diagnosis

- The diagnosis is based on clinical judgment

Differential diagnosis

- The original disease that caused the surgery (including disc disease and spinal tumors)
- Spinal stenosis (clumping due to lack of space)

- Infections
- Post-myelogram or therapeutic injections

History

- Pain and weakness after a spinal procedure. Nonspecific

Exam

- Pain, limited back motion
- Occasional neurological deficit
- Nonspecific findings

Testing

- Classic magnetic resonance imaging (MRI), myelogram, or computed tomography (CT) findings
- No test differentiates clinical syndrome from asymptomatic arachnoiditis
- Electromyography (EMG) confirms neurological deficit, but not the disorder causing it
- MRI Delamarter classification:
  - Type 1: central clumping
  - Type 2: lateral clumping ("empty sac")
  - Type 3: Thecal sac filled with clumped or matted roots

Pitfalls

- Pain and neurological deficit should not be attributed to the common finding of arachnoiditis unless all other etiologies do not exist
- Patients must be counseled about the controversy surrounding diagnosis so they avoid medical misadventure
- Caution about performing a second procedure on someone with severe arachnoiditis

Red Flags

- Infection
- Spinal instability
- Suicide, depression, drug abuse

Treatment

Medical

- Pain management with antidepressant and anticonvulsant medications
- Anti-inflammatory and analgesic medications
- Typically no disease-specific treatment is given

Exercises
- Back stabilization training
- Lower extremity flexibility and strengthening
- Aerobic training and aquatic rehabilitation

Modalities
- Superficial and deep heat modalities
- Transcutaneous electrical nerve stimulation
- Electrical stimulation

Injection
- Limited data in the role of injections
- Steroid injection controversial use
- Injection of scar-reducing chemicals

Surgical
- Note: All invasive treatments listed are uncommon and controversial
- Subarachnoidal endoscopy
- Spinal decompression

Consults
- Multidisciplinary rehabilitation team

- Pain management
- Rarely spine surgeon

Complications/side effects
- Unclear, possibly progressive symptoms
- Suicide, depression, drug abuse

Prognosis
- Among patients with symptoms, ongoing pain, rarely progression of neurological deficit

Helpful Hints
- Don't fester over the one finding (arachnoiditis) just because it is easy to see. Obsess over other causes of pain and whole-patient rehabilitation

Suggested Readings
Guyer DW, Wiltse LL, Eskay ML, Guyer BH. The long-range prognosis of arachnoiditis. *Spine.* 1989;14(12):1332–1341.
Petty PG, Hudgson P, Hare WS. Symptomatic lumbar spinal arachnoiditis: fact or fallacy? *J Clin Neurosci.* 2000;7(5):395–399.

Avulsion Injuries of the Pelvis

Zach Beresford MD ▇ Stuart Willick MD

Description
An avulsion fracture is a failure of bone at the origin or insertion of a tendon, resulting from application of high tensile forces through a musculotendinous unit.

Etiology/Types
- Acute injury in adolescent athletes
- Affects the anterior superior iliac spine (sartorius), anterior inferior iliac spine (rectus femoris), lesser trochanter of the femur (iliopsoas), and ischial tuberosity (hamstrings)
- Some individuals may present with chronic symptoms associated with apophysitis

Epidemiology
- Avulsion fractures are often sports-related (e.g., soccer, gymnastics, dance) and commonly occur in children and adolescents
- Open apophyses are more prone to injury than musculotendinous units
- Pelvic avulsion injuries are far less common in skeletally mature athletes

Pathogenesis
- Acute acceleration (concentric), and deceleration (eccentric) forces applied to the immature skeleton
- The origin or insertion of tendons into bone is the weak link in the adolescent with an open apophysis

Risk Factors
- Participation in sports that involve acceleration and deceleration
- Adolescent age
- Muscle weakness, and imbalances

Clinical Features
- Acute pain following forceful muscle contraction
- Difficulty with walking, and inability to run
- Localized swelling and tenderness

Natural History
- Minimally displaced fractures (<3 mm), heal well with conservative treatment
- Displaced fractures (>5 mm), may require surgical treatment

- Muscle weakness remains if not specifically addressed in rehabilitation

Diagnosis
Differential diagnosis
- Acute muscle strains
- Apophysitis
- Slipped capital femoral epiphysis
- Synovitis

History
- Generally seen in young athletes who describe a mechanism involving an acute muscle contraction or sudden stretch, followed by sudden pain at the muscle origin or insertion
- Less commonly, the patient will report gradual onset of pain with an increase in activity

Exam
- Swelling and local tenderness
- Limited active motion
- Muscle weakness, or pain inhibition
- Pain may be reproduced with passive stretch and resistance testing of the involved muscle
- Antalgic gait

Testing
- Plain radiography is usually diagnostic and allows evaluation of the degree of displacement
- Follow-up films to evaluate healing
- Magnetic resonance imaging (MRI) can frequently show signal change in the area of injury

Pitfalls
- Diagnosis may be initially missed
- Not addressing the involved muscles in management of residual inflexibility or weakness

Red Flags
- Pain that worsens despite treatment
- Residual gait dysfunction
- Pain at night, pain at rest, fever (may be associated with tumor, infection)

Treatment
Medical
- Relative rest

- Protected weight bearing
- Analgesics

Exercises
- Pain-free range of motion (midrange)
- Brief static contractions in pain-free position
- Concentric exercise; as pain decreases progress to full range of motion; eccentric training when pain-free

Modalities
- Cryotherapy
- Superficial heat
- Transcutaneous electrical nerve stimulation, electrical stimulation

Injection
- Not indicated

Surgical
- Referral for displaced avulsion fractures or patients who remain symptomatic despite conservative treatment

Consults
- Orthopedic surgery
- Physical medicine and rehabilitation

Complications/side effect
- Myositis ossificans
- Residual pain
- Muscle weakness

Prognosis
- Good with prompt diagnosis and appropriate treatment
- Return to sports in 6 to 12 weeks following injury

Helpful Hints
- Consider avulsion fracture in any young athlete with acute hip and pelvic pain following sudden muscle contraction
- Compare films to the opposite hip and side of the pelvis

Suggested Readings

Metzmaker JN, Pappas AM. Avulsion fractures of the pelvis. *Am J Sports Med*. 1985;13:349–358.

Rossi F, Dragoni S. Acute avulsion fractures of the pelvis in adolescent competitive athletes: prevalence, location and sports distribution of 203 cases collected. *Skeletal Radiol*. 2001;30:127–131.

Vandervliet EJ, Vanhoenacker FM, Snoeckx A, et al. Sports-related acute and chronic avulsion injuries in children and adolescents with special emphasis on tennis. *Br J Sports Med*. 2007;41(11):827–831.

Biceps Tendinopathy/Tear

Phillip T. Henning DO ■ Jay Smith MD

Description
Degenerative changes within the proximal aspect of the long head of the biceps tendon. First described by Pasteur in 1932.

Etiology/Type
- Several proposed mechanisms, including aging-related tendon degeneration, inflammation from repeated subacromial impingement, instability leading to chronic subluxation/dislocation, trauma, and systemic inflammatory conditions such as rheumatoid arthritis
- Types include tendinosis/tendinopathy, partial thickness tearing, or full thickness tearing, with or without tenosynovitis

Epidemiology
- Eighteen percent to 50% incidence in those with anterior shoulder pain
- Rarely an isolated process, seen in association with rotator cuff tendinopathy/tears

Pathogenesis
- Degenerative process
- Lack of inflammatory component within tendon (i.e., tendinosis/tendinopathy, not tendinitis)
- Many cases associated with instability (subluxation or dislocation) of tendon out of the bicipital groove

Risk Factors
- Advanced age
- High or repetitive mechanical loading
- Bicipital subluxation/dislocation due to concomitant rotator cuff tears
- Stenosis of bicipital groove from degenerative joint disease

Clinical Features
- Anterior shoulder pain
- Pain with overhead activity
- Pain with palpation of biceps tendon
- Weakness or sense of instability with overhead activity
- In cases of tendon rupture, the long head of biceps retracts leading to a visible bulge/deformity (Popeye sign)

Natural History
- Highly variable

Diagnosis

Differential diagnosis
- Rotator cuff tear/tendinopathy
- Superior labral anterior and posterior injury/tear
- Subacromial bursitis
- Adhesive capsulitis
- Coracoid impingement syndrome
- Subacromial impingement syndrome
- Osteoarthritis/rheumatoid arthritis
- Cervical spinal cord syrinx, radiculopathy (C5 and C6), brachial plexopathy, peripheral neuropathy—neurological reasons for dysfunctional neuromuscular control

History
- Anterior shoulder pain
- Deep dull ache
- Occasionally sharp
- Radiation into the arm
- Pain worse with overhead activities
- Sleeping on involved side causes pain
- Deformity, weakness/cramp with active forearm supination in cases of complete biceps tendon rupture

Exam
- Tenderness along the bicipital groove
- Reproduction of pain with Speeds test
- Evidence of concomitant rotator cuff injury
- Tendon tear associated with retraction of the long head (Popeye sign), weakness/pain with supination/flexion of elbow

Testing
- Magnetic resonance imaging (MRI) and ultrasound can be used but are not always indicated
- Sonography examines extra-articular pathology of tendon and tenosynovitis, as well as extent of rotator cuff involvement. Also assesses dynamic stability of the biceps tendon
- MRI can identify tendon tears, tenosynovitis, rotator cuff tears, and intra-articular pathology, and evidence of coracoid impingement (narrowed coracohumeral interval)

- Radiographs of shoulder to assess for osteoarthritis of glenohumeral joint or narrow coracohumeral interval

Pitfalls
- Mistaking biceps tendinopathy over rotator cuff tendinopathy as primary cause of pain

Red Flags
- Night pain
- Unresolving biceps tendinitis may be associated with superior labral tears

Treatment

Medical
- Activity modification
- Nonsteroidal anti-inflammatory medications
- Analgesics

Exercises
- Rotator cuff strengthening leads to humeral head depression, thus reducing tension on biceps tendon within the bicipital groove
- Stretching to eliminate range of motion imbalances
- Scapular stabilizer strengthening

Modalities
- Cryotherapy
- Superficial/deep heat
- Electrical stimulation
- Iontophoresis/phonophoresis (theoretical risk of tendon weakening/rupture)

Injection
- Glenohumeral joint or biceps tendon sheath corticosteroid injection (glenohumeral joint synovial space is continuous with the bicipital tendon sheath)

Surgical
- Biceps tendon repair in younger patients, distal biceps tears
- Tenodesis
- Tenotomy
- Rotator cuff repair

Consults
- Orthopedic surgery

Complications/side effects
- Progressive pain and dysfunction
- Tendon rupture that can lead to deformity, weakness/cramping with forearm supination

Prognosis
- Highly variable

Helpful Hints
- Treating additional underlying pathology (i.e., rotator interval tears or rotator cuff dysfunction) is often needed for resolution of symptoms

Suggested Readings
Ahrens P, Boileau P. The long head of biceps and associated tendinopathy. *J Bone Joint Surg (Br)*. 2007;89-B:1001–1009.
Patton C, McCluskey G. Biceps tendinitis and subluxation. *Clin Sports Med*. 2001;20(3):505–529.

Calcaneal Apophysitis (Sever's Disease)

María A. Ocasio-Silva MD FAAPMR

Description
Calcaneal apophysitis (or Sever's disease) is an inflammation of the apophysis at the posterior aspect of the calcaneus.

Etiology/Types
- Overuse syndrome

Epidemiology
- These patients are primarily in the early phase of accelerated growth; they are most commonly 9 to 12 years of age but may be younger
- Affects boys more frequently than girls
- Sever's disease occurs most frequently in active 10- to 12-year-old boys
- Bilateral presentation in about 60% of cases

Pathogenesis
- Repetitive loading leading to microtrauma from the pull of the Achilles tendon on the unossified calcaneal apophysis
- During the rapid growth surrounding puberty, the apophyseal line appears to be weakened further because of increased fragile-calcified cartilage
- Microfractures are believed to occur because of shear stress, leading to the normal progression of fracture healing

Risk Factors
- Growth spurt
- Tight gastroc-soleus tendon Achilles complex
- Tight plantar fascia
- High impact jumping and running sports such as basketball, running, gymnastics, soccer
- Poor-quality athletic shoes

Clinical Features
- Tenderness at the insertion of the Achilles tendon into the posterior calcaneus
- Recent growth spurt coinciding with increase in high impact recreational or sports activities (preseason or early season)

Natural History
- Self-limited condition
- Symptoms usually resolve within a few weeks or occasionally months with appropriate treatment

Diagnosis
Differential diagnosis
- Insertional Achille's tendonitis
- Calcaneal bursitis
- Calcaneal stress fracture
- Tumor
- Osteomyelitis

History
- Pain in one or both heels
- Pain worsened by activity, especially running and jumping
- Pain relieved by rest

Exam
- Tenderness to palpation at the posterior heel (Figure 1)
- Exquisite heel pain produced by medial and lateral compression ("squeezing") of the heel
- Reduced ankle dorsiflexion
- Pain reproduced with resisted plantarflexion
- Pain reproduced with standing on tiptoe, jumping, and running

Testing
- Radiographs are not required in routine cases
- Radiographs might be needed in patients with refractory symptoms

Pitfalls
- The condition can also be part of an inflammatory arthropathy

Red Flags
- Fever
- Weight loss
- Other constitutional symptoms

Treatment
Medical
- Acetaminophen or nonsteroidal anti-inflammatory drug on as needed basis for pain relief
- Activity modification including relative rest when symptoms arise

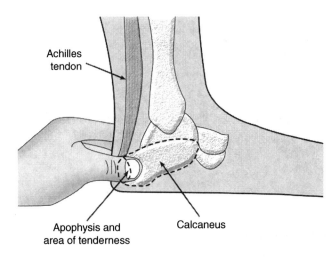

Figure 1. Area of tenderness to palpation in Sever's disease.

- Good-quality shoes with adequate shock absorption
- Orthotic
- Heel cushioning, heel lift
- Heel cups and other forms of custom-molded shock-absorbing insoles
- Short leg cast or walking boot for severe/refractory cases

Exercises
- Flexibility and stretching exercises of the Achilles tendon
- Strengthening of gastroc-soleus complex, ankle dorsiflexors, and quadriceps
- Eccentric exercises

Modalities
- Cold
- Heat (but avoid ultrasound)
- Electrical stimulation

Injection
- Not indicated

Surgical
- Not indicated
- Condition rarely needs surgical intervention

Consults
- Sports medicine or orthopedic surgery if no resolution of symptoms

Complications/side effects
- Usually none
- There have been no reports of long-term sequelae

Prognosis
- Symptoms usually resolve within a few weeks or occasionally months with appropriate treatment
- In patients with refractory symptoms, several weeks of immobilization can relieve severe symptomatology, which can be followed by a formal therapy regimen
- No recurrence after growth plate fuses

Helpful Hints
- Of primary importance are activity modification and flexibility training.
- Patients are counseled to maintain a home baseline stretching program to prevent recurrences, which can occur during periods of rapid growth.

Acknowledgments
The author thanks Kevin Walter, MD, Department of Orthopedics, Medical College of Wisconsin for his advice and comments.

Suggested Readings
Hendrix CL. Calcaneal apophysitis (Sever disease). *Clin Pediatr Med Surg.* 2005;22:55–62.
Micheli LJ, Ireland MO. Prevention and management of calcaneal apophysitis in children: an overuse syndrome. *J Pediatr Orthop.* 1987;7:34–38.

Carpal Tunnel Syndrome

Ralph Buschbacher MD

Description

Carpal tunnel syndrome (CTS) is an entrapment neuropathy of the median nerve in the carpal tunnel of the wrist.

Etiology/Types

- Idiopathic—most common
- Traumatic
- Fluid retention
- Anatomic variant
- Repetitive use/vibration/forceful gripping (possible)

Epidemiology

- Most common compression neuropathy (3.8% of population has clinical symptoms, 4.9% has electromyography (EMG) evidence, 2.7% has both)
- Age 30 to 60 years (peak in late 50s, especially for women; second peak in late 70s—men and women more equal)
- Fifty-five percent to 65% bilateral, more likely in dominant hand
- Increased incidence in late pregnancy
- Genetic factors account for half of risk (especially if present bilaterally)
- Increasing age, female gender, white race, obesity, diabetes (especially Type I, but to some extent Type II)—strong association
- Hormonal level (postmenopausal or postoopherectomy)—some association
- Smoking—minor association
- Occupational factors—debatable or minor association—possibly associated with vibratory tools, continuous or repetitive wrist flexion/extension, high force gripping, repetitive or prolonged nonergonomic hand positions, cold environment
- Keyboarding/computer work not associated with CTS

Pathogenesis

- The carpal tunnel is formed by the carpal bones and the transverse carpal ligament
- Contains nine tendons and median nerve, which is the most susceptible to pressure injury
- Pressure increased by wrist flexion, finger flexion, and especially wrist extension

- Sustained or intermittent pressure increase leads to impaired microcirculation, demyelination, and possibly axonal loss
- Any cause of decreased dimensions of the tunnel or increase in volume of the contents can cause nerve damage

Risk Factors

- Obesity in young persons
- Pregnancy
- More "square" wrist/shorter finger to palm width ratio
- Rheumatoid arthritis, osteoarthritis, diabetes, hypothyroidism, dialysis/end-stage renal disease, surgical or natural menopause, acromegaly

Clinical Features

- Paresthesias in the radial 3½ fingers (variations in symptoms and innervation patterns common— sometimes affects whole hand; pain may extend up the arm)
- Swelling—usually subjective
- Decreased sensation in the median nerve distribution, sparing the thenar eminence, which is innervated by the palmar cutaneous branch, which does not pass through the tunnel (Figure 1)

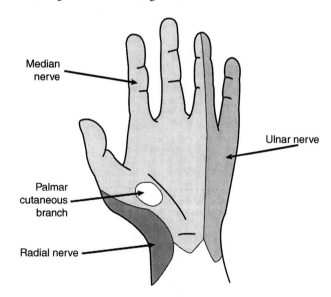

Figure 1. Median nerve sensory distribution in the hand. The thenar eminens is supplied by the palmar cutaneous branch of the median nerve, which branches off in the forearm and does not pass through the tunnel.

- Weakness/wasting of the thenar muscles less common, but seen in more severe cases
- Nighttime symptoms common, possibly due to increased pressure at night

Natural History
- Variable
- In pregnancy usually resolves
- Worse prognosis in the elderly

Diagnosis

Differential diagnosis
- Radiculopathy
- Raynaud's phenomenon
- Trigger finger/tendonitis/Dupuytren's contracture
- Degenerative arthritis
- Other focal neuropathy/peripheral neuropathy
- Syringomyelia
- Multiple sclerosis

History
- Paresthesias/dysesthesias in median nerve distribution
- Nighttime symptoms
- Subjective swelling
- Subjective weakness/dropping things

Physical examination
- Limited by high false positives/negatives; poor sensitivity/specificity
- Phalen's test—significant if reproduces symptoms with wrist flexion, especially <1 minute (or 30 seconds)
- Tinel's sign—paresthesias with tapping the nerve
- Durkan test—paresthesias with carpal compression
- Decreased objective sensation, 2-point discrimination, moving 2-point discrimination, sensory threshold testing
- Motor weakness and thenar atrophy—only positive in severe "obvious" cases

Testing
- EMG—gold standard; excludes other neurological causes
- Ultrasound—shows anatomy, not physiology; in CTS nerve, cross section is increased (can test wrist vs forearm cross-sectional area); cannot evaluate other nerve conditions
- Magnetic resonance imaging (MRI)—poor sensitivity and specificity, but may rarely reveal a space occupying lesion in cases confirmed by EMG

Pitfalls
- Anomalous innervation
- Congenitally absent abductor pollicis brevis
- Other neuropathies

Red Flags
- Denervation or significant conduction block on EMG—consider surgery sooner rather than later

Treatment

Medical
- Splinting in neutral—shown to provide lasting benefit
- Activity modification or removal of external compressive factors
- Nonsteroidal anti-inflammatory drugs (NSAIDs)—not proven but commonly used; some benefit possible
- Vitamin B-6—ineffective or negligible benefit
- Oral steroids—probably beneficial in some cases
- Diuretics—some benefit possible in pregnancy

Exercise
- Multiple treatments have been recommended—none proven
- Some inconclusive evidence of benefit of yoga and nerve glide techniques

Modalities
- Iontophoreses (steroid)—may help temporarily; not as good as injection
- Low-level laser, low-intensity ultrasound—some inconclusive and conflicting evidence

Injection
- Steroid—beneficial, but frequently just temporarily
- Botulinum toxin—no benefit

Surgery
- No significant difference in outcomes between open and endoscopic resection of the traverse carpal ligament, but endoscopic cases may return to work a week or so sooner; surgeon experience more critical in endoscopic technique
- In severe cases, surgery may have limited benefit, as the nerve damage has already occurred
- In mild cases or if EMG normal, consider conservative care first

Consults
- Physical medicine and rehabilitation for conservative management and EMG
- Neurology for EMG

- Orthopedic hand surgery/plastic surgery/ neurosurgery for conservative care or surgery

Complications/side effects
- Injection/surgical complications
- Damage to palmar cutaneous nerve branch (innervates thenar eminence)

Prognosis
- Seventy-five percent symptomatic success rate with surgery; 8% are worse
- Surgical success lower in clinical CTS without EMG evidence
- Slightly worse surgical outcome in older patients

Helpful Hints
- Always do EMG before surgery; if it confirms CTS, there is a better surgical prognosis; if it detects another problem, it can prevent unnecessary/wrong surgery; if negative, or if there are multiple nerve diagnoses (e.g., concurrent radiculopathy), then surgical prognosis may be worse (important for establishing realistic expectations)

Suggested Readings

Bland JDP. Carpal tunnel syndrome. *Curr Opin Neurol.* 2005;18:581–585.

Lozano-Calderon S, Anthony S, Ring D. The quality and strength of evidence for etiology: example of carpal tunnel syndrome. *J Hand Surg.* 2008;33A:525–538.

Cervical Disc Pathology

Michael Furman MD MS

Description
Cervical disc disease is the process of disruption of the normal architecture of the cervical intervertebral disc. This process can represent normal aging or can be related to direct injury to the disc.

Etiology/Types
- Three major types
- Herniated nucleus pulposus (HNP)
- Internal disc disruption (IDD)
- Degenerative disc disease (DDD)

Epidemiology
- Magnetic resonance imaging (MRI) changes have been observed in up to 40% of asymptomatic patients younger than age 40 and 60% of those older than age 60
- Not all disc herniations result in radiculopathy; radiculopathy may be seen in the absence of herniation
- True etiology of radiculopathy is unknown but estimated at 63 to 100 per 100,000

Pathogenesis
- A basic understanding of cervical spine and disc architecture is necessary to understand pathological changes
- There are seven cervical vertebrae, with intervertebral disc between C2 and T1
- There is no disc between the occiput and C1 or axis but there is a synovial joint
- There is no joint between C1 and C2 or atlas, but there is an articulation between these two vertebrae
- The major movement between C1 and C2 is rotational
- Each disc consists of an outer annular ring called the annulus fibrosis, which is made of Type II collagen
- The annulus surrounds the nucleus pulposus, which has Type I collagen
- The nucleus pulposus is a gel-like material with proteoglycans, water, and enzymes
- The disc is metabolically active but has a very poor blood supply; nutrients diffuse through the vertebral endplates
- The outer aspect of each disc is innervated by the vertebral nerve

- HNP implies that nuclear material extends beyond the posterior border of the vertebral body, and usually occurs at the posterolateral aspect of the disc
- HNPs are classified as: disc bulge, protrusion, extrusion, sequestration
- C6 and C7 discs are the most commonly affected. The most common nerve roots affected in descending order are C7, C6, C8, and C5
- DDD occurs most commonly from the normal aging process in the cervical spine
- Tears in the annulus will coalesce into radial tears, which can then lead to disruption throughout the disc
- The disc will then lose height leading to further spondylosis throughout the spine
- The disc will also lose hydration or dessicate along with changes within the nuclear matrix
- Eventually osteophytes and sclerosis will occur
- IDD refers to pathological disruption of the annulus fibrosus without visible external disc disruption
- This can lead to ingrowth of nerve fibers through outer third of the annulus
- The disc then becomes mechanically sensitive leading to pain generation

Risk Factors
- Trauma
- Repetitive stress/trauma
- Smoking
- Age
- Whiplash injuries
- Genetics

Clinical Features
- Axial neck pain only
- Radicular pain radiating to the upper limbs in some cases
- Sensory changes in a dermatomal pattern
- Weakness in a myotomal pattern
- Decreased reflexes
- Myofasical pain in the upper neck and back musculature

Natural History
- Disc degeneration begins as early as the second decade of life

- By the age of 60 years, near 90% of individuals will have spondylitic changes in the cervical spine
- There is no way to predict which disc will become symptomatic later in life
- HNP will usually improve on its own over 2 to 6 months

Diagnosis

Differential diagnosis
- Musculoskeletal pain
- Facet-mediated pain
- Mononeuropathy
- Infection
- Fracture
- Neoplasm
- Sensitization of the central nervous system
- Neurological disease—that is, multiple sclerosis, and so on
- Rheumatologic disease

History
- Progressive neck pain
- Increasing radicular symptoms
- Upper extremity numbness
- Weakness

Exam
- Tenderness in the cervical spine
- Sensory changes in a dermatomal pattern
- Weakness in a myotomal pattern
- Decreased reflexes
- Decreased range of motion in the cervical spine
- Signs of myelopathy (increased tone, increased muscle stretch reflexes, Hoffman's, Babinski signs) if the spinal cord is compressed

Testing
- X-rays reveal spondylitic changes
- Flexion and extension films can identify instability
- Computed tomography (CT) scans give a more detailed look at the bony architecture of the cervical spine
- CT myelography can image far lateral and foraminal stenosis that MRI can miss
- MRI is superior for imaging the intervertebral disc and the soft tissues
- Cervical discography can be used to identify pathological discs that reproduce pain
- Electromyography (EMG) will identify radiculopathies affecting motor fibers
- Somatosensory-evoked potentials (SSEPs) may be used to assess cervical cord compression

Pitfalls
- Imaging alone is not enough to accurately diagnose a patient's pathology and should not supplant a full history and physical
- HNP does not always lead to radiculopathy

Red Flags
- Upper motor neuron signs, Hoffman's reflexes, spasticity
- Atrophy in the upper limb musculature, preserved sensation
- Fever, chills, and night sweats
- New onset gait abnormalities
- Bowel or bladder changes

Treatment

Medical
- Nonsteroidal anti-inflammatory medications
- Oral steroid taper for acute pain and radicular symptoms

Exercises
- General strengthening and stretching
- McKenzie approach
- Cervicothoracic stabilization
- Ergonomic improvements in work space and posture/functional positioning
- Functional training
- Neuromobilization

Modalities
- Heat
- Cold
- Ultrasound
- Transcutaneous electrical nerve stimulation
- Traction (caution with central HNP, Down's syndrome, and rheumatoid arthritis may lead to spinal cord injury)

Injection
- Trigger point injections
- Epidural steroid injection with fluoroscopic guidance for radicular symptoms
- Facet joint injects with fluoroscopic guidance for facet joint-mediated pain and associated referred headaches/shoulder pain

Surgical
- Indications for surgery
- Deteriorating radicular findings
- Bowel or bladder changes
- Myelopathic changes

- Spinal instability
- Chronic axial pain, which is significantly limiting function

Consults
- Physical medicine and rehabilitation
- Neurosurgical or orthopedic-spine surgery

Complications/side effects
- Chronic radicular or axial pain
- Myelopathy
- Quadriplegia

Prognosis
- Generally patients will recover with appropriate conservative therapies

Helpful Hints
- The cervical discs naturally degenerate over time and this is a benign process

- When pathology does occur, treatment should be geared to the specific etiology knowing that most patients will recover
- Deteriorating or worsening symptoms should prompt appropriate imaging and surgical consult

Suggested Readings

Anderson P, Subach B, Riew K. Predictors of outcome after anterior cervical discectomy and fusion—a multivariate analysis. *Spine.* 2009;34(2):161–166.

Carragee E, Hurwitz E, Cheng I, et al. Treatment of neck pain-injections and surgical interventions: results of the bone and joint decade 2000–2010 task force on neck pain and its associated disorders. *Spine.* 2008;33(45):S153-S169.

Furman M, Simon J, Puttlitz K, et al. *Cervical Disc Disease.* www.emedicine.com. Updated 21 February 2007.

Cervical Facet Syndrome

Dave Bagnall MD

Description
Cervical facet syndrome refers to axial neck pain thought to be related to nonspecific involvement of the cervical facet joint and its related structures.

Etiology/Types
- There are a variety of complaints associated with this syndrome, which are inconsistent across the spectrum. It carries no affinity for sex, age, or level of degenerative change
- It is generally associated with a defined episode of noncatastrophic injury affecting the upper quadrant

Epidemiology
- Universal degeneration, usually asymptomatic
- Estimated prevalence between 26% and 65% in patients with chronic neck pain

Pathogenesis
- The facets of C3 to C7 are encapsulated synovial diarthrodial joints
- The fibrous capsules are innervated by mechanoreceptors and accessory nerves originating from overlying muscular or cutaneous tissues to which they provide primary innervation
- The mechanoreceptors may stimulate protective muscular reflexes important to joint stability, whereas the accessory-free nerve endings are involved primarily in pain sensation
- The facet joints are innervated by anterior and dorsal rami of the cervical spinal nerves at and above C3, and by the dorsal rami at and below C3
- The cervical intervertebral disc annulus is susceptible to rotational injury and is innervated by nociceptors
- Damage to the lateral alar ligaments at the dens following whiplash may stimulate mechano- and nociceptors leading to headache, neck pain, and vertigo
- Microdamage to the anterior and posterior longitudinal ligaments, supraspinous and interspinous ligaments, and ligamentum flavum may have an effect on the development neck symptoms
- Cervical segmental motion is complex and couples rotation with lateral flexion
- The atlanto occipital (AO) joint accounts for 13° of cervical flexion and extension
- The atlanto axial (AA) joint accounts for about 50% of cervical rotation
- There is a clear correlation between sclerotomal pain patterns and cervical facet joint level

Risk Factors
- Mechanical neck injury
- Whiplash injury

Clinical Features
- Axial neck pain
- Headache
- Decreased cervical range of motion

Natural History
- Mild or moderate trauma such as motor vehicle accident, sports injury, work-related injury, or fall
- Onset of headache, neck pain, and occasionally pain in the upper back or shoulder regions in a sclerotomal rather than dermatomal pattern
- No clear association with age
- Duration of symptoms lasting over 6 months following the onset

Diagnosis
Differential diagnosis
- Disc herniation
- Ligament disruption
- Musculotendinous injury
- Fracture
- Stenosis
- Cervical disc disruption
- Infection
- Connective tissue disease

History
- History of whiplash or mechanical neck injury
- Dull ache at posterior neck
- Headache
- Occasional radiation into the shoulders or midthoracic region
- Decreased neck range of motion
- Absence of neurological anomaly
- Absence of radicular complaints

Exam

- Palpatory tenderness over the facets or the cervical paraspinal muscles (may be nonspecific)
- Pain with cervical extension or rotation
- Possible exacerbation with cervical compression
- Absence of neurological anomaly
- Absence of nerve root irritation signs

Testing

- Cervical radiographs including flexion and extension views may show evidence of mild intervertebral body displacement
- Degenerative changes are noncontributory as they are equally prevalent in patients with and without neck pain
- Magnetic resonance imaging (MRI), computed tomography, and bone scan are not helpful in making the diagnosis
- Medial branch blocks using image guidance have high sensitivity and moderate specificity for identifying the facets as the pain generator

Pitfalls

- Overinterpretation of imaging studies

Red Flags

- Fracture
- Ligamentous instability
- Neoplasm
- Infection

Treatment

Medical

- Nonsteroidal anti-inflammatory medications
- Analgesics
- Muscle relaxants

Exercises

- Passive to active range of motion in pain-free range
- Isometric to isotonic exercise as pain improves
- Graduation to improving strength, flexibility, neuromuscular control, and endurance of the upper quadrant structures as pain dissipates

Modalities

- Ice
- Heat
- Manual joint therapy
- Ultrasound
- Electrical nerve stimulation
- Massage therapy

Injection

- Radiofrequency neurotomy of medial branches proven to be a source of pain is effective in up to 70% of patients with a mean duration of 6 to 12 months
- Occasionally trigger point injections may be helpful

Surgical

- There is no indication for surgical intervention for cervical facet syndrome, and facet joint pain can occur after cervical fusion

Consults

- Physical medicine and rehabilitation
- Chiropractic (may help for short-term symptomatic relief, unclear long-term benefit)
- Physical therapy

Complications/side effects

- Progressive pain and dysfunction

Prognosis

- Variable

Helpful Hints

- Cervical facet syndrome is rarely a progressive condition
- Encouraging patients to actively participate in their own rehabilitation is the single most effective intervention

Suggested Readings

Lord SM, Barnsley L, Wallis BJ, et al. Percutaneous radio-frequency neurotomy for chronic cervical zygapophyseal joint pain. *N Engl J Med.* 1996;335(23):1721–1726.

Sherman AL, Young JL. Musculoskeletal rehabilitation and sports medicine. 1. Head and spine injuries. *Arch Phys Med Rehabil.* 1999;80(5 suppl 1):S40-S49.

Cervical Myofascial Pain

Marta Imamura MD PhD ■ Rui Imamura MD PhD

Description
Cervical myofascial pain syndrome (MPS) is defined as pain that originates from muscles (including myofascial trigger points [MTrPs]) in skeletal muscle. MPS is usually localized in the neck region, is associated with reproducible pain patterns, and is among the most common causes of musculoskeletal pain.

Etiology/Types
- Regional soft tissue pain
- Associated with trauma
- Insidous in onset
- Commonly involved muscles are the sternocleidomastoid (clavicular belly), anterior and medial scalenes, masseter, and lateral and medial pterigoids in the anterior and medial cervical region. Posterior cervical muscles involved are the levator scapula, posterior scalenes, and the upper trapezius muscle

Epidemiology
- Up to 66% of the adult population will experience cervical pain sometime in their lives
- Twenty percent to 30% of patients in orthopedic and general medical clinics have MPS
- As high as 80% of patients seen in specialty pain clinics may have MPS
- Men and women are equally affected

Pathogenesis
- Unknown; however, theories include:
  - Active MTrPs in the upper trapezius muscle present lower pressure pain threshold when compared with people with no pain or with latent trigger points
  - Increased acetylcholine (Ach) release present at the motor end plate, associated with muscle shortening and possible hypoxia
  - A distinct in vivo biochemical milieu with significant elevated levels of substance P, calcitonin gene-related peptide (CGRP), bradykinin, tumor necrosis factor-α (TNF-α), interleukin-1β (IL-1β),

serotonin, and norepinephrine has been found in the vicinity of active trigger points
  - Overall, pH has been shown to be significantly lower in active trigger points
  - Chronic patients present with central sensitization and amplified pain responses

Risk Factors
- Acute musculoskeletal trauma
- Underlying cervical spine pathology such as disc disease
- Overuse/poor biomechanics or ergonomics
- Chronic pain

Clinical Features
- Muscle aching, stiffness, tightness, and pain in the affected areas
- Pain more commonly located at the C5 and C6 segments usually radiates to the shoulder or upper limb of the involved side
- Distal paresthesias may be seen
- Associated with frontal, parietal, temporal, occipital, and periorbital headache
- Concurrent neurovegetative symptoms may rarely be present, including lacrimation, ocular erythema, dizziness, vertigo, and nausea

Diagnosis

Differential diagnosis
- Cervical radiculopathy
- Cervical facet syndrome
- Rotator cuff tendinopathy
- Fibromyalgia
- Migraine/muscle tension headaches
- Metabolic myopathies/thyroid disease
- Depression

History
- Cervical pain that radiates to the upper extremity, head, or face
- Numbness/paresthesia of the upper extremity, cervical region, or face

- Recent or remote trauma
- Change in activity level, biomechanics, or ergonomics
- Underlying cervical spine problems

Exam
- Limited neck motion
- Taut band with tender spots or trigger points located at the midpoint of the muscle belly
- Focal tenderness and reproduction of the patients' pain with firm palpation of the trigger point
- Twitch response may be present
- Neurological examination should be normal
- Muscle weakness present in shoulder, cervical, and scapular muscles (pain inhibition, disuse weakness?)

Testing
- MPS is a clinical diagnosis; diagnostic studies may be used to rule out associated conditions:
  - X-rays document underlying cervical spine/shoulder degenerative disease or soft tissue calcifications
  - Magnetic resonance imaging (MRI) to evaluate for cervical disc pathology
  - Electrodiagnostic studies to rule out radiculopathy or entrapment neuropathy

Pitfalls
- Missing underlying clinical conditions that merit specific treatments
- Only treating the patients' symptoms and not addressing abnormal biomechanics, and associated stressors

Red Flags
- Worsening pain despite treatment
- Progressive neurological deficits

Treatment

Medical
- Analgesics/anti-inflammatory medications (mixed data)
- Muscle relaxants used short term for patients with associated sleep dysfunction
- Antidepressants, particularly dual (serotonin and norepinephrine) reuptake inhibitors
- Cognitive/behavioral programs

Exercises
- Muscle relaxation techniques
- Stretching the upper trapezius, pectoral and cervical muscles
- Static and dynamic strengthening for cervical, scapular (lower trapezius and serratus anterior), and shoulder girdle muscles
- Cervical stabilization and postural restoration programs
- Aerobic/aquatic exercise program

Modalities
- Superficial heat
- Electrical stimulation
- Massage

Injections
- Steroid/anesthetic injection of tender/trigger points
- Dry needling is also used for the inactivation of the taut band and the trigger points
- Concomitant treatment of the myofascial component using lidocaine 1%, needling, and infiltration of the taut bands and trigger points. MTrPs injection is one of the few therapies that show evidence of benefit in controlling pain in chronic neck disorders. Due to anatomical proximity to large important vessels and nerves of the neck, injections of muscles such as the scalenes should be performed by experienced physicians and/or under imaging guidance
- When peripheral segmental sensitization is present, desensitization of the affected cervical level is recommended by some clinicians, using a paraspinous block (PSB), injecting local anesthetic (1% lidocaine) in the loose subcutaneous tissue along the spinal process. This PSB is theorized to reverse central sensitization by blocking nociceptive impulses from the supra/interspinous ligaments

Surgical
- Not indicated for MPS, may be required for underlying problems such as radiculopathy or rotator cuff tears

Consults
- Physical medicine and rehabilitation
- Pain medicine
- Psychology for biofeedback, muscle relaxation

Complications/side effects
- Chronic pain
- Activity intolerance

Prognosis
- Variable, depends on early intervention
- Worse results in chronic patients

Helpful Hints
- Failure to recognize and diagnose the peripheral and central sensitization of the dorsal horn neurons may lead to transient benefit rather than long-term relief

Suggested Readings

Fischer AA, Imamura M, Dubo H, et al. Segmental sensitization: diagnosis and treatment. In: O'Young BJ, Young MA, Steins SA, eds. *Physical Medicine and Rehabilitation Secrets*. 3rd ed. Philadelphia: Mosby Elsevier; 2008:610–625.

Peloso PM, Gross AR, Haines TA, et al. Medicinal and injection therapies for mechanical neck disorders: a Cochrane systematic review. *J Rheumatol*. 2006; 33(5):957–967.

Shah JP, Phillips TM, Danoff JV, et al. An in-vivo microanalytical technique for measuring the local milieu of human skeletal muscle. *J Appl Physiol*. 2005;99(5):1977–1984.

Cervical Radiculopathy

Gerald Malanga MD

Description
Cervical radiculopathy (*radicula*, little root; *pathos*, disease) by definition is any disease of a nerve root affecting the cervical segments (cervical nerve roots C1 to C8).

Etiology/Types
Pathology of the nerve roots that may result from a myriad of etiologies, including injury from direct trauma or compression by lesions such as tumors, herniated discs, and foraminal stenosis due to spondylosis

Epidemiology
- The average annual age-adjusted incidence rates per 100,000 population are 83.2 total, 107.3 for males and 63.5 for females
- The C7 nerve root is the most frequent affected nerve root, followed by C6
- A confirmed disc protrusion was responsible for cervical radiculopathy in 21.9% of patients; 68.4% were related to spondylosis, disc, or both
- Disc-related etiologies are more likely to be found in younger populations, whereas spondylytic causes predominate in the elderly
- Cervical spinal stenosis increases with aging

Pathogenesis
- Cervical spine annulus is crescent-shaped, thicker ventrally, and thins as it wraps dorsally
- Anterior aspect of the annulus is thick, with multiple layers of interwoven fibers set at oblique angles; posterior aspect consisted of one set of vertically orientated collagen fibers
- The disc is essentially deficient posteriolaterally and supported medially by the posterior longitudinal ligament
- The outer one-third of the annulus is richly innervated by the sinuvertebral nerve and vertebral nerves
- Mechanical factors that may lead to neurological symptoms are classified into static and dynamic
- Static factors are related to primary degenerative processes and include congenital spinal canal stenosis, disc herniation, vertebral body osteophyte growth into the spinal canal, degenerative osteophytes of the uncovertebral and facet joints, hypertrophy of the ligamentum flavum, and degenerative or calcific processes of the posterior longitudinal ligament and the ligamentum flavum
- The dynamic pathological factors that foster radiculopathy are abnormal forces on the spinal column during normal and abnormal movements and loads
- These degenerative changes can lead to loss of or reversal of normal cervical lordosis.
- Irritation of the cervical root by inflammatory mediators can lead to chemical radiculopathy and pain
- Compression of the nerve root may lead to weakness and sensory loss

Risk Factors
- No identifiable risk factors

Clinical Features
- Neck or scapular pain
- Pain that radiates into the scapular region or the upper extremity
- Sensory loss (rare specific dermatomal pattern)
- Muscle atrophy (rare)
- Muscle weakness
- Pain with Valsalva maneuvers

Natural History
- Chronic waxing and waning radicular symptoms may be caused by spondylotic processes, degenerative uncovertebral joints, nerve root sleeve fibrosis, herniated disc, and facet joint disease
- Acute disc herniations and sudden narrowing of the neural foramen may occur from injuries involving cervical extension, lateral bending or rotation, and axial loading
- This is a common mechanism for "burner" injuries, which may involve traction to the brachial plexus or cervical nerve roots or foraminal compression of nerve roots
- Ninety percent of cervical radiculopathy results in a favorable outcome with conservative treatments

Diagnosis

Differential diagnosis
- Myelopathy

- Neuralgic amyotrophy/Parsonage Turner syndrome
- Shoulder impingement syndrome
- Cervical strain/sprain
- Myofascial pain syndrome
- Upper extremity peripheral nerve impingement
- Osteoarthrosis
- Brachial plexopathy
- Malignant compression

History

- The intensity and characteristics (burning) of pain should be noted
- Localization of pain and referral pattern of both myotomal and dermatomal should be noted
- Pain diagrams are helpful in localizing pathology
- Some patients report a reduction in their radicular symptoms by abducting their shoulder and placing their hand behind their head; very specific but not a very sensitive presentation
- Symptoms suggestive of a cervical myelopathy include changes in gait, bowel or bladder dysfunction, lower-extremity sensory changes, and weakness
- Athletes will usually present with performance complaints

Exam

- Inspection for atrophy and attempting to note any myotomal pattern of atrophy in the upper limb, or scapular stabilizer muscles
- Active range of motion will be limited, particularly in extension, rotation, and lateral bending either toward or away from the side
- Spurling's maneuver is a passive lateral flexion and compression of the head with a positive test causing radicular symptoms at a distance from the neck
- Neck distraction may relieve symptoms
- Palpation may show increased myofascial tender and trigger points
- Complete neurological examination including manual muscle testing, sensory examination, as well as an assessment of muscle stretch reflexes and upper motor neuron signs

Testing

- Gold standard is electrodiagnosis (electromyography [EMG]), a physiological test, that detects nerve damage
- Electrodiagnostic studies helpful in localizing a lesion. Needle EMG established test for detection of acute and chronic denervation, a hallmark of radiculopathy
- Although studies show a high false positive rate regarding plain x-rays, cervical AP and lateral x-rays are helpful in determining stability, extent of foraminal stenosis, and alignment
- Magnetic resonance imaging (MRI) provides a direct visualization of neural structures and other soft tissues such as the intervertebral discs, may detect abnormalities at multiple levels (high false positives), need to correlate with clinical and electrodiagnostic findings

Pitfalls

- Malignancy should be ruled out if no response to initial treatment
- Confusing plexopathy or focal neuropathies with radiculopathy
- Relying on imaging abnormalities

Red Flags

- Malignancy
- Myelopathy
- Infectious etiologies

Treatment

Medical

- In the acute setting, nonsteroidal anti-inflammatory medications, muscle relaxants, and heat or cold modalities may be used to reduce pain and improve function
- There is anecdotal evidence supporting the use of oral prednisone with good clinical results; however, there is no scientific evidence for its use acutely
- Opioid therapy may be needed depending on severity of pain
- Anticonvulsants and tricyclic antidepressants may be useful in treating neuropathic pain.
- Lidocaine-medicated patches may provide local symptomatic relief of pain

Exercises

- Physical therapy after acute pain is controlled to work on muscular imbalances and weakness
- Core, and scapular/neck stabilization program
- Trial of manual traction at 24° to 30° of cervical flexion, home traction (caution with central HNP, may cause cord damage)

Modalities

- Heat
- Cold
- Transcutaneous electrical nerve stimulation

Injection

- Tender/trigger point injections
- Epidural steroid injection (ESI)

- There is a significant risk of serious neurological injury after cervical transforaminal ESIs likely due to embolic events
- Fluoroscopy-guided cervical interlaminar ESI is a safe and effective means of treating patients with cervical radiculopathy

Surgical
- Depending on clinical presentation and surgical experience, the approach may include discectomy, discectomy with fusion (anterior and posterior approaches), disc arthroplasty, laminectomy, and neuroforaminotomy
- Usually reserved for those with progressive neurological symptoms, refractory pain that does not improve with treatment including ESIs and/or myelopathy

Consults
- Neurological or orthopedic-spine surgery
- Pain management

Complications/side effects
- Myelopathy
- Chronic pain and disability

Prognosis
- In younger patients without comorbidities, minimal spondylosis with acute disc herniation prognosis is good for complete resolution of symptoms and return to prior function
- In older patients with advanced facet and uncovertebral osteoarthrosis, the prognosis is guarded with potential for chronic waxing and waning pain syndrome

Helpful Hints
- Early and accurate diagnosis will ensure appropriate therapies and medications to reduce pain, disability while allowing for healing

Suggested Readings
Malanga GA. The diagnosis and treatment of cervical radiculopathy. *Med Sci Sports Exerc.* 1997;29:S236-S245.

Polston DW. Cervical radiculopathy. *Neurol Clin.* 2007;25:373–385.

Shedid D, Benzel E. Cervical spondylosis anatomy: pathophysiology and biomechanics. *Neurosurgery.* 2007;60:S1-S7, S1-S13.

Cervical Spinal Stenosis

Michael Furman MD MS

Description

As the cervical spine ages, multiple changes in the bones, ligaments, and soft tissues lead to narrowing or stenosis of the cervical canal. Cervical spinal stenosis is common in the general population and only considered pathological when significant symptoms are present.

Etiology/Types

- Two major types:
  - Central stenosis
  - Foraminal stenosis
- Due to either normal aging in the cervical spine or pathological changes associated with trauma or injury
- Congenital

Epidemiology

- All members of society can be affected
- Prevalence has been estimated between 4.9% and 21.5%
- There are individuals with congenitally narrow cervical canals

Pathogenesis

- The major contributors to reduction of the cervical canal diameter are spondylosis, bony spurring, and congenitally narrow canals
- Cervical spondylosis, the most common progressive disorder of the aging cervical spine, can lead to spinal stenosis
- Spondylosis is noted in 10% of the population by age 20 and 95% by age 65
- The degenerative changes noted with spondylosis begin with cervical disc desiccation
- The cervical intervertebral disc is similar in structure to the lumbar disc, made up of the two distinct parts: the anulus fibrosis and the nucleus pulposus
- The discs are avascular and the vertebral endplates allow diffusion of nutrients and water into the intervertebral disc, which helps maintain overall hydration and health of the disc
- With aging, the vertebral endplates become less permeable, allowing less diffusion of nutrients and water disrupting the normal metabolic state of the disc
- Imbalances in enzyme activity further lead to changes within the nucleus, which increase the loss of water content and shift the balance of protein aggregates
- These degenerative changes eventually lead to a loss of disc space height and abnormal force distribution throughout the cervical spine
- As the nucleus undergoes these degenerative changes, it also loses the ability to take on axial and torsional loads and passes off these forces to the annulus fibrosis
- The annulus is thinner posteriorly and laterally and will fissure and bulge as these increased forces are applied through it
- With disc height loss, the diameter of the cervical spinal canal begins to narrow and bony hypertrophy also occurs
- The facet joints, uncovertebral joints, and vertebral bodies undergo bony (osteophyte) changes that contribute to the compromise of the canal
- The ligamentum flavum undergoes degenerative changes and experiences buckling and hypertrophy, and the posterior longitudinal ligament thickening and calcification also contribute to the diminished size of the cervical canal

Risk Factors

- High or repetitive axial loading
- Aging
- Smoking
- Male sex
- Genetic inheritance
- Congenital narrowing of the spinal canal

Clinical Features

- Neck pain
- Cervical radiculopathy
- Cervical myelopathy

Natural History
- May remain static
- It may progress to significant stenosis and eventual compromise of the cervical canal

Diagnosis

Differential diagnosis
- Disc herniation
- Musculoskeletal pain
- Facet cyst
- Mononeuropathy of the upper limb
- Infection
- Fracture
- Neoplasm
- Sensitization of the central nervous system
- Amyotrophic lateral sclerosis
- Multiple sclerosis
- Normal pressure hydrocephalus
- Syringomyelia

History
- History of neck and/or upper limb symptoms
- Occasionally sharp radiation into the upper limbs with flexion and extension of the neck
- Radiation into the upper back, shoulder, or limbs
- Myelopathic symptoms such as difficulty walking and lower extremity stiffness

Exam
- Tenderness in the cervical spine
- Paraspinal tenderness
- Muscle weakness and/or atrophy in the upper limb
- Decreased reflexes with predominately radicular pathology
- Evidence of upper motor neuron signs including spasticity, hyper-reflexia, and pathological reflexes

Testing
- X-rays in anteroposterior and lateral views can reveal central stenosis but are prone to magnification errors
- Flexion/extension films can reveal instability that static films will miss
- Computed tomography (CT) scans are superior to magnetic resonance imaging (MRI) when looking at bony pathology
- CT with myelography can identify far lateral foraminal stenosis but not commonly used because of risk

- MRI can identify soft tissue pathology-related issues that cannot be identified as accurately as on CT scans and is the standard diagnostic study
- Electromyography (EMG) studies will reveal multilevel radicular findings

Pitfalls
- Overinterpretation of imaging studies
- No definitive cervical canal diameter is an indicator for surgical intervention

Red Flags
- Infection
- Fracture
- Neoplasm
- Significant neurological dysfunction

Treatment

Medical
- Nonsteroidal anti-inflammatory medications
- Analgesics
- Oral steroid taper

Exercises
- Cervical stabilization programs focus on stabilizing the painful pathological region
- Muscle strengthening
- Balance, gait training

Modalities
- Heat
- Ice
- Transcutaneous electrical nerve stimulation
- Ultrasound

Injection
- Tender/trigger point injections
- Epidural injections with fluoroscopic guidance for symptoms related to radiculitis or stenosis

Surgical
- Cervical surgery is warranted for unrelenting pain, weakness, or myelopathy
- The majority of procedures are anterior cervical decompression and fusion (ACDF) or anterior cervical discectomy and fusion
- Patient selection is key for achieving positive outcomes

Consults
- Physical medicine and rehabilitation
- Orthopedic or neurosurgical-spine surgery

Complications/side effects
- Progressive pain and dysfunction
- Myelopathy
- Paralysis

Prognosis
- Highly variable
- Stenosis can be radiographically severe but clinically insignificant
- Positive predictive factors for surgery are higher neck disability index scores prior to surgery and older age
- Negative predictive factors for surgery include litigation and dermatomal sensory deficits

Helpful Hints
- Cervical spinal stenosis is common
- Benign condition managed conservatively
- Cervical myelopathy requires prompt imaging and surgical evaluation

Suggested Readings
Baron EM, Young WF. Cervical spondylotic myelopathy: a brief review of its pathology, clinical course, and diagnosis. *Neurosurgery.* 2007;60(1):S35-S41.

Lee M, Ezequiel H, Riew K. Prevalence of cervical spine stenosis. Anatomic study in Cadavers. *J Bone Joint Surg Am.* 2007;89:376–380.

Shedid D, Benzel E. Cervical spondylosis anatomy: pathophysiology and biomechanics. *Neurosurgery.* 2007;60(1):S1-S7.

Chest Pain, Musculoskeletal

Christine Lawless MD MBA ■ John MacKnight MD

Description
Chest pain is a common complaint in athletes, and may be due to any one of a number of causes. Most often, it is noncardiac in origin. Nonetheless, it is necessary to first consider a potentially life-threatening cause of chest pain before attributing such pain to a noncardiac cause.

Etiology/Types
- Gastrointestinal, musculoskeletal, pulmonary, idiopathic, and psychiatric causes account for the majority of chest pain syndromes in athletes
- Chest pain may occur at rest or with exercise. It may be acute, associated with trauma, or may occur due to overuse such as in the case of costochondritis or a rib stress fracture
- Musculoskeletal causes of chest pain include constochondritis, Tietze's syndrome, slipping rib syndrome, stitch, precordial catch, and cervical-thoracic disc disease

Epidemiology
- The overall incidence of chest pain attributable to cardiac causes is <5%
- Musculoskeletal causes account for at least 20%

Pathogenesis
- *Costochondritis* results in chest pain located at the rib/cartilage junction of the costosternal joints
- It can result from overuse or overload of the chest wall during weight lifting or repeated chest compressing motions
- *Tietze's syndrome* is an inflammatory, nontraumatic disorder manifested by painful nonsuppurative swelling of the second and third cartilaginous articulations of the anterior chest wall
- *Slipping rib syndrome* causes chest pain in adolescent runners and swimmers
- Laxity of the medial fibrous attachments of the lower ribs causes cartilage to slip superiorly and impinge on the intercostal nerve above
- *Stitch* is a common, cramping pain experienced by lesser-trained individuals during vigorous, extended exercise. Etiology most likely results from spasm or

strain of musculoskeletal structures supporting the diaphragm
- *Precordial catch syndrome* (Texidor's twinge) is a sharp, well-localized pain lasting only seconds to minutes, occurring episodically at rest, but may occur with exercise as well. Etiology is unknown but may arise from the pleura
- *Cervical disc disease* (cervical angina) *or thoracic radiculopathy* can be a cause of referred chest pain
- Compression of cervical roots C6 and C7 is the most common source of pain, mediated via medial and lateral pectoral nerves

Risk Factors
- Trauma
- High or repetitive mechanical loading
- Certain sports: weight lifting, running, swimming

Clinical Features
- *Costochondritis* typically affects the second to fifth costal cartilages
- Symptoms typically are one-sided, made worse by breathing, and radiate to the back and abdomen
- On examination, there is localized costochondral tenderness without warmth, redness, or swelling
- *Tietze's syndrome* is distinguished from costochondritis by presence of joint swelling
- The inflammatory nature of Tietze's syndrome is supported by elevated erythrocyte sedimentation rate (ESR) and morning stiffness
- *Slipping rib syndrome* causes the athlete to complain of pain located in the inferior costal areas of the chest or upper abdomen; a "slipping" or "popping" sensation may be experienced
- Performing the "hooking maneuver" (examiner's curved fingers pull the affected rib margin anteriorly) results in a popping sensation and/or pain, thereby confirming the diagnosis
- *Stitch* pain is pleuritic, generally located over the lower chest wall, left side more common than right
- *Precordial catch syndrome* (Texidor's twinge) is described as a sharp, well-localized pain lasting only

seconds to minutes, exacerbated by deep inspiration, and relieved by sitting upright. It generally occurs episodically at rest, but may occur with exercise as well.
■ Cervical disc disease (*cervical angina*) results in pain that may be reproduced via cervical manipulation or the Spurling's maneuver with head rotation to the affected side of the chest

Natural History
■ Costochondritis, Tietze's syndrome, slipping rib syndrome, stitch, and precordial catch are generally self-limited and resolve with rest, analgesics, nonsteroidal anti-inflammatory agents, and, when indicated, exercises and enhanced training
■ Cervical disc disease may become chronic

Diagnosis

Differential diagnosis
■ Costochondritis
■ Tietze's syndrome
■ Slipping rib
■ Precordial catch syndrome
■ Stitch
■ Cervical disc disease
■ Chest wall pain due to blunt chest trauma
■ Traumatic rib fracture
■ Rib stress fractures
■ Sternoclavicular (SC) sprains, dislocations
■ Asthma/exercise-induced bronchospasm (EIB)
■ Pneumothorax
■ Pulmonary contusion
■ Pneumomediastinum
■ Pulmonary embolus
■ Pneumonia
■ Pleurisy
■ Hyperventilation
■ Gastroesophageal reflux disease
■ Dysphagia
■ Psychiatric etiology of chest pain
■ Substance abuse
■ Pericarditis
■ Cardiac angina due to cardiomyopathy or coronary artery disease, or anomalous coronary artery
■ Aortic dissection

History and exam
■ See clinical features

Testing
■ Choose test based on clinical picture

■ Twelve-lead electrocardiogram
■ Chest x-ray
■ ESR
■ Echocardiogram
■ Stress testing
■ Rib x-ray
■ Neck x-ray
■ Magnetic resonance imaging (MRI) cervical spine

Pitfalls
■ Misdiagnosing a cardiac, pulmonary, or gastrointestinal diagnosis
■ Ordering unnecessary tests!

Red Flags
■ Symptoms occurring with exertion, consider cardiac etiology
■ Associated symptoms like syncope, dyspnea, or palpitations
■ Positive family history of sudden death age ≤50 years
■ History of trauma
■ History of overuse
■ Fever or infection
■ Auscultation of pericardial rub
■ Chest wall tenderness
■ Associated swelling of joints
■ Hooking maneuver elicits pain
■ Spurling's maneuver reproduces pain

Treatment

Medical
■ For all diagnoses: relative rest, technique modification, local modalities, and nonsteroidal anti-inflammatory medications
■ Acupuncture, and relaxation techniques may be complementary alternatives

Exercises
■ Stitch and precordial catch: upper torso stretching and enhanced training methods
■ Cervical angina: decompression of the affected nerve roots via traction and rehabilitative exercise with surgery for refractory cases

Modalities
■ Heat
■ Ice
■ Transcutaneous electrical nerve stimulation
■ Ultrasound

Injection
- Trigger point injections
- Injections for symptoms related to slipping rib, cervical radiculitis, or stenosis

Surgical
- For refractory cervical disc disease

Consults
- Cardiology (if history suggests cardiac cause)
- Pulmonary (if history suggests pulmonary cause)
- Gastroenterology (if history suggests gastrointestinal [GI] cause)
- Neurological or orthopedic surgery, for cervical disc disease

Complications/side effects
- Progressive pain and dysfunction

Prognosis
- Highly variable

Helpful Hints
- Cardiac causes of chest pain, although not as common, ought not be missed
- Once musculoskeletal cause is determined, athlete can be reassured that pain is non–life threatening and most diseases are self-limited and/or treatable with analgesics, anti-inflammatories, injections, physical therapy, modalities, and rarely surgery

Suggested Readings

Lawless CE. Return-to-play decisions in athletes with cardiac conditions. *Phys Sports Med.* 2009;37(1):80–91.

MacKnight JM, Mistry DJ. Chest pain in the athlete: differential diagnosis, evaluation, and treatment. In: Lawless C, ed. *Sports Cardiology Essentials: Evaluation, Management and Case Studies.* New York, NY: Springer Science + Business Media; 2010;115–136.

Perron AD. Chest pain in athletes. *Clin Sports Med.* 2003;37–50.

Chronic Exertional Leg Compartment Syndrome

Robert P. Wilder MD FASCM ■ Eric Magrum PT

Description
Chronic exertional compartment syndrome is defined as a condition in which elevated tissue pressure occurs within a noncompliant osseofascial compartment, resulting in reduced perfusion, pain, and compression of neurovascular structures.

Etiology/Types
■ Acute: usually associated with trauma such as tibial fractures or muscle ruptures, rarely seen as a complication of chronic elevation of compartment pressures
■ Chronic: commonly seen in running athletes affecting the lower leg, exertional compartment syndrome has also been described in the thigh and medial compartment of the foot

Epidemiology
■ Associated with running and other endurance sports, as well as military training
■ Prevalence as high as 25% of leg pain with exercise
■ Initially described to affect more men than women; recent literature shows women may be more affected
■ In the lower leg, anterior compartment syndrome is most common (45%), followed by the deep posterior compartment (40%), lateral compartment (10%), and superficial posterior compartments (5%)

Pathogenesis
■ The pathophysiology is not clearly understood
■ During exercise, muscle contraction increases tissue perfusion, which causes an increase in muscle size; fascia surrounding muscle compartment is stiff, resulting in elevated intracompartmental pressures
■ Relative ischemia of involved muscles is postulated to cause pain and neuromuscular symptoms, but its role in causing symptoms is still not clear
■ There are four major compartments in the leg. Each is bound by bone and fascia, and each contains a major nerve and muscles. Symptoms are associated with the structures within each compartment
■ The anterior compartment contains the extensor hallucis longus, extensor digitorum longus, peroneus tertius, anterior tibialis muscles, as well as the deep peroneal nerve
■ The lateral compartment contains the peroneus longus and brevis as well as the superficial peroneal nerve
■ The superficial posterior compartment contains the gastrocnemius and soleus muscles as well as the sural nerve
■ The deep posterior compartment contains the flexor hallucis longus, flexor digitorum longus, and posterior tibialis muscles, as well as the posterior tibial nerve. Some authors believe that the posterior tibialis should be considered a separate compartment, since it is surrounded by its own fascia

Risk Factors
■ Participation in endurance sports
■ Running and landing styles
■ Excessive pronation
■ Lack of conditioning

Clinical Features
■ Characteristic presenting complaint is recurrent exercise-induced leg discomfort that occurs at a well-defined and reproducible point in the run
■ Increases if training persists
■ Relief of symptoms only occurs with discontinuation of activity

Natural History
■ Symptoms usually worsen if training continues
■ Surgery may be required if intensity of exercise is maintained
■ Conservative measures are generally found ineffective
■ Reduction of exercise intensity, correction of biomechanical abnormalities, and use of orthotics may allow continued participation in some sports

Diagnosis
Differential diagnosis
■ Medial tibial stress syndrome
■ Tibial stress fractures
■ Chronic muscle strain

- Lumbar radiculopathy
- Neurological/vascular claudication

History
- Leg pain with activity
- Numbness, tingling, and weakness may be present
- Rest reduces symptoms

Exam
- Examination may or may not demonstrate fascial hernias in the legs
- Muscle tenderness to palpation
- Pronated feet, tight Achilles tendon
- Less commonly focal weakness or numbness affecting the structures in the respective compartments involved. Typically neurological examination is normal

Testing
- X-rays, bone scan, and magnetic resonance imaging (MRI) are negative, and are used to rule out other conditions
- Compartment pressure measurements test of choice
- Criteria consistent with the diagnosis of chronic exertional compartment syndrome (CECS):
  - Pre-exercise pressure ≥15 mm Hg
  - One-minute postexercise pressure ≥30 mm Hg
  - Five-minutes postexercise pressure ≥20 mm Hg
- Clinicians should also be aware that standard exercise protocols often used in the clinical setting may or may not be adequate to raise intracompartment pressure; diagnosis may require the sports-specific activity to induce symptoms and raise intracompartment pressure

Pitfalls
- May miss diagnosis if not clinically suspected, and appropriate testing performed

Red Flags
- Acute severe pain
- Pain that persists at rest
- Progressive weakness or neurological deficits

Treatment

Medical
- Reduction of activity
- Anti-inflammatory medication

- Orthoses

Exercises
- Stretching of heel cords
- Light strengthening of distal lower extremity muscles
- Cross training: swimming, cycling

Modalities
- Cryotherapy
- Superficial heat

Injection
- Not indicated

Surgical
- Indicated if symptoms persist despite conservative treatments and activity modification.
- Fasciotomy is the treatment of choice with 90% success rate
- Failure of surgical treatment may be because of inadequate fasciotomy or involvement of more than one compartment

Consults
- Orthopedic surgery

Complications/side effects
- Inability to return to sports despite treatment

Prognosis
- Good with prompt diagnosis and appropriate treatment

Helpful Hints
- Consider chronic compartment syndrome in athletes, which present with neurological complaints associated with activity
- Examination at rest will usually be normal

Suggested Readings

Glorioso J, Wilckens J. Compartment syndrome testing. In: O'Connor R, Wilder R, eds. *The Textbook of Running Medicine.* New York: McGraw-Hill; 2001:95–100.

Pedowitz RA, Hargens AR, Mubarak SJ, et al. Modified criteria for the objective diagnosis of chronic compartment syndrome of the leg. *Am J Sports Med.* 1990;18(1):35–40.

Wilder R, Sethi S. Overuse injuries: tendinopathies, stress fractures, compartment syndrome, and shin splints. *Clin Sports Med.* 2004;23:55–81.

Coccydynia (Coccygodynia)

Liza M. Hernández-González MD

Description
Coccygodynia is defined as pain in and around the coccyx. It is often triggered by prolonged sitting or when standing from the sitting position.

Etiology/Types
- Trauma (i.e., falls causing contusion or fractures)
- Childbirth
- Immobility, hypermobility, or luxation
- Tumor
- Degenerative sacrococcygeal disease
- Spicules
- Idiopathic

Epidemiology
- Relatively uncommon but data are lacking
- Seen most commonly in females
- Not age-specific
- Associated with increased morbidity and decreased quality of life if severe

Pathogenesis
- Fracture or contusion
- Abnormal sacrococcygeal and coccygeal mobility
- Degenerative disc changes in sacrococcygeal and intercoccygeal intervertebral discs

Risk Factors
- Increased intercoccygeal angle
- Obesity
- Trauma
- Vaginal delivery

Clinical Features
- Localized aching, stabbing pain on the coccyx after a fall on the buttocks, vaginal delivery, or spontaneous origin
- Pain may radiate to buttocks
- Pain worse with prolonged sitting or standing from sitting position

Natural History
- Most patients improve with conservative measures
- In a small subgroup of patients, chronic pain may interfere with functional activities and quality of life

Diagnosis

Differential diagnosis
- Mechanical low back pain
- Lumbar degenerative disc disease
- Ischial bursitis
- Sacroiliac joint pain
- Pudendal neuralgia
- Anismus
- Levator ani syndrome
- Pyriformis syndrome
- Referred pain from reproductive system
- Hemorrhoids
- Malignancy

History
- Coccyx pain with prolonged sitting position
- Pain severity may vary with hard or soft surfaces
- Pain may be related to intercourse or bowel movements

Exam
- Pain upon palpation or manipulation of coccyx or sacrococcygeal junction
- Pain or increased mobility upon coccygeal (anteroposterior) rectal manipulation
- Palpate ischial bursae, posterior superior iliac spine, lumbar facet joints, pelvic floor, and gluteal muscles
- Usually normal neurological examination

Testing
- Standard anteroposterior and lateral lumbosacral x-rays with focused views of the coccyx and sacrococcygeal junction to evaluate the presence of fractures or spicules
- Lateral dynamic x-rays (standing and sitting views) to evaluate sacrococcygeal and intercoccygeal angle and coccyx luxation and mobility
- Magnetic resonance imaging (MRI) with coccygeal visualization or if referred pain is suspected
- Bone scan or computed tomography (CT) if plain x-rays are negative or inconclusive for suspected fracture or pelvic pathology
- Electromyography (EMG) if suspected referred pain from lumbosacral radiculopathy
- Discography for surgical prognosis
- Stool for occult blood to rule out malignancy, bleeding

Pitfalls

- Substantial preinjury anatomic variation of coccyx and sacrococcygeal junction
- Multiple causes of referred pain
- Lack of suspicion and clinical evidence to make appropriate diagnosis
- Psychosocial factors

Red Flags

- Infection
- Neoplasm
- Neurological deficits

Treatment

Medical

- Relative rest and activity modification
- Nonsteroidal anti-inflammatory drugs (NSAIDs)
- Muscle relaxants
- Nonopioid analgesics (*N*-acetyl-*p*-aminophenol [APAP], tramadol, gabapentin)
- Opioid analgesics
- Stool softeners
- Donut or wedge cushions
- Manipulation

Exercises

- Stretching of pelvic floor and pelvic girdle muscles (i.e., levator ani, coccygeus, piriformis, and gluteal muscles)
- Core and pelvic floor muscle strengthening

Modalities

- Cryotherapy
- Heat (hot packs and ultrasound)
- Myofascial release techniques
- Therapeutic massage

Injection

- Fluoroscopically guided to better identify anatomy
- Local sacrococcygeal joint injection

- Caudal or interlaminar epidural steroid injection in combination with local anesthetics
- Ganglion impar block
- Thermocoagulation of coccygeal nerve using radiofrequency ablation
- May attempt with direct palpation of coccyx (variable results)

Surgical

- Partial or total coccygectomy

Consults

- Physical medicine and rehabilitation
- Pain management
- Orthopedic spine surgery
- Obstetrics and gynecology/urogynecology
- Colorectal surgery

Complications/side effects

- Progressive pain and dysfunction
- Infection, wound dehiscence, and fecal incontinence after surgery

Prognosis

- Variable
- More difficult to treat if chronic

Helpful Hints

- Early recognition is important
- Search for red flags

Suggested Readings

Fogel GR, Cunningham PY, Esses SI. Coccygodynia: evaluation and management. *J Am Acad Orthop Surg.* 2004;12:49–54.

Patrick M, Foye MD, Charles J, et al. Successful injection for coccyx pain. *Am J Phys Med Rehabil.* 2006;85(9):783–784.

Wray CC, Eason S, Hoskinson J. Coccydynia aetiology and treatment. *J Bone Joint Surg Br.* 1991; 73(2):335–338.

Complex Regional Pain Syndrome

George Tsao DO MPH ■ Julio A. Martínez-Silvestrini MD

Description

Complex regional pain syndrome (CRPS) is a disease characterized by severe pain, swelling, vasomotor instability, skin changes, and limited limb function, usually following minor trauma.

Etiology/Types

- Type I (reflex sympathetic dystrophy or RSD): there is no evidence of nerve injury
- Type II (causalgia): objective evidence of nerve lesion

Epidemiology

- May occur at any age, with a mean age of 42 years
- Occurs more frequently in females than males with a ratio of 2.3:1
- The lower extremity is more frequently affected in children and adolescents

Pathogenesis

- Unclear, but may include central, autonomic, and peripheral nervous system factors
- Posttraumatic sympathetic dysfunction, resulting in up-regulation of peripheral cathecolamine receptors
- The resulting increased sensitivity to cathecolamines produces exaggerated vasoconstriction of the cutaneous vasculature and vasodilation of deeper limb vasculature, resulting in cold, cyanotic skin with associated limb edema
- Can be precipitated by nerve injury, soft tissue injury, trauma, myocardial infarction (MI), coronary artery disease (CVA), surgery

Risk Factors

- Soft tissue injuries
- Fractures
- Injections
- Surgery
- No precipitating event identified in 35% of patients

Clinical Features

- Allodynia (pain associated with nonpainful stimulus)
- Pain severity disproportionate to injury severity
- Swelling
- Inability to bear weight
- Pain with range of motion

Natural History

- Stage 1: burning, throbbing pain, localized edema, altered color, and temperature
- Stage 2: progression of soft tissue edema, skin and articular tissue thickening, muscle wasting
- Stage 3: contractures, atrophic skin, brittle nails, and bone demineralization

Diagnosis

Differential diagnosis

- Venous thrombosis
- Nerve injuries
- Fractures
- Infection

History

- Soft tissue or nerve injury
- Acute fracture, injection, or surgery
- Pain intensity disproportional to magnitude of trauma

Exam

- Allodynia
- Edema
- Temperature changes
- Vasomotor changes (cyanosis, erythema, edema)
- Loss of motion, in the upper extremity pain with metacarpophalangeal passive flexion

Testing

- To rule out other conditions with similar clinical presentation
- Electrodiagnostic studies to identify nerve injury
- X-rays to evaluate for bone pathology and periarticular osteopenia
- Vascular studies
- Bone scan

Pitfalls

- Failure of early recognition and treatment may lead to permanent dysfunction, loss, and chronic pain

Red Flags

- Infection
- Fracture
- Neoplasm
- Nerve injury
- Venous thrombotic event

Treatment

Medical
- Anti-inflammatory medication
- Anticonvulsants
- Oral steroids
- Analgesics
- Antidepressants
- Psychosocial support
- Topical lidocaine

Exercises
- Stress loading activities/weight bearing exercises/ closed chain exercises
- Desensitization techniques
- Gentle motion
- Gradual strengthening

Modalities
- Contrast baths (1 minute in 50°F water, followed by 4 minutes in 100°F water)
- Transcutaneous electrical nerve stimulation

Injection
- Regional sympathetic nerve block
- Sympathetic ganglion block

Surgical
- Dorsal column spinal cord stimulation
- Sympathectomy

Consults
- Pain medicine
- Physical medicine and rehabilitation
- Neurology

Complications/side effects
- Progressive, chronic pain
- Permanent contracture, loss of function

Prognosis
- Variable
- Early recognition and prompt treatment provide the greatest opportunity for recovery

Helpful Hints
- Goals of CRPS treatment are to reduce pain and to maintain mobility
- Forceful exercise may actually exacerbate symptoms
- Always suspect when pain exceeds what is expected for the injury suffered

Suggested Readings

Harden, RN. Pharmacotherapy of complex regional pain syndrome. *Am J PMR.* 2005;84(2 suppl):S17-S28.

Sharma A, Williams K, Raja SN. Advances in treatment of complex regional pain syndrome: recent insights on a perplexing disease. *Curr Opin Anaesthesiol.* 2006;19(5):566–572.

Compression Fractures of the Thoracolumbar Spine

Ari C. Greis DO ▪ Larry H. Chou MD

Description
Compression fractures are defined as a collapse of the vertebral body.

Etiology/Types
- Can occur when the load applied to the vertebral body exceeds its mechanical resistance
- Acute vs chronic
- Insufficiency/osteoporotic fracture
- Traumatic origin
- Wedge: collapsed anterior border with intact posterior border
- Crush: entire vertebral body is collapsed (vertebra plana)
- Biconcave "codfish deformity": collapsed central portion of the vertebral body
- Burst: fracture involving the posterior vertebral body with possible retropulsion of bony fragments into the spinal canal
- Severity:
  - Grade 1: 20% to 25% loss of vertebral body height
  - Grade 2: 25% to 40% loss of vertebral body height
  - Grade 3: >40% loss of vertebral body height

Epidemiology
- Commonly occur at the thoracolumbar junction (T12-L1) and midthoracic (T7-T8) spine
- Vertebral compression fractures are the most common type of osteoporotic fracture with an incidence of 700,000 per year in the United States
- The lifetime risk of clinically diagnosed vertebral fractures is approximately 15% in white women
- Approximately 19% of patients who have a vertebral compression fracture will have another fracture within a year

Pathogenesis
- Can occur spontaneously or after minor trauma in bone with decreased density or from a traumatic event in normal bone

- Common at the thoracolumbar junction (T12-L1) because the change in zygapophyseal joint orientation alters segmental biomechanics and provides less resistance to anteroposterior displacement at this level

Risk Factors
- Osteoporosis, postmenopausal women over the age of 55 years
- Chronic illnesses, smoking, alcohol use, corticosteroid use
- Prominent thoracic kyphosis, loss of 2" of height
- Trauma

Clinical Features
- Two-third are asymptomatic
- Severe, sharp, localized, axial pain that rarely radiates into the extremities
- Kyphosis, "dowager hump"
- Restrictive respiratory problems
- Costoiliac impingement syndrome

Natural History
- Acute pain from vertebral compression fractures tends to gradually decrease over 4 to 8 weeks
- Chronic pain is common in this patient group
- Pain and disability greater in those with greater height loss and higher degree of kyphosis

Diagnosis
Differential diagnosis
- Disc herniation, degenerative disc disease
- Zygapophyseal joint-mediated pain
- Scoliosis/kyphosis
- Spondylolisthesis
- Myofascial pain
- Post-thoracotomy pain syndrome
- Postherpetic neuralgia
- Rheumatologic/inflammatory disorder
- Spinal infection, discitis, osteomyelitis
- Malignancy, large benign spinal tumors

History
- Can occur without history of antecedent trauma
- Acute back pain after sudden bending, coughing, lifting, or minor trauma
- Known osteoporosis

Exam
- Kyphosis
- Pain with posterior-anterior glide and/or percussion at level of injury
- Decreased thoracic and/or lumbar spine range of motion
- Paravertebral muscle hypertonicity/tenderness
- Normal lower limb strength, sensation, reflexes

Testing
- Plain x-ray of the thoracolumbar spine is usually all that is needed
- Magnetic resonance imaging (MRI) of the spine is most useful in determining fracture age, excluding malignant tumor, and for selecting appropriate treatment
- Urgent MRI or computed tomography (CT) scan should be obtained when neurological abnormalities present, which may demand surgical intervention
- A dual energy x-ray absorptiometry study, performed on a nonurgent basis, to quantify bone density
- Nuclear medicine bone scan considered if multiple fractures are present, to exclude distant metastases, or if MRI is contraindicated

Pitfalls
- Overinterpretation of radiographic findings

Red Flags
- Infection
- Systemic illness
- Neoplasm
- Neurological dysfunction

Treatment

Medical
- Nonopioid drugs should be used initially for pain relief
- Unclear if fracture healing is impaired with nonsteroidal anti-inflammatory drugs in humans
- If opiates are required, consider treatment with oxycodone, at a dose of 5 to 10 mg (often in combination with acetaminophen) every 4 to 6 hours and titrating to a maximal dose of 30 mg/day as needed

- Tricyclic antidepressants may be helpful for chronic pain
- A laxative or stool softener given to prevent straining, which can increase pain and may cause further fractures
- Nasal calcitonin for relief of pain, useful adjunct in the acute setting
- Bisphosphonates treatment of choice for management of osteoporosis
- Bracing provides initial benefit and if used, should be discarded when pain is controlled and fracture is healed, since braces may promote osteoporosis, truncal weakness, and dependence

Exercises
- Early resumption of activity, begin as soon as patients can tolerate the movements
- Spinal extension exercises may relieve pain and limit kyphosis
- Aquatic therapy

Modalities
- Heat
- Ice
- Transcutaneous electrical nerve stimulation

Injection
- Vertebroplasty and kyphoplasty involve the percutaneous injection of bone cement under fluoroscopic guidance into a collapsed vertebra
- Kyphoplasty also involves introduction of inflatable bone tamps into the fractured vertebral body for elevation of the endplates prior to fixation of the fracture with bone cement
- Optimal timing is unclear
- Potential long-term benefits for both procedures include prevention of recurrent pain at the treated level(s) and improved functional capability
- Studies have not conclusively demonstrated one technique to be superior to the other in terms of outcomes or complications (kyphoplasty is more expensive)

Surgical
- Spinal decompression with or without fusion for neurological compromise

Consults
- Physical medicine and rehabilitation/pain management

■ Neurological or orthopedic spine surgery

Complications/side effects
■ Progressive pain, kyphosis, and dysfunction
■ Recurrent vertebral compression fracture at adjacent levels
■ Vertebra plana with neurological sequelae

Prognosis
■ Highly variable

Helpful Hints
■ An asymptomatic compression fracture should not be mistaken for the etiology of a patient's pain

■ Always ordering thoracic x-rays in patients with pain or back trauma

Suggested Readings
Mattern CJ, Lin JT, Lane JM. Osteoporosis. In: Slipman CW, Derby R, Simeone FA, et al., eds. *Interventional Spine: An Algorithmic Approach*. Philadelphia, PA: Saunders Elsevier; 2008:435–444.

Papaioannou A, Watts NB, Kendler DL, et al. Diagnosis and management of vertebral fractures in elderly adults. *Am J Med*. 2002;113(3):220–228.

Watts NB, Harris ST, Genan HK. Treatment of painful osteoporotic vertebral fractures with percutaneous vertebroplasty or kyphoplasty. *Osteoporos Int*. 2001;12:429–437.

De Quervain's Tenosynovitis

Michael J. Gruba MD ■ Jeffrey S. Brault DO

Description
De Quervain's tenosynovitis is characterized by pain, swelling, and crepitus over the first dorsal compartment, which houses the tendons of extensor pollicis brevis (EPB) and abductor pollicis longus (APL).

Etiology/Types
- Rarely traumatic
- Commonly insidious in onset: gradual worsening of pain due to chronic repetitive grasping and ulnar/radial deviation movements of the wrist and thumb
- Classified as stenosing tenosynovitis or tenovaginitis

Epidemiology
- Five times more common in women than in men
- Equal frequency in dominant and nondominant hands
- Associated with various racquet sports, golf, volleyball, fly-fishing
- Associated with holding an infant during breast-feeding

Pathogenesis
- Thickening of the extensor retinaculum over the first extensor compartment
- Thickening of the tendon sheath and proliferation of fiber tissue
- Impaired gliding, mechanical impingement of tendons, and narrowing of the fibro-osseous canal through which they travel
- Variable anatomy in the first dorsal compartment is considered the rule, rather then the exception
- Multiple studies have shown that the vast majority of De Quervain's cases that fail conservative treatment (including blind injections) are found to have separate compartments for the two tendons and multiple APL slips
- Surgically removed tendon sheaths are five times thicker than normal control sheaths due to deposition of dense fibrous tissue and mucopolysaccharides consistent with degenerative changes and not signs of active inflammation

Risk Factors
- Repeated ulnar deviation of the wrist and hand in activities such as piano playing, computer typing, chopping wood, and farm labor
- Hormonal changes associated with pregnancy
- Rheumatoid arthritis

Clinical Features
- Pain located on the radial side of the wrist, first dorsal compartment over the radial styloid
- Pain worsens with repeated thumb movement
- Swelling, warmth, and crepitus

Natural History
- May improve with activity modification, splinting, and medication
- Injections may be required in addition to immobilization
- Some patients may fail conservative treatment and require surgery

Diagnosis

Differential diagnosis
- Osteoarthritis of the thumb carpometacarpal (CMC) joint
- Intersection syndrome
- Dorsal wrist ganglia
- Wartenberg syndrome (superficial radial nerve entrapment)
- Infectious tenosynovitis
- Flexor carpi radialis tendinitis
- Scaphoid or distal radial styloid fractures
- Scapholunate dissociation

History
- Pain with repeated hand activity
- Progressive symptoms, proximal radiation of pain to the elbow
- Swelling and erythema of the wrist
- Difficulty in carrying heavy objects

Exam
- Swelling of the first dorsal compartment
- Tenderness to palpation over the radial styloid
- Pain with resisted thumb abduction and extension

- Positive Finkelstein's test (pain is reproduced by passively flexing the patient's thumb into their palm, creating a fist and then passively moving the wrist into ulnar deviation)
- Finkelstein's test has long been pathognomonic for De Quervain's; however, it can also be positive with osteoarthritis (OA) of the first CMC joint as well as with intersection syndrome

Testing
- X-rays: AP and lateral views of the hand and wrist may be helpful if there is a history of trauma or question of first CMC joint OA
- Magnetic resonance imaging (MRI) can be helpful to document tenosynovitis, but is rarely needed
- Ultrasound may show hypo- or isoechoic thickening of the tendon sheath with diffuse circumferential hypoechoic fluid around the EPB and/or APL tendons at the point of tenderness

Pitfalls
- Not limiting activity after injections and medications
- Missing concomitant problems such as CMC OA

Red Flags
- Fever
- Severe pain
- Crepitus and continued erythema despite treatment

Treatment

Medical
- Nonsteroidal anti-inflammatory drugs (NSAIDs) are successful when combined with splinting in mild cases, but not in more severe cases
- Daytime use of a thumb spica splint
- Activity modification

Exercises
- Passive thumb and wrist range of motion exercises may be helpful in mild cases
- Static thumb and wrist exercises
- Thumb and wrist stretching and tendon gliding as pain improves

Modalities
- Cryotherapy
- Iontophoresis
- Phonophoresis

Injection
- A pooled quantitative literature evaluation of seven studies showed cure rates of 83% after one corticosteroid injection, 61% when injection was combined with splint immobilization, and 14% after splinting only (immobilization may lead to more stiffness; more severe patients may be injected and immobilized, so this needs further study).
- For patients unresponsive to blind injections, experienced clinicians can use ultrasound to diagnose and accurately guide injections into anatomic variations if present.

Surgical
- Surgical release is reserved for cases that are refractory to the above conservative treatments and has been shown to be up to 91% successful

Consults
- Orthopedic/hand surgeon
- Physical medicine and rehabilitation

Complication/side effects
- Continued pain
- Difficulty with lifting and carrying

Prognosis
- De Quervain's is a self-limited disease when associated with breast-feeding and pregnancy
- Good prognosis with early diagnosis and appropriate treatment

Helpful Hints
- Early injection improves treatment results
- Postinjection-immobilization/rehabilitation should emphasize flexibility and thumb mobility as well as appropriate biomechanics of lifting and work activities

Suggested Readings
Avci S, Yilmaz C, Sayli U, et al. Comparison of nonsurgical treatment measures for De Quervain's disease of pregnancy and lactation. *J Hand Surg Am.* 2002;27(2):322–324.

Lane LB, Boretz RS, Stuchin SA. Treatment of De Quervain's disease: role of conservative management. *J Hand Surg Br.* 2001;26(3):258–260.

Richie CA, Briner WW. Corticosteroid injection for treatment of de Quervain's tenosynovitis: a pooled quantitative literature evaluation. *J Am Board Fam Pract.* 2003;16(2):102–106.

Ta KT, Eidelman D, Thomson JG. Patient satisfaction and outcomes of surgery for De Quervain's tenosynovitis. *J Hand Surg Am.* 1999;24(5):1071–1077.

Wainstein JL, Nailor TE. Tendinitis and tendinosis of the elbow, wrist, and hands. *Clin Occup Environ Med.* 2006;5(2):299–322.

Discitis

Andrew J. Haig MD

Description
Inflammation or infection of the intervertebral disc

Etiology/Types
- Infectious, spontaneous, postsurgical
- Typically *Staphylococcus aureus*; methicillin-resistant; more common in iatrogenic cases
- *Streptococcus* if dental or bacterial endocarditis cause
- Tuberculosis or fungus in immunocompromised, homeless, alcoholic, or developing world cases
- Inflammatory, or sterile discitis might just be infectious with false-negative cultures

Epidemiology
- 0.4 to 2.4/100,000/year

Pathogenesis
- Children: septic emboli through arterial channels of immature disc
- Adults: seeding to edge of disc and infection due to lack of blood supply within the disc

Risk Factors
- Age (etiology and mechanism of disease vary in children and adults)
- Diabetes
- Immunosuppression
- Intravenous drug use
- Alcoholism
- Hepatic cirrhosis
- Malignancy
- Renal failure
- Spine surgery
- Endocarditis
- Dental work and other nonsterile procedures

Clinical Features
- Pain and infection, often indolent, but sometimes related to severe instability, sepsis, or neurological deficit

Natural History
- In children sometimes resolves without treatment
- In adults and some children can lead to fusion, occasionally paraspinal abscess, epidural abscess, and progressive neurological deficit, osteomyelitis, draining wound

Diagnosis
- Usually missed—2 to 6 months delay in diagnosing bacterial discitis, over 6 months delay with tuberculosis. Must have a high index of suspicion

Differential diagnosis
- Spondyloarthritis
- Cancer
- Disc herniation
- Compression fracture
- Back pain with coincidental infection elsewhere

History
- Infants and toddlers may avoid walking or standing due to pain
- Older children and adults have unremitting back pain at night
- Fever in 70%, weight loss, occasionally paraparesis
- Recent surgery, especially spine surgery is important

Exam
- Often no back complaint
- Children present with avoidance of walking, or standing, abdominal pain, or stiff gait
- Back tenderness
- Occasional neurological deficits

Testing
- Magnetic resonance imaging (MRI) is highly sensitive and specific, and can detect abscesses and neurological risks
- Sedimentation rate and C-reactive protein elevated in 90% or more. For postsurgical cases, note that usual postoperative elevated sedimentation rate and C-reactive protein normalize at 3 and 2 weeks, respectively
- Leukocytosis in 50%
- In adults, try hard to get pathogen before treatment if not gravely ill (blood cultures × 3), if not positive within 48 hours, computed tomography (CT)-guided disc biopsy and consider open disc biopsy
- X-ray shows disc collapse
- CT can show bone changes

- In children, x-ray is sufficient imaging unless atypical findings, then bone scan (if nonlocalizable) or MRI (if region is localized). Get blood cultures but do not get biopsy unless treatment is failing

Pitfalls
- Must have a high index of suspicion
- MRI in the first weeks of infection may miss it

Red Flags
- Always an urgent problem. Neurological deficit with discitis is acute emergency

Treatment

Medical
- Antibiotics, best if based on cultures. Typically 6 weeks intravenous (IV) plus 6 weeks oral. Some pediatric cases do well not treated

Exercises
- Bed rest is advocated, though not proven beneficial

Modalities
- Caution about ultrasound or other deep heating
- Orthotics often used for deformity or impending deformity, but also for pain

Injection
- Percutaneous biopsy
- Drainage of abscess

Surgical
- Open biopsy
- Drainage of abscesses
- Spinal decompression
- Fusion for deformity

Consults
- Infectious disease for diagnosis and antibiotics
- Spine surgery or radiology for biopsy
- Spine surgery for surgical management

Complications/side effects
- Pain
- Paralysis
- Death
- Ten percent recurrent infection (typically within 6 months of treatment)

Prognosis
- Many have complete cure
- Others asymptomatic fusion, deformity causing pain, neurological deficit
- Up to one-third have ongoing functional deficits, apparently less in persons who had surgery

Helpful Hints
- If you haven't ordered a sedimentation rate this month, you are probably not paying attention. It's OK to have 100 negative sedimentation rates for the one severe disease detected.

Suggested Readings
Cottle L, Reardon T. Infectious spondylodiscitis. *J Infect.* 2008;55:401–412.

Early SD, Kay RM, Tolo VT. Childhood diskitis. *J Am Acad Orthop Surg.* 2003;11:413–420.

Elbow Dislocations

Leslie Milne MD

Description

An uncommon injury in which there is disruption of the ulnohumeral articulation. The elbow is normally very stable in the flexion-extension plane. Dislocation may be complete or it may be "perched," meaning the humerus is subluxed with the coronoid impinging on the trochlea. "Perching" is associated with less severe injury to the supporting ligaments. Rehabilitation is more effective and overall prognosis is better than with a complete dislocation.

Etiology/Types

- Complete or perched
- Anterior—uncommon (1%–2%)
- Posterior
  - Posterior
  - Posterolateral—most common
  - Posteromedial—least common
  - Lateral

Epidemiology

- Two to 2.5 times more common in males (70% males in pediatric population)
- More common in the nondominant arm (60%)
- Mean age 30 years (13–14 years in pediatrics)
- Six to 13 cases per 100,000 population

Pathogenesis

- Fall on outstretched hand, usually with arm extended backward or in slight flexion with abduction
- Tearing of the lateral ligament complex and capsule from extension varus forces or tearing of medial collateral complex if the elbow is in flexion at the time of impact
- Complete dislocation implies a complete disruption of both the medial and lateral collateral ligaments with stretching or tearing of the anterior capsule and brachialis muscle

Risk Factors

- Forty percent of elbow dislocations occur during sports

- Motor vehicle accidents and injury during play account for 10%

Clinical Features

- Elbow held in 45° flexion
- Pain and swelling around joint
- Exaggerated prominence of the olecranon
- Possible neurovascular compromise in ulnar or median nerve and/or brachial artery distribution

Natural History

- This should be assessed and reduced as soon as possible to avoid missing arterial injuries and to prevent flexion contractures

Diagnosis

Differential diagnosis

- Fracture (supracondylar fracture in children)
- Fracture dislocation
- Soft tissue injury
- Nursemaids elbow (occurs in children younger than 5 years; elbow or wrist pulled, usually followed by pain, crying; associated with elbow subluxation or dislocation)

History

- Fall on an outstretched arm, usually with arm extended backward

Exam

- Elbow swelling with prominent olecranon
- Limited elbow motion
- Neurovascular examination
- Varus or valgus instability

Testing

- Radiography
  - Anteroposterior
  - Lateral
- Arteriography, if vascular injury suspected
- Postreduction radiographs
- Computed tomography (CT) may be helpful for evaluating fractures in complex dislocations

Pitfalls

- Missed brachial artery injury. Arterial injury occurs in 8% of those with significant trauma. Pulse alone does not exclude injury
- Elbow dislocation may spontaneously reduce prior to being evaluated. If history and examination are consistent with this, make sure to fully evaluate neurovascular status despite negative radiographs
- Median nerve entrapment at the time of reduction

Red Flags

- Median nerve symptoms may occur days to weeks postreduction—think of missed entrapment at the time of reduction

Treatment

Medical

- Closed reduction with conscious sedation or general anesthesia and intra-articular lidocaine
- Complete posterior dislocation
  - Patient lies supine
  - Supinate the forearm
  - Longitudinal traction on wrist and forearm
  - Countertraction on humerus by assistant
  - Downward pressure on the proximal forearm to disengage coronoid process from olecranon fossa
  - Use thumb to help coronoid clear the trochlea
  - Flex the elbow as distal traction is continued
  - Feel for "clunk"
- Perched dislocation
  - Direct pressure over the olecranon with elbow slightly extended and axial distraction
- Reassess neurovascular status and range of motion (ROM) postreduction
- Immobilize with sling or 90° posterior splint (axilla to fingers) for 2 to 3 days, then begin ROM—avoid prolonged immobilization
- Consider admission for observation of vascular compromise if suspicion high
- Anti-inflammatory or pain medication

Exercises

- Active and active-assisted ROM by day 3
- Strengthening exercises at 3 weeks

Modalities

- Cryotherapy

- High-voltage galvanic stimulation

Injection

- Intra-articular anesthetic injection may be helpful during closed reduction

Surgical

- No indication for surgical repair of ligaments in uncomplicated dislocations
- Surgery is indicated:
  - If unable to reduce in closed manner
  - If associated fracture such as radial head fracture becomes malpositioned or medial epicondyle fracture displaced >1 cm
  - Suspected brachial artery injury
  - Repair of the ulnar component of the lateral collateral ligament for chronic, recurrent elbow dislocation or subluxation

Consults

- Orthopedic surgery
- Vascular surgery

Complications/side effects

- Twenty-five percent to 50% of dislocations are associated with fractures
  - Medial epicondyle avulsion—most common in children
  - Radial head fractures—most common in adults (10%)
- Neurovascular injury 8% to 21%
  - Brachial artery—most common vascular injury
  - Ulnar nerve—most common nerve injury
  - Median nerve entrapment postreduction
- Heterotopic ossification from repeated attempts at reduction resulting in injury to soft tissue
- Compartment syndrome
- Chronic pain, possibly due to ongoing joint laxity
- Loss of motion, particularly extension (30° at 10 weeks, 10° at 2 years)
  - Most common sequela of elbow dislocation
- Recurrent instability
  - Gross instability uncommon (1%–2%)
  - Mild laxity in one-third of children/adolescents, 20% of adults

Prognosis

- Perched dislocations have normal motion in 6 to 8 weeks
- Complete dislocations regain 80% to 90% of normal function at 3 months

- Most athletes can return to sports in 3 to 6 weeks postreduction in their nondominant arm. Throwers will need rest for up to 3 months before starting a full strengthening program

Helpful Hints

- Early reduction is critical
- Adequate anesthesia to help avoid repeated attempts at reduction
- To assess for chronic instability, determine if patient has difficulty doing a push-up or rising up from a

chair. These maneuvers require use of the ulnar component of the lateral collateral ligament

Suggested Readings

Kuhn MA, Ross G. Acute elbow dislocations. *Orthop Clin North Am.* 2008;39(2):155–161.

Morrey BF. Elbow dislocation. In: DeLee JC, Drez D, eds. *De Lee & Drez's Orthopedic Sports Medicine Principles and Practice.* 2nd ed. Philadelphia, PA: Elsevier Saunders; 2003:1311–1321.

Epiphyseal Injuries of the Ankle

María A. Ocasio-Silva MD FAAPMR ■ Joanne Snow MD

Description

Epiphyseal injuries are injuries that occur at the epiphyseal plate or growth plate of the skeletally immature patient.

Etiology/Types

- Salter and Harris first described these injuries according to the pattern on x-ray appearance, which also corresponded to their severity. This anatomical classification is the most commonly used (Figure 1)
- Salter and Harris classification:
  - Type I: complete separation of epiphysis from the shaft through calcified cartilage (growth zone) of growth plate. No bone actually fractured; periosteum may remain intact. May be missed on x-rays
  - Type II: line of separation extends partially across deep layer of growth plate and extends through metaphysis attached to epiphyseal fragment
  - Type III: intra-articular fracture through epiphysis, across deep zone of growth plate to periphery
  - Type IV: fracture line extends from articular surface through epiphysis, growth plate, and metaphysis
  - Type V: fracture line along epiphysis. Minimal or no displacement makes radiographic diagnosis difficult

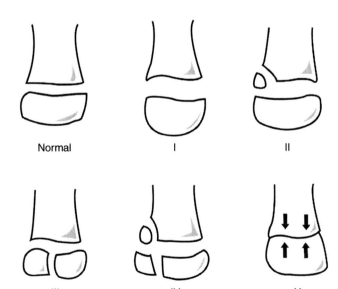

Figure 1. Salter and Harris classification.

  - Rang modification—Type VI: portion of growth plate sheared or cutoff

Epidemiology

- Epiphyseal injuries in general occur in the ratio of 2:1 in boys to girls
- Peak incidence in males aged 12 to 16; in females aged 8 to 13
- Sports lead to 10% of all physeal injuries
- Ankle is the most common site for physeal injuries in adolescents
- Distal tibia Type II injury: most common growth plate injury in ankle

Pathogenesis

- Mechanism of injury is, most commonly, acute mechanical overload
- Cartilaginous physis represents weakest biomechanical link in the growth plate and is the most susceptible to shear forces. This area lacks inherent mechanical strength and is therefore more susceptible to trauma than the surrounding ossified bone
- Ankle injuries result from inversion or eversion; however, eversion injuries are rare due to the strength of deltoid ligament, bony configuration of ankle, and bony alignment at heel strike

Risk Factors

- Younger children sustain greater number of pure physeal separations without bone fractures
- Most common during periods of rapid skeletal growth

Clinical Features

- Range from subtle pain to obvious deformity
- Pain and swelling at the physis
- Decreased ankle motion
- An acute inversion injury strongly suggests a growth plate fracture if tenderness and swelling are located over the physis

Natural History

- Early diagnosis and management of type I and II injuries lead to healing

- Type III-VI injuries may result in ankle deformity and growth arrest

Diagnosis

Differential diagnosis
- Ankle sprain (ligamentous injury)
- Tendon injury

History
- The patient should be asked about the position of the ankle and the direction of forces at the time of injury
- Twisting injury of the foot and/or ankle
- Inversion is frequently encountered
- Inquire about repetitive stress

Exam
- Deformity and location of swelling and ecchymosis should be noted
- Point tenderness over physis, located within 2 cm of the most distal tip of the tibia and fibula
- Decreased ankle range of motion (ROM)
- Assess ligament integrity
- Evaluate contralateral ankle that provides a basis for comparison

Testing
- Plain radiographs including anteroposterior, lateral, and mortise views
- Obtain comparison views of contralateral extremity
- If no obvious physeal disruption is seen on initial radiographs, and examination suggests ligamentous laxity, stress radiographs should be taken to look for occult physeal fractures
- Computed tomography (CT) scanning has been reported to be helpful in evaluation of joint articular surface injury
- Magnetic resonance imaging (MRI) has the potential to provide more detailed information about injury to the growth plate

Pitfalls
- Fractures not always discovered on imaging, especially Types I and V

Red Flags
- Acutely, neurovascular compromise
- Types I and II fractures refractory to immobilization

Treatment

Medical
- Nonsteroidal anti-inflammatory drugs and/or acetaminophen for pain control

Exercises
- Rest initially
- Once activity restrictions liberated, start rehabilitation with goals of pain-free range of motion including dorsiflexion, plantar flexion, inversion, and eversion
- Pain-free weight bearing and strengthening of surrounding musculature
- Focus on restoring the ankle ROM, strength, balance, propioception, and endurance

Modalities
- Type I: splint immobilization, intermittent icing, and elevation for 48 to 72 hours
- Type II: if no angulation or significant displacement of fracture fragment, splint immobilization, intermittent icing, and elevation for 48 to 72 hours
- After surgical intervention: splint immobilization or casting, and elevation
- Superficial heat
- Transcutaneous electrical nerve stimulation/electrical stimulation following surgery or immobilization

Injection
- Not indicated

Surgical
- Types III and IV ankle fractures (intra-articular): open reduction and internal fixation are often indicated
- Surgery is also recommended to prevent displacement of the growth plate that can lead to physeal arrest or growth disturbance

Consults
- Types I and II: orthopedic surgery and/or sports medicine
- Types III, IV, V, and VI: emergency room orthopedic surgery evaluation

Complications/side effects
- Bone growth arrest and limb-length discrepancies
- Asymmetrical growth
- Malalignment of joint
- Ankle joint arthritis
- Avascular necrosis

Prognosis
- Types I and II: rapid healing and normal bone growth

- Type III: guarded prognosis for normal bone growth; the chance for growth disturbance is related to preservation of blood supply of epiphyseal bone fragment
- Type IV: future growth disturbance at risk, dependent on degree of blood supply disruption from epiphysis
- Type V: most likely injury to result in focal bone growth arrest

Helpful Hints
- Growth plate is the weakest biomechanical link; therefore, physeal injuries are far more common than dislocations and ligament tears in growing children
- Ankle injuries in the young athlete are quite different from those of an adult. Because the epiphyseal plates

of the distal tibia and fibula are significantly weaker than surrounding ligaments, failure on stress occurs through the growth plates rather than through soft tissue
- All children with physeal injuries should be followed at regular intervals for at least 2 years or to skeletal maturity
- Treatment of physeal injuries of the ankle must be individualized but should always be based upon classification, potential pitfalls, and prognosis

Suggested Readings
Gladden PB, Wilson CH, Suk M. Pediatric orthopedic trauma: principles of management. *Semin Pediatr Surg.* 2004;13:119–125.
Perron AD, Miller MD, Brady WJ. Orthopedic pitfalls in the ED: pediatric growth plate injuries. *Am J Emerg Med.* 2002;20(1):50–54.

Extensor Carpi Ulnaris Tendinitis

Michael J. Gruba MD ■ Jeffrey S. Brault DO

Description

The extensor carpi ulnaris (ECU) tendon is involved in a constellation of clinical syndromes from tendinitis/tenosynovitis to tendon subluxation and rupture. The ECU tendon rests in the ulnar osseous groove as it courses through the sixth dorsal compartment.

Etiology/Types

- ECU tendinitis often presents insidiously in patients who perform chronic repetitive movements
- In a case of ECU tendon subluxation, there is often a history of initial trauma and often a painful snap when the patient supinates

Epidemiology

- Second most common sports-related overuse syndrome
- Frequently seen in racquet sports, which require repetitive wrist motion

Pathogenesis

- ECU tendinitis is a variant of stenosing tenosynovitis
- In pronation, the ECU tendon follows a straight path across the wrist and attaches onto the base of the fifth metacarpal
- When the wrist is in full supination, the ECU tendon is forced to adopt approximately a 30° angle as it exits the sixth dorsal compartment and this angle creates significant strain on the ECU subsheath
- This repetitive friction is believed to cause tendinitis and with extreme tension this may be a site of tendon rupture
- If the ECU subsheath ruptures, the tendon may slide freely under the intact dorsal retinaculum and the tendon subluxes volarly out of the ulnar groove causing a painful snapping sensation with supination and pronation

Risk Factors

- Racquet sports

Clinical Features

- Ulnar wrist pain
- Sixth dorsal compartment swelling

- Wrist trauma (tennis players hitting a low forehand, baseball players swinging a bat) followed by painful snapping of the wrist

Natural History

- Tendinitis responds to activity modification and injection
- ECU subluxation may require surgical treatment

Diagnosis

Differential diagnosis

- Dorsal radioulnar joint (DRUJ) instability or arthritis
- Triangular fibrocartilage complex injury
- Ulnar impaction syndrome
- Lunotriquetral instability
- Ulnar styloid fracture
- Kienböck disease
- Midcarpal instability
- Fourth and fifth carpometacarpal arthritis
- Pisiform or triquetral fracture
- Flexor carpi ulnaris tendinitis
- Ganglion cyst

History

- Pain with repeated upper extremity use, particularly ulnar deviation
- Participation in racquet sports
- Pain in nondominant wrist when hitting a backhand stroke in tennis
- Ulnar wrist swelling, crepitus, and snap

Exam

- Patients present with pain and possible crepitus when palpating the sixth dorsal compartment
- Passive wrist flexion and supination may be painful
- Resisted wrist extension with ulnar deviation or supination and pronation will cause pain over the dorsal ulnar wrist

Testing

- X-rays: anteroposterior and lateral of the hand and wrist to evaluate for fracture, avascular necrosis (as in Kienböck disease), instability, or degenerative changes
- Ultrasound and magnetic resonance imaging (MRI) can show changes of ECU tendinitis and subluxation while the wrist is in supination

- MRI is more sensitive than ultrasound for other ligament and bony pathology

Pitfalls
- Missing a subluxing ECU tendon

Red Flags
- Pain that worsen with activity
- Pain at rest
- Fever, erythema

Treatment

Medical
- Nonsteroidal anti-inflammatory drugs
- Modified rest
- Acute tendinitis may respond to a short course of splinting
- Patients with acute ECU tendon subluxation or chronic tendinitis should be immobilized for 6 weeks in a long-arm cast with the wrist pronated and slightly extended

Exercises
- Gentle wrist range of motion and tendon gliding exercises
- Static wrist strengthening following initial injury immobilization or surgery
- Dynamic strengthening, progressive resistance, and full range of motion as tissue heals following immobilization or surgical repair

Modalities
- Cryotherapy
- Paraffin bath
- Electrical stimulation

Injection
- A combination of rest, wrist immobilization, and local corticosteroid injections was successful in 93% of patients in one study

Surgical
- Palmaris longus tendon graft for ECU tendon rupture and surgical repair of a ruptured ECU subsheath can be beneficial for chronic refractory subluxation cases

Consults
- Orthopedic hand surgery
- Physical medicine and rehabilitation

Complications/side effects
- Chronic ulnar wrist pain
- Inability to participate in racquet sports

Prognosis
- Good with early diagnosis and appropriate treatment

Helpful Hints
- Suspect ECU tendinitis in tennis and racquet ball players with ulnar wrist pain
- Painful snapping usually associated with a subluxating tendon

Suggested Readings
Futami T, Itoman M. Extensor carpi ulnaris syndrome: findings in 43 patients. *Acta Orthop Scand.* 1995;66(6):538–539.

Montalvan B, Parier J, Brasseur JL, et al. Extensor carpi ulnaris injuries in tennis players: a study of 28 cases. *Br J Sports Med.* 2006;40(5):424–429.

Failed Back Surgery Syndrome

Dave Bagnall MD

Description
Disabling lower back and/or lower extremity pain following lumbar spinal surgery.

Etiology/Types
There are many etiologies and it is worthwhile to broadly categorize patients as having predominantly low back or predominantly lower extremity pain.

Epidemiology
- Younger than 60 years
- One or more surgeries intended to correct disc herniation, lateral recess stenosis, or axial spine pain
- May include discectomy, laminectomy, foraminotomy, or fusion

Pathogenesis
A structural cause of failed back surgery syndrome (FBSS) has been estimated to occur 90% of the time
- Foraminal stenosis (25%–29%) can occur from loss of disc height or zygapophysial hypertrophy-osteophytosis or insufficient decompression
- Discogenic pain (20%–22%) may occur at or adjacent to the level of surgery
- Pseudoarthrosis (14%) from failed fusion due to poor healing or surgical technique
- Neuropathic pain (10%) resulting from incomplete neural decompression, misplaced or migrated pedicle screws, spinal nerve trauma, neural compression from scar tissue
- Recurrent disc herniation (7%–12%), insufficient removal of, or unrecognized second disc herniation
- Iatrogenic instability (5%) usually after decompression of spondylolisthesis or nonunion of interbody fusion
- Zygapophysial pain (3%)
- Sacroiliitis (2%)
- Wrong segment surgery or unrecognized sequestered disc
- Discectomy syndrome: epidural fibrosis, local arachnoiditis, segmental microinstability
- Centralized neuropathic pain unrelated to objective nerve impingement

- Successful rates of surgical reintervention descend from 50% after the first attempt at repeat surgery to 30% after the second, 15% after the third, and 5% after the fourth

Risk Factors
- Poor compliance with presurgical rehabilitation
- Tobacco use
- Laborer
- Liability-based injury
- Personality disorder
- Pre-existing psychiatric history
- History of substance, physical, or sexual abuse

Clinical Features
- Unrelieved pre-existing pain or new pain following lumbar surgery
- May include axial, radicular, or referred symptoms

Natural History
- The history will vary; primary complaint will help to clarify the diagnosis
- Predominantly axial symptoms generally reflect potential discogenic pain, zygapophysial pain, segmental instability, pseudoarthrosis
- Predominantly radicular symptoms generally reflect foraminal stenosis, recurrent or residual disc herniation, or neuropathic pain
- Temporal considerations should also be utilized to make the correct diagnosis
- Immediate failure or continuation of presurgical symptoms reflects possible wrong presurgical diagnosis, technical error, or psychosocial overlay
- Temporary relief of a few weeks followed by pain suggests infection
- Relief for months preceding recurrence suggests recurrent disc herniation, spinal nerve trauma, or discectomy syndrome
- Recurrence after a year or more should lead to suspicion of segmental instability or stenosis
- Biopsychosocial issues must be considered as secondary gain, liability, litigation, personality disorders, and psychiatric disorders will influence the perception and reporting of symptoms and disability

Diagnosis

Differential diagnosis
- Infection
- Fracture
- Neoplasm
- Arachnoiditis
- Residual radiculopathy
- Fibromyalgia/chronic pain syndrome

History
- History of presurgical axial or radicular symptoms leading to surgical intervention in the lumbar spine
- Maintenance or recurrence of presurgical symptoms following surgical recovery
- Development of new lumbar axial, radicular, or referred pain following surgery
- Failure of nonsurgical methods to achieve symptom relief

Exam
- Axial pain with weight bearing, lumbar extension, or side bending, or evidence of segmental instability with lumbar range of motion testing
- Radicular pain with lumbar range of motion testing
- Radicular pain with neurodynamic testing in the standing, seated, supine, or prone positions
- Tenderness with lumbar segmental testing or palpation
- Reduced or absent reflexes
- Myotomal motor loss
- Dermatomal sensory changes
- Sclerotomal hypersensitivity

Testing
- Image testing should be applied based on symptoms, presurgical diagnosis, surgical intervention, and postsurgical symptoms
- Standing radiographs, including flexion, extension, and lateral bending views, can evaluate extent of segmental instability
- Computed tomography (CT) with multiplanar reconstruction may reveal evidence of pseudoarthrosis
- Magnetic resonance imaging (MRI) with sagittal, coronal, and axial views with suspicion of discogenic pathology or foraminal encroachment (contrast enhancement may not be necessary depending on the capacity of the MRI)
- CT myelography is rarely of value

- Provocation discography is controversial, but when utilized to assess for discogenic pain, performed appropriately reflecting at least one legitimate painless control disc, can be useful
- Image-guided diagnostic spinal nerve blocks when performed appropriately can elucidate symptomatic spinal nerves
- Image-guided diagnostic medial branch blocks when performed appropriately can elucidate symptomatic zygapophysial joint levels
- Electrodiagnostic testing is rarely valuable unless coincidental extraspinal neuropathology is suspected

Pitfalls
- Over-reliance on surgical options to correct the symptoms
- Overinterpretation of imaging studies
- Ignorance of biopsychosocial influences

Red Flags
- Infection
- Fracture
- Neoplasm
- New neurological dysfunction

Treatment

Medical
- Nonsteroidal anti-inflammatory medications
- Sustained release opioid analgesics
- Nonopioid analgesics
- Nerve membrane stabilizers
- Tricyclic antidepressants
- Antitonic muscle relaxants (baclofen/tizanidine)

Exercises
- Lumbo-pelvic stabilization exercises focused on painful segments and restoration of normal movement patterns
- Neuromobilization exercises to diminish neuropathic pain
- Intensive functional restoration once segmental areas are stabilized and movement patterns restored

Modalities
- Heat
- Ice
- Transcutaneous electrical nerve stimulation

Injections
- Image-guided transforaminal epidural steroid injections for radicular symptoms
- Rarely, image-guided sympathetic blockade

Surgical
- Correction of underlying objective evidence of reversible nerve compression
- Correction of underlying evidence of segmental instability amenable to surgical stabilization/fusion
- Spinal cord stimulation for predominantly radicular pain
- Implantation of an intrathecal morphine pump

Consults
- Physical medicine and rehabilitation
- Neurology
- Psychology
- Social worker

Complications/side effects
- Progressive pain and dysfunction
- Worsens with multiple surgeries

Prognosis
- Poor, but variable

Helpful Hints
- FBSS is a multifactorial process dependent on many variables, objective and occult; a flexible, thorough evaluation incorporating pre- and postsurgical symptoms, type of surgery performed, and biopsychosocial influences must be pursued

Suggested Readings
Hazard RG. Failed back surgery syndrome: surgical and nonsurgical approaches. *Clin Orth Rel Res.* 2006;443:228–232.

Onesti ST. Failed back syndrome. *Neurologist.* 2004;10(5): 259–264.

Schofferman J, Reynolds J, Herzog R, et al. Failed back surgery: etiology and diagnostic evaluation. *Spine J.* 2003;3:400–403.

Female Athlete Triad

Albert Gunjan Singh MD ■ Shashank J. Dave DO

Description

Female athlete triad refers to the detrimental effects of energy deficits on the reproductive and skeletal health of physically active women. Triad components includes energy deficiency, with or without disordered eating; abnormal menstrual cycles, referred to as functional hypothalamic amenorrhea; and bone loss, the most severe cases of which are called osteoporosis.

Etiology/Types

- Associated to endurance or intense sports
- Athletes in endurance sports present with endocrine abnormalities
- These abnormalities affect energy availability, menstrual function, bone mineral density (BMD; Figure 1)
- Athletes travel along these spectrums depending on their diet and exercise habits

Epidemiology

- Eating disorders are more common in "thin-build" sports (e.g., gymnastics) and in those athletes participating in endurance, aesthetic, and weight-class sports
- Prevalence of secondary amenorrhea varies widely with sport, age, training intensity, and body weight; can be as high as 69% in dancers and 65% in long-distance runners
- Prevalence of primary amenorrhea is >22% in cheerleading, diving, and gymnastics compared with <1% in the general population
- Disordered eating (i.e., irregular eating habits or patterns), eating disorders (e.g., anorexia nervosa, bulimia nervosa), and amenorrhea (both primary and secondary) occur more frequently in sports that emphasize leanness, such as ballet, gymnastics, and long-distance running
- The simultaneous occurrence of disordered eating, menstrual disorders, and low BMD in elite athletes is similar to that of the general population

Pathogenesis

- Low energy availability, with or without eating disorders, is the key disorder affecting the other two components (menstrual function and bone health)

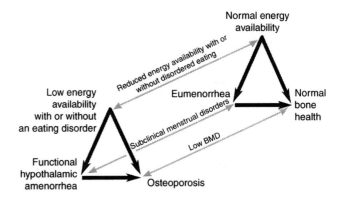

Figure 1. Female athlete triad. The spectrums of energy availability, menstrual function, and bone mineral density along which female athletes are distributed. Modified from Female Athlete Triad Coalition. http://www.femaleathletetriad.org/for-athletes-coaches/what-is-the-triad/

- Energy availability can be reduced by either decreasing caloric intake or increasing energy expenditure
- Decreased energy availability impairs bone health and development both indirectly and directly
  - Indirectly, deficits in energy availability cause a disruption in the pulsatile secretion of luteinizing hormone (LH), menstrual dysfunction, and a decrease in estrogen, which removes the suppression on osteoclastic activity
  - Directly, low energy availability acts through an estrogen-independent mechanism to impair bone formation by affecting hormones that regulate bone formation (e.g., insulin, T3, insulin-like growth factor-I)
- Failure to match energy intake to activity may be inadvertent, as prolonged exercise and a high-carbohydrate diet may suppress appetite

Risk Factors

- Restricted dietary energy intake
- Exercise for prolonged periods
- Early childhood start of sports-specific training and dieting
- Sudden increase in training volume
- Low body weight is a risk factor for amenorrhea

- Risk factors for stress fracture include low BMD, late menarche, biomechanical abnormalities, and training errors

Clinical Features
- Weight loss
- Sensitivity to cold
- Fatigue and impaired ability to concentrate
- Brittle hair and/or nails
- Dental caries
- Menstrual dysfunction
- Stress fractures
- Muscle injury

Natural History
- Athletes will present with stress fractures if not properly diagnosed
- Identification and correction of energy deficits will result in improved menstrual function and BMD

Diagnosis

Differential diagnosis
- Eating disorders (anorexia nervosa/bulimia)
- Endocrine disorders such as thyroid disease
- Osteopenia/osteoporosis
- Pregnancy/gynecologic disorders

History
- Information on energy intake, dietary practices, weight fluctuations, eating behaviors, and exercise energy expenditure
- Current and past menstrual status, including menarche, amenorrhea
- Prior stress fractures

Physical examination
- Bradycardia and orthostatic hypotension
- Cold, discolored hands and feet
- Vaginal atrophy on pelvic examination
- Yellowing of the skin (associated with hypercarotenemia often seen due to consumption of low-calorie foods such as carrots, squash, and spinach)
- Lanugo hair in anorexics with decreased body fat
- Unilateral or bilateral parotid gland enlargement seen with multiple emetic episodes

Testing
- Serum electrolytes, chemistry profile, complete blood count with differential, erythrocyte sedimentation rate, thyroid function tests, and urinalysis

- Electrocardiography (EKG) may occasionally show a prolonged QT interval, despite the presence of normal serum electrolytes
- Pregnancy test
- Follicle-stimulating hormone (FSH), LH to rule out ovarian failure
- LH/FSH ratio to rule out polycystic ovarian syndrome
- Prolactin levels to rule out lactotropic secreting tumor
- Bone densitometry (DXA) in disordered eating, or eating disorders for a cumulative total of ≥6 months and/or history of stress fractures/fractures from minimal trauma
- Diagnosis of low BMD or osteoporosis is based on lowest BMD Z-score of either posterior-anterior (PA) spine or hip
- Bone loss detected by declining Z-scores in two or more measurements at intervals of ≥6 months

Pitfalls
- Lack of suspicion may lead to missed diagnosis
- Accepting menstrual dysfunction as a normal part of some sports

Red Flags
- Continued weight loss
- Recurrent stress fractures

Treatment

Nonpharmacological
- Should employ a team approach consisting of physician/healthcare provider, registered dietician, and mental health practitioner; additional valuable team members may include certified athletic trainer, exercise physiologist, coach, and parents/family members
- Modify diet and exercise behavior to increase energy availability by increasing energy intake, reducing energy expenditure, or a combination of both
- Athletes should be referred for nutrition counseling
- Cognitive-behavioral therapy, group therapy, and/or family therapy may also be helpful
- Athletes with disordered eating and eating disorders, who do not comply with treatment may need to be restricted from training and competition

Pharmacological
- Antidepressants are often used for anorexia nervosa, bulimia nervosa, eating disorder not otherwise specified (ED-NOS)
- Oral contraceptives for restoration of menstrual cycles

- To restore fertility, clomiphene citrate and exogenous gonadotropins may be used to induce ovulation
- Adequate amounts of bone-building nutrients such as calcium (1000–1300 mg/day), vitamin D (400–800 IU/day), and vitamin K (60–90 µg/day)
- Bisphosphonates approved for treatment of postmenopausal osteoporosis should NOT be used in the young athlete with functional hypothalamic amenorrhea as there is unproven efficacy in women of child-bearing age. In addition, bisphosphonates may reside in a woman's bone for many years, potentially causing harm to the developing fetus during pregnancy

Exercises
- Weight-bearing exercise, cycling/reduced training intensity
- Dynamic strengthening exercise
- Aquatic rehabilitation for individuals with stress fractures

Modalities
- Cryotherapy for acute injury

Injections
- Not indicated

Surgical
- High-risk stress fractures such as anterior tibia, tarsal navicular, or fifth metatarsal may require surgery

Consults
- Obstetrics and gynecology
- Psychiatry/psychology

- Orthopedic surgery
- Sports medicine/physical medicine and rehabilitation

Complications/side effects
- Osteopenia/osteoporosis
- Inability to return to sports
- Eating disorders that do not respond to treatment

Prognosis
- Good with early identification, education, and treatment

Helpful Hints
- Female athletes will not always present with full-blown eating disorders, amenorrhea, and osteoporosis, so high level of suspicion is necessary
- An athlete's condition varies according to her diet and exercise habits. Only in the pathological extreme, the triad may present as three inter-related clinical disorders (eating disorder, functional hypothalamic amenorrhea, and osteoporosis)

Suggested Readings
Loucks A, Thuma J. Luteinizing hormone pulsatility is disrupted at a threshold of energy availability in regularly menstruating women. *J Clin Endocrinol Metab.* 2003;88:297–311.

Nattiv A, Loucks A, Manore M, Sanborn C, Sundgot-Borgen J. The female athlete triad position stand. *Am Coll Sports Med.* 2007;1867–1882.

Fibromyalgia

David A. Cassius MD ■ Marta Imamura MD PhD

Description

Fibromyalgia is a clinical syndrome of chronic widespread pain and reduced pain threshold to palpation associated with chronic fatigue, cognitive dysfunction, sleep disturbances, postexertional pain, and morning stiffness. There appears to be a central sensitization, causing an amplification of sensory impulses.

Etiology/Types

- Primary: occurs in the absence of other rheumatic disorders
- Secondary: associated with other rheumatic or pain disorders
- Associated with psychiatric comorbidities such as anxiety and depression
- Medical comorbidities include irritable bowel syndrome, migraine, interstitial cystitis, and pelvic floor pain

Epidemiology

- Two percent prevalence in adults in the United States
- International data more variable results
- Three times more common in women than in men
- Age of onset typically 30 to 50 years
- Peak incidence in middle age

Pathogenesis

- Unknown pathophysiology
- Abnormal central processing of pain considered an important component of the disease process
- Abnormalities in serotonin and norepinephrine neurotransmission also described

Risk Factors

- Genetic/familial predisposition
- Repeated exposure to stressful situations
- Rheumatic disorders
- Anxiety and depression

Clinical Features

- Chronic generalized pain of 3 months duration
- Axial and appendicular pain involving left and right sides
- Chronic fatigue
- Sleep dysfunction
- Diffuse soft tissue tenderness
- Associated gastrointestinal, genitourinary, and neurological symptoms

Natural History

- Chronic course with persistent symptoms
- Young patients and individuals in which early diagnosis is made may have better prognosis
- Some patients improve with treatment but difficult to predict

Diagnosis

Differential diagnosis

- Rheumatoid arthritis
- Polymyalgia rheumatica
- Systemic lupus erythematosus
- Inflammatory/metabolic myopathy
- Depression
- Chronic fatigue syndrome

History

- Chronic generalized pain
- Fatigue, sleep dysfunction, and morning stiffness
- Soft tissue tenderness
- Exacerbations following trauma or injury
- Difficulty with concentration and memory
- Female patient with family history of pain

Exam

- Multiple tender points, at least 11 of possible 18 points, identified by the American College of Rheumatology (ACR) criteria (Figure 1). Pressure on points equivalent to 4 kg/cm^2, measured by algometer or documented by blanching of the nail bed
- Myofascial trigger points may coexist
- No neurological deficits or focal weakness unless associated with other conditions such as radiculopathy, peripheral neuropathy, or entrapment neuropathy

Testing

- Diagnosis of exclusion
- CBC, CPK, ESR, ANA test, RA latex test, and other laboratory studies to rule out rheumatic disease
- X-rays to look for arthritis, soft tissue calcification, disc abnormalities

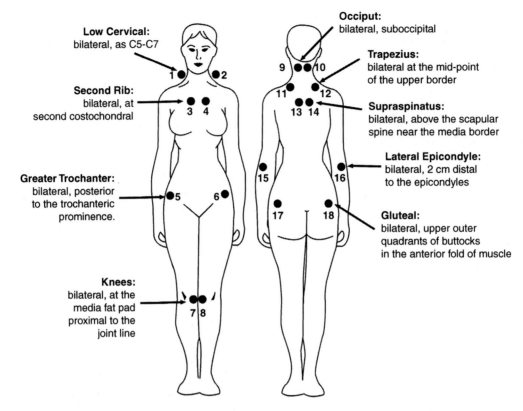

Low Cervical:
bilateral, as C5-C7

Second Rib:
bilateral, at
second costochondral

Greater Trochanter:
bilateral, posterior
to the trochanteric
prominence.

Knees:
bilateral, at the
media fat pad
proximal to the
joint line

Occiput:
bilateral, suboccipital

Trapezius:
bilateral at the mid-point
of the upper border

Supraspinatus:
bilateral, above the scapular
spine near the media border

Lateral Epicondyle:
bilateral, 2 cm distal
to the epicondyles

Gluteal:
bilateral, upper outer
quadrants of buttocks
in the anterior fold of muscle

Figure 1. Schematic representation of the location of the tender points for diagnosis of fibromyalgia.

- Magnetic resonance imaging to rule out disc herniations, degeneration, or spinal stenosis
- Electrodiagnostic studies to rule out neuropathy, myopathy, or radiculopathy

Pitfalls
- Missing other disease entities that require specific treatment
- Treating the symptoms separately and not as a specific clinical entity

Red Flags
- Progressive weakness
- Severe pain unresponsive to treatment

Treatment

Medical
- Medications
  - Low-dose tricyclic antidepressants (TCA): amitryptiline at doses of 10 to 25 mg at night effective in treating pain and sleep dysfunction in some patients. Higher doses lead to side effects, and contraindicated in the elderly
  - Muscle relaxants: Cyclobenzaprine may be used at night for patients with sleep dysfunction. Chemical structure similar to TCAs
  - Selective norepinephrine reuptake inhibitors (SNRI) appear to be more effective than selective serotonin reuptake inhibitors (SSRI) in pain control, reducing anxiety, and associated depression. Duloxetine and milnacipram indicated in management of fibromyalgia
  - Anticonvulsants such as pregabalin effective in reducing pain, fatigue, sleep dysfunction, and quality of life
  - Analgesics rarely effective as single agents. Tramadol may be used, particularly in patients with neuropathic type pain. Opioids may be required for patients with severe pain but should not be first-line agents
  - Anti-inflammatory medications usually not recommended, but may be effective in combination with other agents, for patients with joint pain or coexisting arthritis
- Cognitive remediation therapy
- Muscle relaxation techniques

- Acupuncture
- Patient education

Exercises
- Light aerobic exercise program
- Aquatic rehabilitation
- Stretching exercises
- Light dynamic strengthening

Modalities
- Superficial heat
- Cryotherapy
- Massage

Injection
- Trigger point injections of coexisting myofascial trigger points may be beneficial
- Localized pain that affects function may improve with local injections. Lateral epicondylitis, rotator cuff tendinopathy, or trochanteric pain syndrome respond to steroid injections or prolotherapy

Surgical
- Surgery not indicated
- Need to be vigilant not to miss other conditions such as entrapment neuropathies, disc herniations, spinal stenosis, or rotator cuff tears that merit surgical evaluation

Consults
- Physical medicine and rehabilitation
- Rheumatology
- Psychiatry/psychology
- Neurology

Complications/side effects
- Chronic pain and fatigue
- Deconditioning and muscle weakness
- Activity limitation

Prognosis
- Chronic illness with episodes of exacerbation
- Patients of younger age and educated about their condition do better

Helpful Hints
- High level of suspicion required for early diagnosis.
- Treatment should integrate medications, exercise, patient education, and cognitive therapy for best results.

Suggested Readings

Busch AJ, Schachter CL, Overend TJ, Peloso PM, Barker KA. Exercise for fibromyalgia: a systematic review. *J Rheumatol.* 2008;35(6):1130–1144.

Carville SF, Arendt-Nielsen S, Bliddal H, et al. EULAR evidence-based recommendations for the management of fibromyalgia syndrome. *Ann Rheum Dis.* 2008;67(4):536–541.

Hauser W, Bernardy K, Uceyler N, et al. Treatment of fibromyalgia syndrome with antidepressants a meta-analysis. *JAMA.* 2009;301(2):198–209.

Mease P. Fibromyalgia syndrome: review of clinical presentation, pathogenesis, outcome measures and treatment. *J Rheumatol.* 2005;(suppl 75):6–21.

Gastrocnemius Tear (Tennis Leg)

Phillip T. Henning DO ▪ Jonathan T. Finnoff DO

Description
Tennis leg or tennis calf is a partial- or full-thickness tear of the medial head of the gastrocnemius at its distal myotendinous junction. It was first described by Powell in 1883.

Etiology/Types
- Occurs with a sudden forced dorsiflexion of the ankle with the knee located in an extended position
- Types include partial- or full-thickness tears

Epidemiology
- Most common in middle-aged recreational athletes involved in sports requiring sudden deceleration and/or direction changes

Pathogenesis
- Tears occur at the distal myotendinous junction of the medial head of the gastrocnemius, in part due to the medial head generating higher force

Risk Factors
- Middle age, prior injury, tight gastrocnemius-soleus complex, suboptimally conditioned athletes

Clinical Features
- Acute presentation with pain, swelling, and difficulty walking
- May be confused with deep vein thrombosis

Natural History
- No specific distinguishing trends
- Improves with rest, and treatment, but may recur

Diagnosis

Differential diagnosis
- Achilles tendon rupture
- Plantaris tendon rupture
- Deep vein thrombosis
- Fracture (rare)

History
- Sudden onset of pain at the medial calf during activity involving sudden stopping or change in direction
- Patients describe a sense of tearing or pop followed by immediate pain, swelling, weakness, bruising, and difficulty with weight bearing

Exam
- Tenderness to palpation at site of tear
- May have palpable defect within the muscle
- Ecchymosis, localized edema
- Pain with active plantar flexion or passive dorsiflexion
- Weakness with resisted plantar flexion
- Assure continuity of Achilles tendon as well as normal neurovascular exam distally

Testing
- Ultrasound or magnetic resonance imaging (MRI) is only required for severe injuries and/or to rule out other conditions (e.g., Achilles tendon rupture or deep vein thrombosis)

Pitfalls
- Enlarging hematoma may lead to worsening pain and disability, compartment syndrome, or venous thrombosis

Red Flags
- Pain out of proportion to the injury, pallor of the lower leg and foot, paresthesias on the plantar aspect of the foot, paralysis of the calf and foot musculature, and decreased posterior tibial artery pulse (compartment syndrome)
- Diffuse leg swelling or increased swelling (venous thrombosis)
- Positive Thompson test and Achilles tendon defect (Achilles tendon tear)

Treatment

Medical
- Protected weight bearing: initially non-weight bearing to partial weight bearing, progress to full as tolerated
- Rest
- Ice
- Compression
- Elevation
- Analgesics/nonsteroidal anti-inflammatory drugs

Exercises
- Active motion starting with knee bent

- Isometrics, light strengthening as pain improves
- Stretching when pain resolves

Modalities
- Cold (acutely)
- Moist heat (after edema resolves)
- Electrical stimulation for pain modulation

Injection
- Not indicated

Surgical
- No surgical correction necessary, even for complete medial head tears
- Fasciotomy or tendon repair for compartment syndrome and Achilles rupture, respectively

Consults
- Orthopedic surgery if compartment syndrome or Achilles tendon rupture is present
- Medical consultation as necessary for venous thrombosis

Complications/side effects
- Compartment syndrome
- Deep vein thrombosis

Prognosis
- Usually have gradual resolution of pain and improvement in function
- Large tears may result in permanent deformity and/or atrophy of the muscle
- Risk of reinjury

Helpful Hints
- Early use of compressive stocking may lead to smaller hematoma development and earlier return to play

Suggested Readings
Flecca D, Tomei A, Martinelli M, et al. US evaluation and diagnosis of rupture of the medial head of the gastrocnemius (tennis leg). *J Ultrasound.* 2007;10:194–198.

Kwak HS, Kwang BL, Han YM. Ruptures of the medial head of the gastrocnemius ("tennis leg") clinical outcome and compression effect. *J Clin Imag.* 2006;30:48–53.

Glenoid Labral Injury

Francisco J. Otero-López MD ■ Omar Morales-Abella MD

Description

A separation of the anterior inferior labral complex from the glenoid rim.

Etiology/Types

- Associated with traumatic anterior shoulder dislocation
- Present in approximately 85% of anterior shoulder dislocations
- A bony Bankart lesion (fracture of the anterior-inferior glenoid) has an associated glenoid avulsion
- Causes anterior shoulder instability
- In the throwing athlete, anterior shoulder instability is more commonly caused by a stretched anterior-inferior capsule and labrum as opposed to an avulsion

Epidemiology

- The shoulder is the most common dislocated joint
- A Bankart lesion is commonly seen in 20- to 40-year-old patients with a traumatic anterior shoulder dislocation
- Seen in throwing/overhead sports associated with repeated activity

Pathogenesis

- The inferior glenohumeral ligament complex is the major shoulder static anterior stabilizer during abduction and external rotation
- As it originates from the inferior labrum and attaches on the humeral neck, a force to the abducted/externally rotated shoulder causes an avulsion of this complex, which may include the glenoid
- Generalized ligamentous laxity or repeated overhead activity with attritional changes to the shoulder capsule or inferior glenohumeral ligament allows superior migration of the humeral head with throwing; this may result in secondary damage to the superior, anterior, and posterior glenoid labrum (SLAP lesion)

Risk Factors

- Contact sports
- Familial generalized laxity
- Repetitive overhead activities

Clinical Features

- Guarding against combined abduction external rotation of the shoulder
- Recurrent instability
- Superior shoulder pain
- Pain with overhead activity

Natural History

- Recurrence of shoulder dislocation in patients 20 years or younger has been reported to be as high as 95%
- Overall incidence of recurrence is 60% for patients younger than 25 years of age
- Management should be guided by age at presentation
- SLAP lesions may result in chronic pain, loss of velocity, and control in throwers

Diagnosis

Differential diagnosis

- Hill-Sachs lesion (compression deformity of the superior-posterior humeral head associated with shoulder dislocation)
- Humeral avulsion of the glenohumeral ligaments (HAGL lesion)
- Superior labrum anterior and posterior lesions (SLAP tears especially in overhead athletes)

History

- Acute traumatic dislocation commonly followed by recurrent dislocation(s)
- Apprehension to combined shoulder abduction external rotation
- Shoulder pain with athletic activities (overhead)

Exam

- Apprehension test (hallmark of anterior instability), relocation test
- Load and shift test (evaluates anterior and posterior migration of the shoulder with the arm at side)
- Pain with abduction and external rotation, instead of apprehension, following these maneuvers is commonly found in overhead athletes

Testing

- X-rays including anteroposterior, lateral West Point, and Stryker notch views

- Magnetic resonance imaging (MRI) (arthrogram increases sensitivity)
- Examination under anesthesia shows increased anterior excursion at abduction of 45° or greater
- Arthroscopic evaluation (most sensitive and specific). The glenoid is measured to identify bony Bankart lesions; capsular and ligamentous laxity allows "Drive-Through" (of the arthroscopic instrumentation) sign present with Bankart or SLAP lesions

Pitfalls

- Bankart lesions lead to recurrent instability of the affected shoulder, which can limit sports participation or the patient's quality of life

Red Flags

- Multidirectional instability (voluntary dislocator)
- Deltoid muscle weakness associated with axillary nerve compression with recurrent dislocations

Treatment

Medical

- Nonsteroidal anti-inflammatory drugs (NSAIDS)
- Shoulder brace (after acute anterior dislocation remember to immobilize in external rotation)

Exercises

- Forward elevation (overhead pulley can assist)
- Internal rotation stretching
- Scapular strengthening and posture program
- Plyometrics (final stage of rehabilitation)

Modalities

- Cryotherapy
- Heat
- Electrical stimulation
- Ultrasound

Injection

- Intra-articular steroid injections, lidocaine/bupivacaine injections

Surgical

- Arthroscopic vs open repair
- Arthroscopic repair recommended if no associated glenoid bone loss; arthroscopic repair with suture anchor yields the best results (Figure 1)

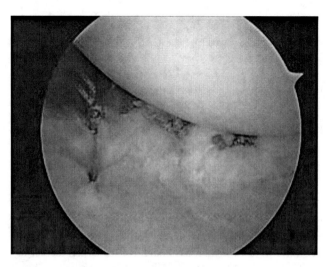

Figure 1. Arthroscopic view of glenoid labral injuries.

- Open repair is done with transosseus tunnels. Glenoid deficiency is addressed through open repair

Consults

- Orthopedic surgeon
- Physical medicine and rehabilitation

Complications/side effects

- Recurrent instability
- Loss of motion
- Subscapularis tendon failure (following surgery)

Prognosis

- Up to 75% of patients improve with an adequate and early rehabilitation protocol
- Adequate shoulder function is expected

Helpful Hints

- Age at presentation of acute shoulder dislocation is the most important factor in predicting a Bankart lesion (<40 years) vs a rotator cuff lesion (>40 years)
- In throwers with shoulder pain and laxity, suspect labral tears

Suggested Readings

Brian S, Levine WN. Arthroscopic Bankart repair. *J Am Acad Orthop Surg.* 2005;13:487-490.

Keener JD, Brophy RH. Superior labral tears of the shoulder: pathogenesis, evaluation, and treatment. *J Am Acad Orthop Surg.* 2009;17(10):627-637.

Hamstring Strain

Michael Henrie DO ▪ Stuart Willick MD

Description

Hamstring strain is an injury that affects the semimembranosus, semitendinosus, and biceps femoris muscles of the posterior thigh, results in localized damage, which could be acute or chronic, and leads to loss of function as well as inability to participate in sports.

Etiology/Types

- Acute/macrotrauma: associated with stretch, eccentric overload, and seen in sports that require acceleration, deceleration, and change of direction
- Chronic/microtrauma: seen in repetitive activities such as long distance running; may be associated with muscle weakness, fatigue, and abnormal biomechanics

Epidemiology

- Hamstring injuries are common among individuals participating in ballistic activities
- Hamstring injuries tend to heal slowly and have a high rate of recurrence

Pathogenesis

- The hamstring group includes the short and long heads of biceps femoris laterally, and the semitendinosus and semimembranosus medially
- Acting concentrically across the knee, the primary function of the hamstring group is knee flexion. Acting eccentrically across the knee, the primary function is to control terminal knee extension. Via their origin at the ischial tuberosity, the hamstrings act as secondary hip extensors and pelvic stabilizers in the closed kinetic chain environment
- Acute hamstring injuries most commonly occur with forceful eccentric contraction
- Young athletes present with avulsion injuries of the ischial tuberosity
- Adults present with injuries localized at the muscle side of the muscle-tendon junction
- The risk of acute hamstring strain is increased when the muscle group is placed at a mechanical disadvantage near full flexion or extension, and when the muscle is weak or fatigued
- The hamstring muscle group is also vulnerable to repetitive overload injury

- The hamstring muscle group may be associated with chronic lumbosacral root injury

Risk Factors

- Participation in high-velocity sports
- Muscle weakness
- Poor flexibility
- Lack of conditioning

Clinical Features

- Acute and chronic hamstring injuries may be symptomatic at the origin at the ischial tuberosity, within the muscle belly, and along the distal tendons
- Young athletes may present with gluteal or proximal thigh pain associated with avulsion of the ischial tuberosity
- Adults usually present with pain in the posterior thigh seen in injury at the muscle tendon junction
- Difficulty with activity, including running and jumping

Natural History

- Symptoms improve with rest initially, but high rate of recurrence if not rehabilitated
- Poor flexibility and muscle weakness remain after injury
- Athletes in specific sports such as sprinting, soccer, basketball, and football prone to recurrent injury

Diagnosis

Differential diagnosis

- Avulsion fractures
- Lumbar radiculopathy
- Sacroiliac joint dysfunction
- Myofascial pain

History

- Acute injuries: the patient typically describes a mechanism involving acute overload. There is sudden onset of pain and tenderness, and they may report hearing a "pop"
- Repetitive overload injuries: the patient usually reports gradual onset of pain after an increase in exercise activities

Exam

- Pain is usually reproduced with passive knee extensor stretch, and resistance to knee flexion
- Ecchymosis at and distal to the injury site may be seen after an acute, severe strain
- A palpable defect may be present following a large tear
- Hamstrings, gluteal, and core muscle weakness in chronic cases
- Neurological deficits in underlying radiculopathy

Testing

- Usually not necessary to make diagnosis. Plain films should be obtained if there is concern for an avulsion fracture or joint injury
- Magnetic resonance imaging is the modality of choice for severe injuries in which muscle tears are suspected
- Ultrasound is also a good imaging option to identify hematomas and large tears

Pitfalls

- Not identifying proximal injuries, avulsion fractures
- Missing tears that may require surgical evaluation
- Allowing rapid return to sports that results in recurrent injury

Red Flags

- Severe pain and limited motion despite treatment
- Marked muscle weakness despite rehabilitation
- Numbness, distal lower extremity weakness

Treatment

Medical

- Relative rest
- Analgesics
- Short course of anti-inflammatory medications (concerns for increased bleeding, and delayed healing)

Exercises

- Early, gentle pain-free range of motion
- Carefully progressive strengthening exercises focusing on the hamstring and other muscles along the kinetic chain, increasing resistance as tolerated. Start with static exercises, back stabilization, and progress to midrange concentric exercise
- Transition to ballistic and sports-specific activities
- Eccentric training to improve muscle-loading capability
- Restoration of quadriceps-hamstring force couple

Modalities

- Cryotherapy
- Superficial heat
- Transcutaneous electrical nerve stimulation, electrical stimulation
- Laser in subacute stages

Injection

- Steroid injections should be avoided in acute cases
- Soft tissue injections (trigger point needling), prolotherapy, and botulinum toxin use are considerations for chronic injury with localized muscle tenderness and scar tissue (limited scientific evidence)
- The role of platelet-rich plasma injections needs to be defined in acute/chronic strains

Surgical

- Surgical referral for displaced ischial tuberosity avulsions (>5 mm)
- Consideration of repair of large muscle tears in competitive athletes

Consults

- Orthopedic surgery
- Physical medicine and rehabilitation
- Sports medicine

Complications/side effects

- Residual pain and weakness
- Myositis ossificans
- Inability to return to high-level sports

Prognosis

- Good with prompt diagnosis and appropriate treatment
- Recurrence of injury with incomplete rehabilitation

Helpful Hints

- Suspect avulsion in young athletes with proximal pain
- Emphasize eccentric strengthening exercise to prevent recurrence

Suggested Readings

Croisier J, Forthomme B, Namurois MH, et al. Hamstring muscle strain recurrence and strength performance disorders. *Am J Sports Med.* 2002;30(2):199–203.

Mason DL, Dickens V, Vail A. Rehabilitation for hamstring injuries. *Cochrane Database Syst Rev.* 2007;(1):CD004575.

Tornese D, Bandi M, Melagati G, et al. Principles of hamstring strain rehabilitation. *J Sports Traumatol.* 2000;22(2):70–85.

Hip Adductor Strain

Anton Wicker MD PhD ■ Sebastian Edtinger MD

Description
- Hip adductor strains can present as acute injuries or overuse syndromes. These injuries occur at the muscle-tendon junction and sometimes in the muscle belly. The lesions in the muscle belly tend to be less severe
- The hip adductors include the adductor magnus, adductor brevis, and adductor longus, as well as the pectineus and the gracilis

Etiology/Types
- Adductor strains are generally classified as Degrees I to III
  - Degree I strains are painful without loss of function or mobility
  - Degree II strains have a loss of strength and mobility without complete loss of function
  - Degree III strains will have complete loss of function

Epidemiology
- Adductor strains are frequently seen in all sports activities requiring changes of direction or propulsion. These activities are necessary in soccer, alpine skiing, high jump, gymnastics, ice hockey, water skiing, and swimming
- Ten percent of injuries in ice hockey; 5% to 9% of injuries in high school athletes

Pathogenesis
- Very often an imbalance in strength between the abductor and adductor muscles is the predisposing factor. Two joint muscles are more susceptible to these lesions
- Poor conditioning; overtraining predispose athletes to adductor strains
- The common mechanism of injury involves a sudden stretch caused by forced external rotation of an abducted leg. Stretching of this muscle group in a similar position without an adequate warm-up period also may trigger this type of injury
- Inflammation, ruptures, and strains of the musculotendinous units

Risk Factors
- Abnormal hip abductor-adductor strength ratios
- Loss of adductor and psoas flexibility
- Core muscle weakness
- Sudden mechanical loading
- Sacroiliac joint dysfunction
- Smoking
- Previous injury

Clinical Features
- Progressive groin pain
- Progressive gait disorders
- Progressive weakness
- Loss of flexibility

Natural History
- The structures in this region are extremely vulnerable to both tensile overload and direct trauma, and recurrence is high if not rehabilitated
- The vulnerability to sudden mechanical loading increases with age

Diagnosis

Differential diagnosis
- Stress fracture of the femoral neck
- Hip labral tears
- Osteitis pubis
- Inguinal hernia/sports hernia
- Osteoarthritis
- Neoplasm
- Genitourinary causes
- Obturator nerve entrapment
- Inguinal nerve injury

History
- Groin or pelvic girdle pain
- Increasing weakness of hip muscles
- Decreased flexibility of pelvic girdle
- Radiation from groin into the quadriceps

Exam
- Pain with resisted adduction and forced abduction of the hip
- Tender points at the origin of the adductor tendons at the os pubis
- Irritation of the sacroiliac joint
- Tenderness along the course of the adductor muscles

Testing

- X-rays may demonstrate pathology in the hips and pelvic bones; always should be taken
- Ultrasound can be used to evaluate muscle and tendon injuries and to rule out more serious conditions
- Magnetic resonance imaging (MRI) and computed tomography (CT) are effective in diagnosing the extent of the tears, and to evaluate for other possible etiologies of pain

Pitfalls

- Incarceration of an inguinal hernia, gynecologic pathology, a testicular tumor, or testicular torsion may result in irreversible complications

Red Flags

- Infection
- Fracture
- Neoplasm
- Increasing neurological dysfunction
- Testicular torsion

Treatment

Medical

- Nonsteroidal anti-inflammatory medications
- Analgesic drugs

Exercises

- Reduce sports training intensity/cross training
- Establish a gradual strengthening program for the adductor group, the hamstrings, and the quadriceps; after pain control start flexibility training
- Stabilization of the trunk in functional movement patterns
- Sports-specific proprioceptive training focusing on balance on unstable surfaces
- Dynamic exercise program focused on concentric, eccentric, and functional strengthening of adductor muscles with the clinical goal of adductor strength at 80% of abduction

Modalities

- Ice
- Heat
- Massage
- Ultrasound

- Electrical stimulation
- Transcutaneous electrical nerve stimulation
- Shock-wave therapy (in chronic cases)
- Low-level laser (may be used as a treatment option for soft tissue injury; some evidence in the medical literature, primarily in Europe)

Injection

- Trigger point injections
- Prolotherapy and platelet-rich plasma need further study in acute and chronic injury

Surgical

- Surgical intervention is only recommended in total tears (all adductors have been torn from symphysis) and very seldom in refractory chronic strains

Consults

- Orthopedic surgery
- General surgery
- Urology
- Gynecology
- Physical medicine and rehabilitation

Complications/side effects

- Progressive pain and continued weakness
- Reduced sports performance

Prognosis

- Continued normal function is possible, if assessed and treated early

Helpful Hints

- For prevention, adductor to abductor ratio strength should not be less than 80%
- Adductor strains should not be ignored—early diagnosis and treatment are necessary to avoid complications

Suggested Readings

Corrado G, d'Hemecourt PA. In: Frontera WR, Herring SA, Michelli LJ, Silver JK, eds. *Clinical Sports Medicine. Medical Management and Rehabilitation*. Philadelphia, PA: Saunders-Elsevier; 2007.

Maffey L, Emery C. What are the risk factors for groin strain injury in sports? A systematic review of the literature. *Sports Med.* 2007;37(10):881–884.

Nicholas SJ, Tyler TF. Adductor muscle strains in sport. *Sports Med.* 2002;32(5):339–344.

Hip Avascular Necrosis

William Micheo MD

Description

Avascular necrosis (AVN) (also known as osteonecrosis, bone infarction, aseptic necrosis, and ischemic bone necrosis) is a disease where interruption of blood supply leads to bone death. It usually affects the epiphysis of the hip, leading to pain, loss of motion, and arthritis.

Etiology/Types

- Associated with trauma (fracture, dislocation)
- Related to medical conditions (collagen vascular disease) or treatments (corticosteroids)
- Ten percent to 20% of cases are idiopathic

Epidemiology

- Hip, the most common site of AVN
- About 10,000 to 20,000 cases per year in the United States
- Affects people in the third and fourth decade of life; mean age of presentation around 38 years

Pathogenesis

- Not clearly known, involves loss of blood supply to the hip
- Because of intracapsular fractures; affects branches of the profunda femoris artery
- Arterial insufficiency or extravascular compression may be seen in systemic diseases
- Fat emboli postulated as a cause in alcoholism
- Corticosteroids may inhibit angiogenesis and are associated with stenotic vessels

Risk Factors

- Hip fracture (subcapital, femoral neck) or dislocation (delay in reduction)
- Developmental hip dysplasia
- Alcoholism
- Use of corticosteroids
- Collagen vascular disease, vasculitis
- Sickle cell anemia
- Gaucher's disease (lipid storage disease, accumulation of glucocerebroside, associated with bone infarctions, AVN)

Clinical Features

- Pain in the groin, buttock, or knee
- Difficulty with gait, weight bearing exercise
- Loss of hip range of motion
- Early radiological changes may be minimal; osteopenia present in the involved hip
- History of alcohol or corticosteroid use; history of trauma to the hip

Natural History

- Early diagnosis may improve treatment outcome
- Moderation of activity and protected weight bearing may reduce symptoms in the early stages
- If diagnosed after hip collapse and osteoarthritis develops, functional limitations will be present
- Surgical treatment required for severe AVN

Diagnosis

Differential diagnosis

- Hip osteoarthritis
- Hip dysplasia
- Transient osteoporosis of the hip
- Hip flexor/adductor strain/tendinopathy
- Hip trochanteric pain syndrome
- Lumbar radiculopathy

History

- Groin or buttock pain that worsens with activity
- History of asthma, immune-mediated diseases, inflammatory arthritis that required use of corticosteroids
- Hip fracture or dislocation
- Limp with ambulation

Exam

- Pain to palpation over the hip and groin (associated with secondary soft tissue overload)
- Reduced hip motion, particularly internal rotation
- Weak gluteal muscles
- Normal neurological examination
- Pain with hip rotation, may have positive Patrick's (FABERE) test with pain reproduced over the groin
- Gait evaluation reveals lateral trunk lean toward the involved side

Testing

- Radiographs may reveal patchy osteopenia, sclerosis, and lucency in the early stages

- As the disease progresses, a crescent sign (collapse of the trabeculae beneath the subchondral bone), hip collapse, and deformity of the femoral head can be identified
- Magnetic resonance imaging (MRI) is the test of choice if AVN is suspected (highly sensitive and specific, 88%–100%); radiographic abnormalities may take up to 3 months to develop after the onset of symptoms

Red Flags
- Progressive pain despite minimal abnormalities on x-rays

Treatment
Medical
- Analgesics and nonsteroidal anti-inflammatory drugs
- Protected weight bearing with crutches or the use of a cane in the opposite upper extremity

Exercises
- Gentle range of motion of the affected hip
- Stretching of hip muscles
- Light strengthening of the hip and gluteal muscles
- Aquatic exercises
- Bicycle

Modalities
- Cryotherapy
- Superficial heat
- Transcutaneous electrical nerve stimulation/electrical stimulation

Injection
- Trigger point injections may be used to treat overloaded and painful gluteal and hip muscles (secondary pain generators)
- Trochanteric injections with local anesthetics, and low dose of corticosteroids may be used to improve symptoms and allow rehabilitation

Surgical
- In the early stages, core decompression is attempted (variable results)
- Vascularized bone graft (fibula) has also been recommended for young patients, athletes, following

pregnancy, and infection, particularly in early stages of the disease
- Hip arthroplasty treatment of choice in older patients with hip collapse (bipolar prosthesis insertion does not have favorable results in patients with AVN)
- In younger patients with severe symptoms and hip collapse, resurfacing (ceramic-on-ceramic, or metal-on-metal) arthroplasties and the newer generation total hip replacement arthroplasties are treatment options with good results

Consults
- Orthopedic surgery
- Physical medicine and rehabilitation

Complications/side effects
- Chronic hip pain
- Difficulty with walking
- Postoperative infection
- Loosening or fracture of the hip prosthesis

Prognosis
- Variable
- May be managed without surgery in the early stages in selected patients who modify their activity, control their weight, and strengthen the hip muscles
- Surgery required in majority of patients because of increased pain and disability

Helpful Hints
- Suspect AVN in patients who present with groin pain and have history of high alcohol intake, treatment with corticosteroids, and history of hip trauma
- Order MRI early if symptoms persist, even in patients with normal plain radiographs

Suggested Readings
Aldridge JM, 3rd, Urbaniak JR. Vascularized fibular grafting for osteonecrosis of the femoral head with unusual indications. *Clin Orthop Rel Res.* 2008;466(5):1117–1124.

Bachiller FG, Caballer AP, Portal LF. Avascular necrosis of the femoral head after femoral neck fractures. *Clin Orthop Rel Res.* 2002;399:87–109.

Seyler TM, Cui Q, Mihalko WM, et al. Advances in hip arthroplasty in the treatment of osteonecrosis. *Instr Course Lect.* 2007;56:221–233.

Hip Labral Injury

Heidi Prather DO ■ Devyani Hunt MD

Description
The acetabular labrum of the hip is a fibrocartilage ring that surrounds the joint. Hip labral tears are a frequent cause of anterior hip and groin pain.

Etiology/Types
- Labral fraying
- Labral tears
- Labral detachment

Epidemiology
- Occurs more frequently in women than in men
- Age range for isolated tears is 15 to 60 years

Pathogenesis
- Acetabular labral tears can occur in association with a traumatic event such as a motor vehicle accident
- The labrum can be damaged with overuse injuries and is commonly seen in specific sports such as soccer, hockey, golf, and dance. Sporting activities with repetitive, torsional force, or end range of flexion, adduction, or abduction can damage the labrum
- Labral tears are linked to osseous abnormalities of the hip and occur more commonly in individuals with developmental dysplasia of the hip (DDH), femoroacetabular impingement (FAI), Legg Calves Perthes disease, and slipped capital femoral epiphysis

Risk Factors
- Trauma
- Repetitive pivoting, hip flexion, and rotation
- Osseous structural abnormalities of the hip such as DDH, FAI, acetabular retroversion, coxa vara, coxa valga, aspherical femoral head

Clinical Features
- Majority of patients describe anterior hip or groin pain
- Small minority with lateral hip, anterior thigh, or posterior hip pain
- Mechanical symptoms such as locking, clicking, or catching

- Pain worsened with walking, pivoting, and impact activities (running)
- Night pain
- Significant functional limitations such as limping and difficulty with stairs

Natural History
- The acetabular labrum protects and seals the hip joint (Figure 1)
- It deepens the socket 21%, therefore improving stability
- It increases the surface area by 28%, therefore distributing the load and decreasing contact stress on the articular surfaces
- Without a functioning labrum, the hip joint will sustain increased pressure
- This increased pressure is believed to start the degenerative cascade and cause early secondary osteoarthritic changes
- Due to poor vascular supply, labral tears are difficult to heal

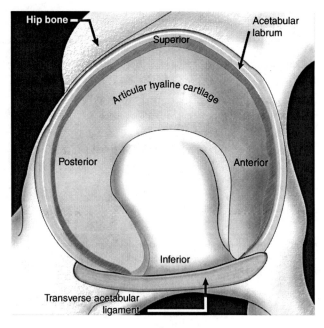

Figure 1. The acetabular labrum. Modified from Primal Pictures Limited.

Diagnosis

Differential diagnosis

- Hip flexor tendonitis
- Illiopsoas bursitis
- Cartilage abnormality
- Bony abnormality
- Arthritis
- Inguinal hernia
- Spine disorder
- Sacroiliac joint disorder
- Pubic symphysis disorder
- Fracture
- Neoplasm

History

- Groin pain, underlying aching, occasionally sharp
- Worsens with activity
- Clicking, popping, or locking
- Traumatic event
- Childhood history of hip problems

Exam

- Antalgic to normal gait
- Normal to decreased hip flexion and rotation
- Positive hip impingement test (pain with hip flexion to 90°, internal rotation, and adduction in the supine position)
- Patients can have a positive log roll test (hip rotation with extended hip and knees)
- Patients can have a positive FABER/Patrick's test

Testing

- X-rays are performed to assess for associated osseous abnormalities
- Diagnostic intra-articular hip injection performed with image guidance can help determine if the disorder is related to an intra-articular process
- In many imaging centers, MR arthrogram is more specific and sensitive than plain MRI to detect labral abnormalities

Pitfalls

- Fifteen percent to 20% of labral tears are not seen with an MR arthrogram
- X-rays can be normal
- Patients can have coexisting conditions that limit progress or impede the diagnosis. Examples include pelvic floor pain and lumbar spine disorders

Red Flags

- Fractures
- Neoplasm
- Infection
- Avascular necrosis

Treatment

Medical

- Relative rest with avoidance of aggravating activities such as pivoting and high-impact activities on the lower extremities
- Nonsteroidal anti-inflammatory medications
- Analgesics as indicated

Exercises

- A focused, specific physical therapy program is the recommended first treatment option for hip labral injuries
- Physical therapy protocols focus on decreasing the anterior glide of the femur and improving the overall functioning of the hip
- Individualization is important to address muscle imbalances and weaknesses
- It is important to emphasize only pain-free range of motion of the hip
- The exercise prescription needs to fit within the range-of-motion limitations, if the patient has related osseous deformity

Modalities

- Heat
- Ice
- Ultrasound

Injections

- Fluoroscopically guided hip injections can be useful as a diagnostic tool to discern between an intra-articular and extra-articular source of pain. This is especially true when the clinical picture points toward a labral tear, but the imaging is negative
- Caution should be used when considering injecting steroid into a young joint with no arthritic changes due to the adverse effects that steroids and anesthetics have on the cartilage

Surgical

- Arthroscopic debridement or repair of the labrum should be considered if conservative measures have failed
- Associated osseous abnormalities may also need to be addressed at the time of surgery, possibly

necessitating a more extensive surgery and/or open approach

Consults
- Orthopedic surgeon specializing in arthroscopy of the hip

Complications/side effects
- Secondary osteoarthritis
- Progressive pain and dysfunction
- Secondary dysfunction in the pelvis or spine due to compensatory mechanisms

Prognosis
- Improved prognosis when recognized and treated early

Helpful Hints
- It is important to have a high level of suspicion for labral abnormalities in adolescents and young adults who present with anterior groin pain and mechanical symptoms such as locking
- A trial of conservative measures is recommended prior to considering labral debridement or repair

Suggested Readings
Burnett S, Della Rocca G, Prather H, et al. Clinical presentation of patients with tears of the acetabular labrum. *J Bone Joint Surg Am.* 2006;88(7):1448–1457.

Mason JB. Acetabular labrum tears: diagnosis and treatment. *Clin Sports Med.* 2001;20:779–790.

Humeral Epiphyseal Injury, Proximal

Brian J. Krabak MD MBA ■ Alison C. Welch MD

Description

The proximal epiphysis is one of two growth plates in the humerus where new bone is formed to contribute to longitudinal growth of the bone. This growth plate typically ossifies between 17 and 18 years of age. In the immature athlete, proximal humeral epiphyseal injuries result from repeated stress to the growth plate that leads to widening of the growth plate.

Etiology/Types

- Overuse injury from repeated stress on the growth plate of the proximal humerus
- Common in high-level overhead adolescent athletes
- Referred to as "little league shoulder," "adolescent athletes shoulder," and proximal humeral epiphyseal osteonecrosis

Epidemiology

- Adolescent athletes between 11 and 15 years of age
- Males greater than females
- Increased incidence in adolescents involved in sports involving high levels of overhead activity, especially baseball (especially pitchers and catchers), swimming, volleyball, and tennis

Pathogenesis

- Type I Salter-Harris physeal fracture with separation of the metaphysis from the epiphysis
- Thought to be due to the repetitive microtrauma of shear forces and rotational torque to the relatively weak epiphysis
- Some theories include interruption of vascular supply as a contributing factor

Risk Factors

- Overtraining without adequate rest between seasons
- High force and frequency of overhead activity
- In baseball: high number of pitches (>75 per game, >600 per season), type of pitches (curve ball and sliders), and months per year of pitching (>8 months/year). Highest risk factor is overall number of pitches
- Improper biomechanics and sports-specific technique
- Higher levels and frequency of competition

Clinical Features

- Superior-lateral shoulder pain during overhead activity
- Pain-free at rest

Natural History

- Progressive pain—initially only with high levels of activity, then progressively worsening to consistent pain with continued activity
- Can eventually lead to decreased level of performance, especially deterioration of pitching technique due to pain
- Swimmers may initially only have pain during competition, which may progress to pain even during light swimming

Diagnosis

Differential diagnosis

- Rotator cuff tendinopathy
- Acromioclavicular joint injury
- Impingement syndrome
- Shoulder instability
- Fracture
- Infection
- Tumor
- Bone cyst

History

- Gradual onset and progressively worsening shoulder pain, particularly at point of maximum shoulder external rotation (ER) and extension. However, symptoms can occur through all phases of throwing
- Report of high level of athletic involvement, particularly overhead activity
- Adolescent

Exam

- Typically, full and pain-free passive range of motion
- Tenderness to palpation over proximal humerus

- Pain in superior-lateral shoulder with dynamic and resisted overhead activity
- No impingement, shoulder instability, or labral signs

Testing
- Anteroposterior radiographs of the bilateral shoulders in internal rotation (IR) and ER for comparison
- X-rays demonstrate widened and irregular lateral physis on ER view (Figure 1), whereas IR demonstrates two narrow radiolucent lines
- Lateral fragmentation, calcification, sclerosis, and cyst formation may be present on x-rays, as this a chronic stress injury
- Magnetic resonance imaging (MRI) shows physeal widening, with focal extension into the metaphysis on T1-weighted images. Increased T2-weighted signal in metaphysic consistent with marrow edema

Pitfalls
- Failure to image both shoulders may lead to missing the diagnosis

Red Flags
- Constitutional symptoms concerning for neoplasm or infection
- Neurological deficits
- Red, warm, swollen joint

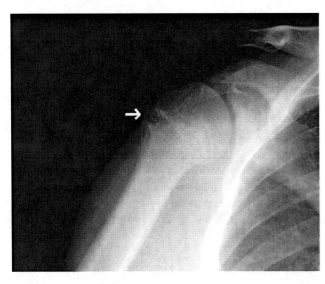

Figure 1. X-ray demonstrating widening (white arrow) of the lateral physis consistent with a physeal injury.

Treatment

Medical
- First-line treatment is activity modification, including:
  – Relative rest
  – Avoidance of activities causing pain
- Pitchers will need to stop pitching for at least 3 months
- Pitchers and catchers can often play infield positions
- Swimmers may need to decrease yardage or change strokes
- Patient should avoid any activity that causes pain
- Progressive return to play once overhead activity is pain-free by using an Interval Throwing Program with progressive increase of distance and number of throws per session. This program should progress over at least 8 weeks to full distance and intensity of throws

Exercises
- Strengthening of shoulder external rotators and scapular stabilizers
- Stretching of shoulder internal rotators
- Review of proper sports-specific technique, especially throwing technique

Modalities
- Sling if needed to keep arm inactive, initially

Injection
- Should be avoided in the skeletally immature athlete

Surgical
- Unusual, unless evidence of premature closure of the growth plate

Consults
- Orthopedic surgery
- Sports medicine
- Physical medicine and rehabilitation

Complications
- Rare premature closure of growth plate

Prognosis
- Good; most patients are able to return to previous level of activity
- Average rest time 3 months
- Average time to return to full play 7 to 8 months
- Prolonged symptoms require referral to a sports medicine physician for further evaluation

Helpful Hints

- Prevention is important, including education of coaches, parents, and children about the risk of overuse injuries
- Limiting the number of pitches per week, and games per season in little league can be helpful in prevention
- Importance of variety of activity to prevent overuse injury
- Focus on progressive skill development in adolescent athletes
- Radiographic evidence of healing can take 6 to 12 months, and does not need to be followed clinically

Suggested Readings

Caine D, DiFiori J, Maffulli N. Physeal injuries in children's and youth sports: reasons for concern? *Brit J Sports Med.* 2006;40:749–760.

Krabak BJ, Alexander E, Henning T. Shoulder and elbow injuries in the adolescent athlete. *Phys Med Rehabil Clin North Am.* 2008;19:271–285.

Lyman S, Gleisig GS, Andrews JR, Osinski ED. Effect of pitch type, pitch count, and pitching mechanics on risk of elbow and shoulder pain in youth baseball pitchers. *Am J Sports Med.* 2002;30:463–468.

Iliopsoas Tendinopathy

Christopher J. Visco MD ■ Joshua D. Rittenberg MD

Description

The iliopsoas muscle is the prime mover of hip flexion and also assists with external rotation of the femur. A tendinopathy affecting the insertion of the iliopsoas on the femur can occur with biomechanical deficits and repetitive hip flexion, resulting in chronic degenerative changes of the tendon.

Etiology/Types

Structurally, tendinopathy is an alteration in the normal fibrillar architecture of tendon. Generally, this is thought to occur from a chronic overuse of the tendon causing microtrauma. The exact etiology is unclear.

Epidemiology

- Occurs more commonly in kicking athletes, including soccer players
- May occur in the nonathletic population
- Peak age group is in 30s

Pathogenesis

- Flexibility or strength deficits may lead to alterations in body mechanics, causing overload of the iliopsoas tendon
- Chronic repetitive overload leads to architectural tendon changes
- Histopathologically, mucoid degeneration with increased interfibrillar glycosaminoglycans disrupting collagen fiber structure
- Pain results from chronic microtearing and tendon degeneration

Risk Factors

- Insidious onset
- Repetitive hip flexion

Clinical Features

- Deep aching pain in the groin
- Clicking or catching sensation
- Inflexibility of the lumbar spine
- Tightness of hip flexors

Natural History

- Nonremittent deep aching groin pain
- Symptoms worsen with activity

Diagnosis

Differential diagnosis

- Hip labral tear
- Sports hernia
- Iliopsoas bursitis
- Inguinal hernia
- Osteitis pubis
- Abdominal muscle tendinopathy/strain
- Adductor tendinopathy
- Osteoarthritis
- Obturator nerve entrapment
- Neoplasm

History

- Deep aching groin pain
- Intermittent
- Worse with activity, especially kicking
- Pain may radiate to anterior thigh
- Improves with rest

Exam

- Tenderness at the distal insertion of iliopsoas tendon
- Tightness of iliopsoas tendon
- Positive Thomas test (evaluation for hip flexion contracture by flexing the contralateral hip and assessing the ability to maintain ipsilateral hip extension)
- Abdominal and groin examination/palpation
- Normal neurological examination

Testing

- Radiograph of the affected hip is normal
- Magnetic resonance imaging (MRI) may reveal increased fluid around the iliopsoas tendon
- Musculoskeletal ultrasound can be helpful for identifying thickened tendon when compared with unaffected side

Pitfalls

- Failure to identify underlying strength or flexibility deficits

Red Flags

- Infection
- Fracture
- Neoplasm
- Neurological dysfunction

Treatment

Medical
- Nonsteroidal anti-inflammatory medications
- Analgesics

Exercises
- Correct underlying strength and flexibility deficits
- Range of motion and hip flexibility
- Lumbar spine and pelvic mobilization
- Core strengthening
- Anterior hip mobilization (see Figure 1)

Modalities
- Deep heat
- Therapeutic ultrasound

Injection
- Diagnostic anesthetic injection

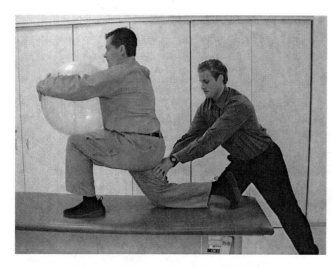

Figure 1. Assisted anterior hip mobilization.

- Local steroid injection to the iliopsoas bursa or tendon sheath injection

Surgical
- Rarely needed

Consults
- Orthopedic surgery for chronic recalcitrant cases
- Manual therapy for mobilization of capsule or flexibility deficits

Complications/side effects
- Delayed return to play
- Snapping hip syndrome
- Chronic intermittent groin pain

Prognosis
- Good with correction of underlying biomechanical deficits

Helpful Hints
- Keep differential diagnosis in mind (i.e., labral tear)
- Early identification of biomechanical deficits can prevent development of chronic symptoms
- Return to play with full, pain-free range of motion

Suggested Readings

Geraci MC. Rehabilitation of the hip, pelvis, and thigh. In: Kibler WB, Herring SA, Press JM, eds. *Functional Rehabilitation of Sports and Musculoskeletal Injuries.* Philadelphia, PA: Lippincott Williams & Wilkins; 1998:226–243.

Johnston CA, Wiley JP, Lindsay DM, Wiseman DA. Iliopsoas bursitis and tendinitis. A review. *Sports Med.* 1998;25(4):271–283.

Iliotibial Band Friction Syndrome

Michael Fredericson MD FACSM

Description
Iliotibial band friction syndrome (ITBFS) is the most common cause of lateral knee pain in runners. The syndrome results from repetitive friction of the iliotibial band (ITB) sliding over the lateral femoral epicondyle, moving anterior to the epicondyle as the knee extends and posterior as the knee flexes, and remaining tense in both positions.

Etiology/Types
- ITBFS is caused by excessive rubbing of the band over the lateral epicondyle of the femur during sporting activity, which produces pain and inflammation
- Debate exists as to which structure lies underneath the ITB: bursa or synovial tissue with a capsular origin

Epidemiology
- The most common cause of lateral knee pain in runners, with a reported incidence as high as 22.2% of all lower extremity injuries

Pathogenesis
- The ITB is a continuation of the tendinous portion of the tensor fascia lata (TFL) muscle with some contributions from the lateral gluteal muscles. Distally, the ITB spans out and has attachments to the lateral border of the patella and lateral patellar retinaculum before its insertion on Gerdy's tubercle of the tibia
- During the running cycle, the posterior edge of the ITB impinges against the lateral femoral epicondyle of the femur just after foot strike. This "impingement zone" occurs at, or at slightly less than, 30° of knee flexion
- Repetitive irritation can lead to chronic inflammation, especially beneath the posterior fibers of the ITB, which are thought to be tighter against the lateral femoral epicondyle than the anterior fibers

Risk Factors
- Leg-length discrepancy (with the syndrome developing in the shorter leg)
- Increased forefoot varus

- Increased Q angles (measured angle between the anterior superior iliac spine, the center of the patella, and the tibial tuberosity), compared with controls
- Excessive running in the same direction on a track
- Downhill running
- Lack of running experience or abrupt increase in running distance or frequency
- Running long distances

Clinical Features
- Sharp pain or burning in the lateral knee
- Patients start running pain-free, but develop symptoms after a reproducible time or distance
- Initially, symptoms subside shortly after a run, but return with the next run
- Patients often note that running downhill and lengthening their stride aggravate the pain
- In more severe cases, pain can be present even with walking or when descending stairs

Natural History
- Progressive symptoms with continued running
- Improves with activity modification, and treatment
- Some patients may require surgical treatment

Diagnosis

Differential diagnosis
- Patellofemoral stress syndrome
- Early degenerative joint disease
- Lateral meniscal pathology
- Superior tibiofibular joint pain
- Popliteal or biceps femoris tendinitis
- Common peroneal nerve injury
- Referred pain from the lumbar spine

History
- Increasing lateral knee pain
- Increasing inability to run

Exam
- Tenderness on palpation of the ITB 2 to 3 cm superior to the lateral joint line
- Sometimes local edema or crepitation
- Noble compression test often positive (patient supine with knee flexed to 90°, pressure applied to the lateral femoral condyle as the knee is passively extended,

pain reproduction with knee extended approximately to 30°)
- Ober's test to assess tightness of the ITB (patient lies on the unaffected side with hip flexed to 90°; the affected hip is abducted, extended, and subsequently adducted; inability to adduct the hip to the examination table is a positive test)
- Modified Thomas test to evaluate for flexibility deficits in the iliopsoas, and the rectus femoris (patient lies supine with contralateral hip flexed, whereas the symptomatic hip is extended and the knee flexed, inability to fully extend the hip, and to flex the knee to 90° indicates tight iliopsoas and rectus femoris muscle)
- Testing of gluteus medius muscle strength
- Leg-length discrepancies assessment

Testing
- Routine imaging is rarely indicated; radiograph results are usually normal
- Note the prominent lateral condyle in chronic cases
- Magnetic resonance imaging (MRI) may be requested if there is doubt about the diagnosis and to exclude an intra-articular problem such as a lateral meniscal tear

Pitfalls
- Common cause of lateral knee pain in runners or cyclists. Identify overuse history
- Not thinking about the differential diagnosis

Red Flags
- Worsening pain, symptoms at rest
- The patient not understanding the need to rest in the acute phase

Treatment

Medical
- Nonsteroidal anti-inflammatory medications (during the first week of injury)

Exercises
- Elimination of myofascial restrictions along the lateral hip and thigh
- Stretching exercises increasing the length of the TFL/ITB complex

- Contraction-relaxation exercises to lengthen shortened muscle groups
- Strengthening the gluteus medius muscle, especially the posterior fibers that function as abductors and external rotators
- Gradual return to running. Starting with easy sprints on level ground and avoiding any downhill running for the first few weeks

Modalities
- Ice
- Iontophoresis

Injection
- Local corticosteroid injection over the lateral femoral condyle, at the point of maximal tenderness of the ITB

Surgical
- Various surgical techniques in the rare refractory case
- Resecting a triangular piece of the ITB from the area overlying the lateral epicondyle
- Z-lengthening of the ITB

Consults
- Physical medicine and rehabilitation
- Sport medicine
- Orthopedic surgery

Complications/side effects
- Persistent and severe pain
- Inability to run

Prognosis
- Good; return to running if appropriately managed

Helpful Hints
- Repetitive running can lead to irreversible painful irritation and inflammation of the ITB so early treatment is important.

Suggested Readings

Fredericson M, Weir A. Practical management of iliotibial band friction syndrome in runners. *Clin J Sport Med.* 2006;16(3):261–268.

Fredericson M, Wolf C. Iliotibial band syndrome in runners: innovations in treatment. *Sports Med.* 2005;35(5):451–459.

Orchard JW, Fricker PA, Abud AT, et al. Biomechanics of iliotibial band friction syndrome in runners. *Am J Sports Med.* 1996;24:375.

Jersey Finger: Avulsion of the Flexor Digitorum Profundus Tendon

Derek S. Buck MD DC ▪ Gary P. Chimes MD PhD

Description

"Jersey finger" is a rare injury involving avulsion of the flexor digitorum profundus (FDP) from the distal interphalangeal joint (DIP). Described in sports such as football in which the finger flexors are contracted to grab an opponent's jersey while the digit is forcefully extended.

Etiology/Types

- Traumatic event involving resisted flexion of the DIP of the fingers
- Fourth digit is most commonly involved (75%)
- Classified into four types in Leddy and Packer classification scheme:
  - Type I: FDP tendon retracted into palm
  - Type II: FDP tendon remains in sheath
  - Type III: accompanied by avulsion fracture, which keeps distal FDP tendon fixed distal to the A4 or A5 pulley
  - Type IV: accompanied by avulsion fracture, but the FDP tendon separates from the bony fragment and retracts into the palm

Epidemiology

- Incidence of 4.83 per 100,000
- Accounts for 4.5% of tendon or ligament injuries
- Male to female ratio 4:1
- Most common in young athletes

Pathogenesis

- Traumatic avulsion of the FDP tendon at its insertion at the base of the distal phalanx during resisted flexion
- The fourth digit is commonly involved, which may be related to loosening of the grip from the other fingers, which dramatically increases the force placed on the fourth digit

Risk Factors

- Tackling sports
- Rock climbing

Clinical Features

- Usually normal radiograph unless associated avulsion fracture
- Inability to flex the DIP joint actively
- Inability to resist hyperextension of the DIP joint
- Palmar mass at the base of the affected digit (for Types II and IV injuries)

Natural History

- Persistent loss of finger flexion if not addressed

Diagnosis

Differential diagnosis

- Mallet finger
- Flexor digitorum superficialis injury
- DIP sprain
- Proximal IP joint sprain ("finger jam")
- Trigger finger

History

- History of grasping trauma in young athlete
- Inability to make a fist with affected digit
- Inability to flex the DIP of the affected digit
- Persistent pain and swelling of the involved digit
- Palmar mass in the affected digit

Exam

- Inability to flex the DIP of the affected digit
- Palmar mass in the affected digit

Testing

- X-ray may be normal or show avulsion of the palmar portion of the distal phalanx
- Magnetic resonance imaging may be helpful in locating the detached tendon as well as evaluate the distal phalanx cortex
- Some recent literature suggests that ultrasound may be used as an alternative imaging modality
- Clinical evaluation is still the gold standard (isolating the DIP and asking the patient to flex it)

Pitfalls

- Clinically dismissed as minor closed hand tendon injury, resulting in permanent loss of function and deformity

Red Flags

- Unresolving tenderness and swelling with persistent loss of function

Treatment

Medical

- Rapid surgical evaluation
- Range of motion (ROM) should be avoided until surgically evaluated

Exercises

- Postoperative occupational/hand therapy only
- ROM exercises
- Grip-strengthening exercises
- Tendon-gliding exercises (later stages)

Modalities

- Cold
- Paraffin bath
- Ultrasound

Injection

- Not indicated

Surgical

- Injuries with retracted tendons (Types I and IV) should be seen within 7 to 10 days.

- Injuries without retracted tendons (Types II and III) are not quite as emergent, but can progress, and therefore should be seen promptly.

Consults

- Hand surgery (either orthopedic or plastic)

Complications/side effects

- Loss of DIP function
- Permanent deformity
- Tendon necrosis without early intervention

Prognosis

- Poor return of ROM of the affected DIP joint
- Good return to equal hand grip strength when compared with contralateral side

Helpful Hints

- Early diagnosis is critical with referral to hand specialist (plastics or orthopedics) with repair typically needed to be done within 10 days of onset.

Suggested Readings

Clayton RAE, Court-Brown CM. The epidemiology of musculoskeletal tendinous and ligamentous injuries. *Injury.* 2008;39(12):1338–1344.

Lehfeldt M, Ray E, Sherman R. MOC-PS(SM) CME article: treatment of flexor tendon laceration. *Plast Reconstr Surg.* 2008;121(4 suppl):1–12.

Tuttle HG, Olvey SP, Stern PJ. Tendon avulsion injuries of the distal phalanx. *Clin Orthop Relat Res.* 2006;445:157–168.

Lateral Epicondylitis

Edwardo Ramos-Cortes MD

Description
Overuse syndrome of the extensor tendon origin of the forearm and wrist. It is sometimes called tennis elbow.

Etiology/Types
- Overuse injury that involves the origin of the wrist extensors at the lateral epicondyle
- Associated with repetitive wrist extension, and forearm supination in work and sports activity
- Angiofibroblastic hyperplasia, chronic tendinopathy of the extensor carpi radialis brevis (ECRB) tendon

Epidemiology
- Annual incidence of 1% to 3%; the conditions affect men and women equally
- Seen 2- to 4-fold in tennis players older than 40 years, and those who play over 2 hours per week
- Job-related symptoms associated with repetitive activity, lifting loads over 20 kg, and carrying tools

Pathogenesis
- Overuse of extensor tendons of the forearm that can progress
  - Periosteal tearing of the ECRB
- Tissues excised in surgery have shown
  - Mucopolysaccharide infiltration
  - Bone formation
  - Vascular proliferation
- "Angiofibroblastic tendinosis" due to the lack of inflammatory cells
- Vascular cause
  - Repetitive eccentric forces on a region with decreased healing potential due to hypovascularity

Risk Factors
- Repetitive motion of the forearm muscles with wrist extension
- Racquet sports
- Weak shoulder muscles (compensate with wrist movement)

Clinical Features
- Elbow pain with lifting, and gripping
- Loss of grip strength
- Point tenderness at the lateral epicondyle
- Pain that increases with resisted wrist dorsiflexion and passive wrist flexion

Natural History
- Occurs in individual with ages between 35 and 50 years, with a history of repetitive activity during work or recreation
- Usually progresses if not treated, self-limited condition in some individuals
- Nirschl classification:
  - Mild pain after exercise, lasting less than 24 hours
  - Pain after exercise, lasting greater than 48 hours, resolves with warm-up
  - Pain with exercise, does not alter ability to exercise
  - Pain with exercise that alters ability to exercise
  - Pain caused by heavy activities of daily living
  - Pain caused by light activities of daily living; intermittent pain at rest that does not interfere with sleep
  - Constant pain at rest, interferes with sleep

Diagnosis

Differential diagnosis
- Lateral collateral ligament sprain or insufficiency
- Radial tunnel syndrome
- Fracture
- Intra-articular pathology
- Triceps tendonitis
- Referred pain from cervical, shoulder, or wrist injuries

History
- A history of occupational- or activity-related pain
- Pain in the lateral elbow that radiates down the forearm

Exam
- Point tenderness over the lateral epicondyle and extensor tendon origin
- Pain with passive wrist flexion and resisted wrist extension
- Weak grip
- Swelling in the area can be present

Testing
- Imaging studies are rarely required
- X-rays of the elbow

- Studies have shown 16% have positive radiographic findings; in form of calcification
- Ultrasound
  - Calcification
  - Focal hypoechoic regions within the tendon
  - Complete or partial discrete cleavage tears
  - Diffuse heterogeneity
- Magnetic resonance imaging
  - Increased T1 signal within the extensor tendon
  - Tendon thickening
  - Edema of the common extensor origin

Pitfalls
- Pain in the proximal forearm associated with radial nerve injury confused with lateral epicondylitis

Red Flags
- Presence of neurological deficits along radial nerve distribution
- Failure of conservative treatment indicates the need of further evaluation, including the cervical spine

Treatment

Medical
- Topical nonsteroidal anti-inflammatory drugs (NSAIDs) provide short-term relief
- Conflicting evidence with the use oral NSAID
- Little evidence from well-designed clinical trials
- "Watchful waiting": one ramdomized controlled trial showed that approach was comparable with physical therapy and superior to corticosteroid injection
- Orthosis
  - Multiple systematic reviews have been unable to prove benefits of orthoses
  - May decrease pain and increase grip strength after 3 weeks

Exercise
- Strength training with emphasis in eccentric component of wrist extensors
- Stretching of wrist flexors and extensors
- Strengthening of shoulder and core muscles is required for return to overhead sports

Modalities
- Heat
- Ultrasound has thermal and mechanical (nonthermal) effects (mixed results in the medical literature)

- Electrotherapy
- Iontophoresis
- Electromagnetic field therapy
- Mobilization
- Deep transverse friction massage
- Extracorporeal shock wave therapy (has shown promising results for recalcitrant cases)

Injection
- Corticosteroid injection has shown short-term benefits; however, these benefits do not persist beyond 6 weeks
- Prolotherapy and plasma-rich platelets (PRP) injections have recently been used with some reports of good results particularly in chronic patients
- Botulinum toxin (used with variable results, possible change in muscle firing or analgesic effects, effect of needling?)

Surgical
- For patients with pain refractory to nonoperative management
- Numerous surgical techniques but no comprehensive review or consensus
- No surgical techniques appear superior to other

Consults
- Hand surgeon or orthopedic surgeon in cases refractory to conservative treatment

Complications/side effects
- Weakness of the elbow and hand
- Persistent pain

Prognosis
- Takes time to heal, may be self-limited in some individuals (difficult to predict)
- Depends on eliminating risk factors

Helpful Hints
- Early control of pain with modalities and injections allows participation in an eccentric exercise program
- Patients who fail conservative treatment may benefit from PRP prior to surgery being considered

Suggested Readings
Faro F, Wolf JM. Lateral epicondylitis: review and current concepts. *J Hand Surg.* 2007;32A:1271–1279.

Johnson GW, Cadwallader K, Scheffel SB, et al. Treatment of lateral epicondylitis. *Am Fam Physician.* 2007;76:843–853.

Little League Elbow

William Micheo MD ▪ Manuel Velez MD

Description

Little league elbow (LLE) is a valgus overload injury to the medial elbow that occurs as a result of repetitive throwing motions. It affects young athletes. Because of the chronological order of development of secondary ossification centers, LLE is an age-dependent injury.

Etiology/Types

- Childhood: medial apophysitis (the apophysis is the weakest medial structure)
- Early adolescence: avulsion fracture of the medial epicondyle associated with an increase in muscle strength
- Late adolescence-young adulthood: medial epicondylitis and injuries of the ulnar collateral ligament (UCL) become more common

Epidemiology

- Associated with participation in overhead sports
- Baseball-related overuse injuries 2% to 8% per year
- Associated with year-round single sports participation

Pathogenesis

- A general understanding of the varying biomechanical stresses that occur during each phase of throwing is helpful in identifying the mechanisms involved in elbow injuries
- The throwing phases include windup, early cocking, late cocking, early acceleration, late acceleration, deceleration, and follow-through
- Medial side injuries occur during the cocking and acceleration phases.
- During late cocking and early acceleration, the majority of LLE symptoms develop. More stress is to be placed on the medial elbow and anterior shoulder in these phases
- Valgus stress during the throwing motion results in tension on the medial elbow structures, and compression to the lateral structures
- Recurrent microtrauma leads to medial epicondylar fragmentation, apophysitis, and finally stress fractures
- Fusion of the common epiphysis occurs between 14 and 16 years of age

Risk Factors

- High intensity of sports participation
- High volume of pitches
- Participation in sports competition at a young age

Clinical Features

- Progressive medial elbow pain
- Progressive weakness
- Loss of flexibility, elbow extension, elbow locking

Natural History

- Pain is the most common presenting complaint
- Acute onset of symptoms may indicate avulsion type injury
- Chronic symptoms may indicate overuse injury

Diagnosis

Differential diagnosis

- Medial epicondyle apophysitis
- Avulsion fracture
- Fragmentation
- Growth disturbance
- UCL injury
- Ulnar nerve neuritis
- Osteochondritis dissecans (OCD)

History

- Young patient with immature skeleton
- Participates in throwing sports year round
- Initial pain during activity
- Progression to pain at rest
- Commonly affects pitchers
- Increased intensity of play, starting to throw "curve balls"

Exam

- On inspection evaluate for flexion contractures
- Evaluate for muscle atrophy or hypertrophy, bony deformities, or the presence of swelling and ecchymosis
- Palpation of bony structures: epicondyles, the olecranon process, the capitellum, and the radial head
- Soft tissue palpation should include the UCL, the biceps tendon, the triceps tendon, and the flexor-pronator and extensor-supinator muscle complexes
- Ulnar stress testing at 30° of elbow flexion

- Conduct a complete examination of the neck, shoulders, wrist, and hand

Testing
- Up to 85% of patients will have normal radiographs. Initial evaluation includes anteroposterior, lateral, and oblique views
- Skeletally immature athlete comparison with unaffected elbow to evaluate integrity of the apophyses
- Valgus stress views for UCL instability
- Magnetic resonance imaging (MRI) is often indicated to evaluate displacement of fractures, delineate the extent of OCD, or identify the presence of loose bodies inside the joint. MRI can also be diagnostic for medial collateral ligament avulsions or isolated disruptions
- Rarely, ultrasound or three-phase bone scan can be helpful

Red Flags
- Infection
- Fracture
- Neoplasm
- Paresthesias

Treatment

Medical
- Nonsteroidal anti-inflammatory medications
- Analgesics
- Emphasis is placed initially on rest, starting with 4 to 6 weeks of no throwing

Exercises
- Strengthening exercises are performed in a gradual fashion
- Initially isometrics are performed, then light dynamic strengthening of the scapular, shoulder, and upper extremity muscles
- Lower extremity and core strengthening
- No heavy lifting is permitted for 12 to 14 weeks
- An interval throwing program is initiated when symptoms subside, and progressed if no recurrence of pain

Modalities
- Ice
- Transcutaneous electrical nerve stimulation
- Ultrasound

Injection
- Not indicated in the child and adolescent athlete
- May be considered in the older athlete for UCL injury and medial epicondylitis

Surgical
- There is still controversy on when to use ORIF if there is a displaced avulsion fracture
- If surgical management is undertaken, it must be done in a way that allows for early range of motion (ROM)

Consults
- Orthopedic surgery

Complications/side effects
- Residual limitation of motion
- Inability to return to pitching

Prognosis
- Good if diagnosed early
- Need to address the pitching motion and the complete kinetic chain for good results

Helpful Hints
- Increase awareness among coaches, parents, and athletes
- Use proper warm-up, stretching, and strengthening
- Use proper pitching technique/mechanics
- Limit pitches thrown during games and practice (and home)
- Prohibit breaking balls such as curves until the mid- to late-teenage years
- Rehabilitate previous injuries including the shoulder

Suggested Readings
Aditim TA, Cheng TL. Overview of injuries in the young athlete. *Sports Med.* 2003;33(1):75–81.
Benjamin HJ, Briner WW, Jr. Little league elbow. *Clin J Sport Med.* 2005;15:37–40.
Kocher MS, Waters PM, Micheli LJ. Upper extremity injuries in the pediatric athlete. *Sports Med.* 2000;30(2):117–135.

Lumbar Degenerative Disc Disease

Carlos Rivera MD

Description

Degeneration of the lumbar spine is a process associated with aging. It is assumed to happen in all spines. The disc is composed of three major components: the nucleus, the annulus, and the end plates. The function of the lumbar spine is to efficiently transfer weight, provide stability, and allow motion. The stresses experienced are compressive, tensile, and/or shear. A disc can resist high compressive loads but is poorly constructed to combat tensile/torsional loading.

Etiology

- Specifics are unknown. Influenced by genetic inheritance, history of repetitive mechanical loading (like in bending, stooping, sitting, and vibration), smoking
- Athletes have more radiographical abnormalities, but no difference in pain or symptoms has been consistently reported

Epidemiology

- Universal age-related condition that can be symptomatic or asymptomatic

Pathogenesis

- The discs are the largest avascular structures in the body and depend on diffusion from a specialized network of end plate blood vessels for nutrition. The limited blood supply is associated with poor healing potential, making any structural failure irreversible
- Inside the disc annulus fissures develop, causing an inflammatory response with invasion of nociceptive nerve terminals that can produce pain
- These changes begin at the end of the first decade. End plate alterations precede changes in the nucleus, and the nucleus is more severely affected than the annulus

Risk Factors

- Genetic inheritance
- Increasing age
- Smoking
- History of lumbar spine loading

Clinical Features

- In most individuals, degenerative disc disease (DDD) is not associated with pain
- The painful syndrome associated with DDD is called internal disc disruption

Natural History

- Under excessive compressive loads, the end plates bulge into the vertebral bodies and can cause fractures in the end plates
- These microfractures prompt a process in which decreased permeability of the end plate initiates the degenerative cascade
- Episodes of axial back pain followed by radicular symptoms
- Disc degeneration accompanied by zygoapophyseal joint arthritis
- Some patients develop spinal stenosis and neurological claudication

Diagnosis

Differential diagnosis

- Spinal stenosis
- Radiculopathy
- Facet joint syndrome
- Infection
- Fracture
- Neoplasm
- Intra-abdominal and pelvic conditions

History

- Dull ache in the lower back with associated stiffness that can radiate to the buttocks
- Pain increases with prolonged sitting, bending, leaning
- Occasional episodes of debilitating pain can be described

Exam

- Limited lumbar range of motion (ROM) (flexion more than extension)
- Muscle guarding
- Normal neurological examination
- No specific test is reliable

Testing

- X-rays can identify loss of disc height, osteophyte formation, and facet hypertrophy, as well as any segmental instability.
- Magnetic resonance imaging (MRI) is very sensitive for disc abnormalities, including annular tears and disc herniations.
- Discography is the only technique that can correlate the structural abnormalities of the disc seen on MRI with patient pain response.

Pitfalls

- Treating radiographic studies instead of the patient
- Promoting sedentary lifestyle and seated positions (will lead to increased disc pressures, reduced physical condition)

Red Flags

- Fever
- Weight loss
- Severe nocturnal pain
- Neurological deficits in the physical examination

Treatment

Medical

- Analgesics
- Anti-inflammatory medications
- Education and reassurance

Exercises

- Back stabilization
- Core-strengthening exercises
- Hip flexibility and mobilization

Modalities

- Cryotherapy
- Superficial heat
- Electrical stimulation

Injections

- Epidural injections

Surgical

- Lumbar fusion for chronic cases (results variable, may not improve axial pain)
- Disc replacement (promising in younger patients, needs more scientific study)

Consults

- Pain medicine
- Neurosurgery or orthopedic spine surgery

Complications/side effects

- In general, this is a benign condition; in advanced conditions, functional limitations can occur
- Mental disorders such as depression and somatoform disorders can occur in patients with chronic pain

Prognosis

- Prognosis is favorable. The natural history is benign. The vast majority of patients (>90%) have resolution of symptoms within 6 weeks and only 1% have symptoms for longer than a year
- Recurrences occur in 20% to 67% of patients

Helpful Hints

- Radiological imaging does not correlate with symptoms
- Encourage patients to stay active and avoid sedentary environments

Suggested Readings

Crock HV. Internal disc disruption: a challenge to disc prolapse fifty years on. *Spine.* 1986;11(6):650–653.

Schaufele MK. Lumbar degenerative disc disease. In: Frontera WR, Silver JK, Rizzo TD, eds. *Essentials of Physical Medicine and Rehabilitation.* 2nd ed. Philadelphia; Saunders-Elsevier; 2002:229–235.

Lumbar Facet Syndrome

Luis Baerga MD ▪ Ricardo E. Colberg MD

Description
Pain due to inflammation, degeneration, and/or injury of the zygapophyseal joints (also known as facet joints).

Etiology/Types
- Mostly due to degenerative changes, but also due to inflammation, trauma, or repetitive movement
- Difficult to diagnose due to the poor correlation between history and physical examination
- May or may not present with radiating symptoms

Epidemiology
- The source of pain in about 15% to 40% of patients with chronic low back pain
- One of the most common causes of disability in persons younger than 45 years
- Most patients recover in about 6 weeks
- Prevalence of 23% in elderly (>60 years)

Pathogenesis
- May or may not be associated with disc herniation, but degenerative disc changes such as height loss and segmental instability lead to increasing loads across the facet joints with resulting cartilage alteration
- Pain due to degeneration, inflammation, or trauma of the joint causes a decrease in range of motion (ROM)
- Repeated lumbar extension may cause trauma or inflammation of the facet joint

Risk Factors
- High or repetitive mechanical loading
- Discogenic disease
- Lumbar facet degenerative changes

Clinical Features
- Acute or progressive back pain
- Loss of flexibility
- Pain with lumbar extension or posterior element loading
- May be referred to pain in buttocks and thighs

Natural History
- Usually begins in early adulthood
- Peak incidence at around 45 years old
- May be continuous or intermittent the rest of their lives

Diagnosis

Differential diagnosis
- Herniated nucleus pulposus
- Sacroiliitis
- Muscle strain
- Ligamentous sprain
- Spondylolysis/spondylolisthesis
- Lumbar spinal stenosis
- Infection (i.e., osteomyelitis, discitis)
- Compression/pathological fracture
- Neoplasm

History
- History of low back pain
- Repetitive and/or compressive forces to the extended spine
- Deep dull ache/occasionally sharp
- Radiation into the buttock or posterior thighs
- Morning stiffness

Exam
- Physical examination findings not very specific for this diagnosis
- Tenderness over the facet joints
- Pain reproducible with lumbar extension and side bending
- Relief with flexion
- Normal neurological examination

Testing
- X-rays demonstrate degenerative disc changes in 90% of patients screened with low back pain, but not sensitive or specific for the facet joint syndrome
- Computed tomography may demonstrate osteophytosis at the facets and joint space narrowing
- Magnetic resonance imaging shows facet degeneration, hypertrophy, or intra-articular effusion
- There is no correlation between the radiological findings and degree of pain
- Diagnostic medial branch block is the most sensitive for diagnosis

Pitfalls
- Diagnosis only by radiological findings
- Strict bed rest proven to worsen symptoms

Red Flags
- Fever, chills, recent weight loss
- Neurological changes
- Bowel or bladder changes
- Night pain

Treatment
Medical
- Acetaminophen
- Nonsteroidal anti-inflammatory drugs

Exercises
- Core strengthening
- Low back ROM with avoidance of painful extension
- Hip flexor stretching
- Aerobic exercise

Modalities
- Superficial heat
- Transcutaneous electrical nerve stimulation
- Massage/deep tissue massage
- Acupuncture and manipulations (limited evidence)

Injection
- Intra-articular/periarticular injections

- Medial branch blocks
- Radiofrequency facet denervation

Surgical
- Fusion for unremitting mechanical pain with associated segmental instability

Consults
- Physical medicine and rehabilitation
- Interventional pain management
- Neurosurgery or orthopedic-spine surgery

Complications/side effects
- Progressive pain and dysfunction

Prognosis
- Highly variable but good with proper treatment
- Only 1% of patients are permanently disabled

Helpful Hints
- High level of suspicion in axial low back pain that worsens with extension

Suggested Readings
Malanga GA. *Lumbosacral Facet Syndrome.* http://www.emedicine.com/sports/topic65.htm, July 15, 2008.
Manchikanti L, Singh, V. Review of chronic low back pain of facet joint origin. *Pain Physician.* 2002;5(1):83–101.

Lumbar Myofascial Pain

Marta Imamura MD PhD ■ Satiko Tomikawa Imamura MD PhD

Description
Muscle pain or tension syndrome affecting the low back and pelvic region.

Etiology/Types
- Associated with trauma
- Insidious onset
- Indirectly caused or associated with other pathology (disc disease, facet syndrome)
- Muscles commonly involved are the quadratus lumborum, gluteus medius, gluteus minimus, lumbar paravertebrals, piriformis, tensor fascia lata, and proximal hamstrings

Epidemiology
- Isolated myofascial pain accounts for less than 9% of cases of low back pain

Pathogenesis
- There are no specific anatomical or pathological findings specific to myofascial pain syndrome.
- Increased acetylcholine release in the muscle end plate, muscle contracture, and hypoxia have been hypothesized as causative fictions
- Abnormal biochemical milieu with elevated levels of substance P, bradykinins, and other pain mediators may also be involved
- Active trigger points are hypothesized to be dynamic peripheral nociceptive stimulators that can initiate, amplify, and maintain central sensitization

Risk Factors
- Musculoskeletal injury
- Overuse/abnormal biomechanics (leg length discrepancy) and ergonomics
- Underlying lumbar spine disorders

Clinical Features
- Low back and gluteal pain, possibly with a specific pattern of pain radiation
- Insidious in onset or resulting from localized trauma

Natural History
- Variable progression. Symptoms may resolve with early identification and treatment

- Failure to inactivate an active trigger point before central neuroplastic changes occur is hypothesized to be the major cause of chronic myofascial pain

Diagnosis

Differential diagnosis
- Lumbar radiculopathy
- Lumbar facet syndrome
- Sciatic neuropathy
- Trochanteric pain syndrome
- Meralgia paresthetica
- Sacroiliac joint dysfunction

History
- Low back pain, possibly with peripheral radiation
- Worsening of symptoms following activity and trauma
- Lower extremity paresthesias/numbness

Exam
- Limited back and hip motion
- Localized trigger or tender points
- Local taut bands and twitch responses can be seen
- Normal neurological examination

Testing
- Diagnosis by history and physical examination; diagnostic studies to rule out associated pathology that may require different treatments
  - X-rays to evaluate for arthritis and degenerative disc disease
  - Computer tomography or magnetic resonance imaging to assess the lumbar discs, facet joints, and spinal canal
  - Electrodiagnostic studies to evaluate for radiculopathy or focal neuropathy

Pitfalls
- Treating the incorrect pain generator
- Not addressing biomechanical and functional deficits—both intrinsic (leg length discrepancy, etc.) and extrinsic (equipment, shoes, etc.)

Red Flags
- Worse pain despite treatment
- Progressive neurological deficits

Treatment

Medical
- Analgesic/anti-inflammatory medications
- Muscle relaxants
- Anticonvulsants sometimes used, more in chronic pain
- Antidepressants
- Cognitive behavioral therapy

Exercises
- Spray and stretch, strain and counterstrain maneuvers
- Isometric contractions followed by muscle stretch (proprioceptive neuromuscular facilitation [PNF], contract relax)
- Dynamic strengthening of hip, pelvic, and abdominal muscles (core strengthening)
- Back stabilization
- Aerobic exercise/aquatic rehabilitation

Modalities
- Superficial heat
- Transcutaneous electrical nerve stimulation
- Ultrasound
- Massage/soft tissue mobilization

Injection
- Local anesthetic injection commonly used; steroids/local anesthetic, saline injections on dry needling may also work (may be effect of needling, not necessarily substance injected)
- Botulinum toxin injections
- Prolotherapy sometimes advocated but unproven

Surgical
- Surgery not indicated

Consults
- Physical medicine and rehabilitation
- Pain medicine

Complications/side effects
- Chronic pain
- Limited activity tolerance

Prognosis
- Variable; improved long-term outcomes can be achieved by removal of perpetuating and etiological factors, specific muscle strengthening, and aerobic conditioning
- Improved results with early diagnosis

Helpful Hints
- High level of suspicion required
- Beware of overinterpreting diagnostic studies
- Take into account previous physical activity level, severity of pain, and tolerance to activity in order to prescribe a gradual exercise and postural retraining program

Suggested Readings

Fischer AA. New injection techniques for treatment of musculoskeletal pain. In: Rachlin ES, Rachlin IS, eds. *Myofascial pain and Fibromyalgia. Trigger Point Management.* 2nd ed. Saint Louis: Mosby; 2002:403–419.

Gerwin RD, Dommerholt J, Shah JP. An expansion of Simon's integrated hypothesis of trigger point formation. *Curr Pain Headache Rep.* 2004;8(6):468–475.

Rygh LJ, Svendsen F, Fiska A, et al. Long-term potentiation in spinal nociceptive systems—how acute pain become chronic. *Psychoneuroendocrinology.* 2005;30(10):959–964.

Van Tulder M, Koes B, Bombardier C. Low back pain. *Best Pract Res Clin Rheumatol.* 2002;16(5):761–775.

Lumbar Radiculopathy

Christopher J. Visco MD ■ Joel Press MD

Description

Lumbar radiculopathy is compression, damage, or chemical irritation of a lumbar nerve root causing pain and neurological deficit. Pain most commonly radiates in a dermatomal distribution, and the affected myotome may result in reflex and strength deficits. Symptoms may or may not include low back pain and may present suddenly or more insidiously.

Etiology/Types

- Nerve root compression causes radiating pain in dermatomal distribution of the nerve with deficits on neurological examination
- Irritation of the nerve root without neurological deficits may be termed radiculitis

Epidemiology

- Incidence approximately 3% in general population
- Affects men at a younger age
- Younger individuals may present with herniated nucleus pulposus; in older patients, radiculopathy may be secondary to spinal stenosis
- Smoking increases risk

Pathogenesis

- Pathogenesis of lumbar radiculopathy may be multifactorial
- Annulus fibrosus normally contains the nucleus pulposus inside the disc with lamellar collagen fibers that are painful if torn or ruptured
- Nucleus pulposus may herniate through torn annulus causing a bulge, protrusion, or extrusion of disc material
- Large herniated nucleus pulposus may cause local trauma or compression to nerve root, occurring more frequently in younger individuals
- Disc material may also cause local inflammation and nerve root irritation acutely
- Narrowing of the neural foraminae or central canal occurs with subarticular disc material
- Other causes of foraminal narrowing include hypertrophy of the ligamentum flavum or zygapophyseal joints and capsule
- Pain may radiate in a dermatomal or myotomal distribution, respective to the affected level

Risk Factors

- Torsional movements, especially weighted in flexion
- Congenital spinal canal narrowing
- Smoking

Clinical Features

- Sharp radiating pain in the lower limb in a dermatomal distribution
- Worse with certain positions
- Dural tension signs
- Neurological deficits in distribution of nerve root
- Usually presents with back pain in addition to radicular symptoms

Natural History

- Improvement with conservative care
- Most improve within 6 to 8 weeks
- Reabsorption of disc occurs over several months
- Ten to twenty percent of patients may need further treatment

Diagnosis

Differential diagnosis

- Spinal stenosis
- Sacroiliac joint pain
- Spondylolisthesis
- Zygapophyseal arthritis/facet syndrome
- Peripheral nerve entrapment
- Neoplasm
- Shingles (Herpes zoster) in elderly

History

- Lancinating or sharp pain
- Band distribution radiating to lower limb
- Aggravating and relieving positions, often worse with flexion or valsalva maneuvers

Exam

- Straight leg raise or slump test positive in lower lumbar radiculopathies
- Neurological examination may reveal strength, sensation, or reflex deficits at the affected nerve root level
- Femoral nerve stretch positive in upper lumbar radiculopathies
- Restricted lumbar range of motion

- Segmental motion abnormalities
- May be tenderness of the paraspinals or spinous process
- Restricted flexibility of hip flexors, hamstrings, or quadriceps

Testing
- Radiograph if >6 weeks of symptoms or trauma
- Radiograph may reveal decreased disc height
- Magnetic resonance imaging if red flags present or treatment planned
- Computed tomography scan if boney structures involved
- Electromyography to document nerve root damage, to localize the level involved, and in some cases to assess chronicity

Pitfalls
- Failure to identify red flags
- Biomechanical contribution may lead to recurrence if not addressed. These include postural analysis and workplace ergonomic evaluation if needed

Red Flags
- Saddle anesthesia
- Weight loss
- History of cancer
- Bowel or bladder incontinence
- Progressive neurological deficit

Treatment

Medical
- Nonsteroidal anti-inflammatory medications
- Analgesics, including opioids and gabapentin
- Muscle relaxants

Exercises
- Only very brief rest if needed (<48 hours)
- Mechanical diagnosis and therapy
- Avoid movements that worsen pain, exercise in direction of preference
- Stabilization exercises
- Posture and balance training
- Low-level aerobic exercises

Modalities
- Minimal use if concomitant low back pain
- Superficial heat

- Transcutaneous electrical nerve stimulation
- Ultrasound (precaution not to use over inflamed roots)

Injection
- Selective nerve root block if diagnosis is in question
- Lumbar epidural steroid injection if radicular symptoms persist

Surgical
- Progressive neurological deficit
- Recalcitrant severe pain
- Early referral if red flags, cauda equina syndrome
- Resection of large or extruded disc material if symptomatic
- Enlarge affected neuroforamina
- Decompressing neural structures, and/or fusion

Consults
- Orthopedic or neurosurgical referral if red flags are present or persistent or progressive neurological deficit despite treatment
- Workplace evaluation if appropriate
- Pain medicine for injections

Complications
- Neuropathic pain along affected dermatome
- Deficits in proprioception, balance, and strength
- Chronic back pain or failed back surgery syndrome

Prognosis
- Generally very favorable

Helpful Hints
- Symptoms often improve regardless of intervention
- Avoid exacerbating positions and begin activity early
- Correct abnormal biomechanics and predisposing factors to prevent recurrence

Suggested Readings
Bogduk N. *Clinical Anatomy of the Lumbar Spine and Sacrum.* 4th ed. Edinburgh: Churchill Livingstone; 2005.

Rhee JM, Schaufele M, Abdu WA. Radiculopathy and the herniated lumbar disc. Controversies regarding pathophysiology and management. *J Bone Joint Surg Am.* 2006;88(9):2070–2080.

Wetzel FT, Donelson R. The role of repeated end-range/pain response assessment in the management of symptomatic lumbar discs. *Spine J.* 2003;3(2):146–154.

Lumbar Spinal Stenosis

Liza M. Hernández-González MD

Description

Lumbar spinal stenosis is a clinical syndrome where the compression of neural and vascular structures within the lumbar spinal canal, lateral recess, and/or neural foramina results in pain in the back, buttocks, and/or lower extremities.

Etiology/Types

- Classified as central stenosis and lateral stenosis; the latter including lateral recess and neural foramina
- Congenital causes may be subdivided into hereditary and achondroplastic
- Acquired stenosis occurs due to degenerative, iatrogenic, posttraumatic, and metabolic causes

Epidemiology

- Estimated to occur in five of every 1000 Americans over 50 years of age
- Onset is usually in the sixth and seventh decades due to acquired degenerative joint disease
- A subset of patients present in their third to fourth decades due to hereditary or congenital stenosis
- Frequently associated with spinal surgery in adults older than 65 years of age

Pathogenesis

- Not entirely understood
- Most commonly due to degenerative changes, including intervertebral disc degeneration, facet joint degeneration and hypertrophy, degenerative spondylolisthesis, and ligamentum flavum hypertrophy or calcification, alone or in combination
- Postural, ischemic, and venous stasis theories have been developed to explain the clinical symptoms of neurogenic claudication
- Postural theory suggests that a transient compression of the cauda equina occurs with erect posture and increased lumbar lordosis at rest or activity
- Ischemic theory proposes that an increased metabolic demand to supply ratio of the lumbosacral nerve roots occurs with activity, especially with ambulation
- Venous stasis theory explains that venous engorgement occurs in two or more consecutive levels of stenosis inhibiting a reflex vasodilation response and increased metabolite accumulation during activity

Risk Factors

- Advanced age
- Congenital disease (i.e., achondroplasia)
- Metabolic disease (i.e., Paget's disease)
- Scoliosis
- Trauma
- Surgery

Clinical Features

- Progressive back pain exacerbated with walking, especially downhill
- Pain relieved with stooped posture, sitting, and lumbar flexion

Natural History

- Nearly half of patients with mild to moderate lumbar stenosis have favorable outcomes
- Earlier disease progression is seen in congenital and hereditary cases

Diagnosis

Differential diagnosis

- Intermittent (vascular) claudication (relieved by rest, regardless of back position)
- Degenerative disc disease
- Facet joint degeneration
- Spondylolisthesis
- Malignancy
- Infection
- Referred visceral pain or aortic aneurysms

History

- Morning stiffness associated with back and lower extremity pain
- Pain is characterized as crampy, burning, numbness, or tingling sensation
- Pain worse with extension, standing, walking
- Pain relieved with flexion and sitting
- Weakness may be present, depending on the segments involved

Exam

- Stooped posture, decreased lumbar lordosis, and difficulty standing upright or erect
- Pain symptoms increase with back extension and improve with flexion and sitting

- Neurological examination usually normal, with decreased or absent muscle stretch reflexes
- Wide-based gait
- Romberg's test positive if severe stenosis

Testing

- Anteroposterior/lateral/oblique and flexion/extension x-ray views to evaluate for scoliosis and spondylolisthesis, respectively
- Magnetic resonance imaging (MRI) for better visualization of soft tissues
- Computed tomography (CT) scan used for osseous canal changes
- CT-myelogram useful for patients with contraindications for MRI
- Electromyography (EMG) to evaluate for nerve root damage or other disorders
- Exercise treadmill test allows for dynamic testing

Pitfalls

- Overinterpretation of imaging studies
- Poor correlation between clinical symptoms and diagnostic tests

Red Flags

- Fever/chills
- Weight loss/anorexia/nighttime pain
- Trauma
- Neurological deficits

Treatment

Medical

- Relative rest, activity modifications
- Nonsteroidal anti-inflammatory drugs considering renal and gastrointestinal comorbidities
- Muscle relaxants
- Nonopioid and opiod analgesics
- Anticonvulsants
- Antidepressants
- Calcitonin
- Orthosis (flexion bias)

Exercises

- Education on posture and body mechanics
- Flexibility program for pelvic girdle muscles
- Flexion-based lumbar exercises
- Stabilization program
- Core-strengthening exercises
- Manual therapy

- Cardiovascular training
- Home program

Modalities

- Heat
- Cold
- Transcutaneous electrical nerve stimulation
- Traction

Injection

- Trigger point injections
- Fluoroscopically guided epidural injections and facet joint injections

Surgical

- Considered for progressive neurological deficits, cauda equina syndrome, or unrelenting pain despite conservative treatment
- Decompression and/or fusion if instability present
- Interspinous process decompression system

Consults

- Physical medicine and rehabilitation
- Pain management
- Neurosurgery or orthopedic-spine surgery

Complications/side effects

- Progressive chronic unrelenting pain
- Progressive neurological symptoms and cauda equina syndrome

Prognosis

- Mild to moderate has favorable prognosis
- Poor for severe cases

Helpful Hints

- Imaging studies do not correlate clinically with lumbar stenosis severity
- Treatment decisions should take into consideration both clinical symptoms and imaging tests

Suggested Readings

Rademeyer I. Manual therapy for lumbar spinal stenosis: a comprehensive physical therapy approach. *Phys Med Rehabil Clin N Am.* 2003;(14):103–110.

Rittenberg J, Ross A. Functional rehabilitation for degenerative lumbar spinal stenosis. *Phys Med Rehabil Clin N Am.* 2003;(14):11–120.

Watters WC, Baisden J, Gilbert TJ, et al. Degenerative lumbar spinal stenosis: an evidence-based clinical guideline for the diagnosis and treatment of degenerative lumbar spinal stenosis. *Spine J.* 2008;(8):305–310.

Mallet Finger

José Correa MD

Description
Deformity of the distal interphalangeal (DIP) joint, caused by rupture of the extensor tendon on the dorsum of the joint, which can be accompanied by an avulsion fracture; also called as baseball, drop, or hammer finger. Many treatments have been tried, varying from no therapy to conservative splints and surgery.

Etiology/Types
- Classic mechanism of injury is forced flexion of the tip of the finger, whereas DIP is held in full extension when a softball, volleyball, or basketball hits the tip of the finger

Epidemiology
- Most common closed tendon injury in athletes
- Less common than DIP sprains but more common than proximal interphalangeal (PIP) fractures or dislocations
- Also common in nonathletes after mild trauma to the finger tip
- A family predisposition has been described
- Most common injured finger is the long finger, followed by ring, index, little finger, and thumb
- Occurs more often in men than in women
- Most women with this injury are about 10 years older than men with this injury
- Associated with various types of mallet fractures at dorsal surface of the distal phalanx

Pathogenesis
- The rate of loading can determine if tendon ruptures or bony avulsion occurs
- Rapid load causes rupture of tendon
- Slower rate cause more avulsion fractures since bone is more viscoelastic than tendon

Risk factors
- Male
- Household tasks
- Ball-associated sports (eg, baseball, softball, volleyball, and basketball)

Clinical Features
- After forced DIP joint injury, patient is unable to actively extend the distal joint
- Passive extension is normal
- Dorsum of the joint has mild swelling and tenderness
- Patients continue to be active but may present with loss of active extension the following day
- Many patients look for help weeks or months after injury

Natural History
- Active extension is lost after 1 day
- If not treated early, extension permanently lost

Diagnosis

Differential diagnosis
- Jammed finger/DIP sprain
- Phalangeal fracture
- Swan/neck deformity

History
- Athletes with history of a direct blow to a finger
- Usually in ball sports (baseball, basketball, volleyball, or softball) or often a mild trauma

Exam
- Localized swelling and tenderness at the affected DIP joint
- Inability to actively extend the injured DIP joint

Testing
- Anteroposterior; lateral and oblique x-rays of involved digit
- Three patterns of fracture:
  - Small piece of bone with less than 25% of articular surface
  - Large piece of bone of more than 30% of articular surface
  - Avulsion of any size with palmar subluxation of distal phalanx

Pitfalls
- Hyperextension of PIP joint can be seen in untreated injuries (swan/neck deformity)
- Delay in treatment may produce permanent disability

Red Flags
- Pain and swelling could mean avulsion fracture (mallet fracture)

- Painless injury can occur with tendon rupture and lead to delayed treatment

Treatment

Medical

- Tendinous mallet finger splint DIP in full extension for 6 to 8 weeks with PIP free to move
- Stable mallet fracture (less than 30% of articular surface) 4 to 5 weeks splint in full extension
- Do not remove splint, maintain extension at all times
- Hyperextension can cause ischemia to dorsal skin and lead to pressure sores
- Aluminum splint with foam pad can be used in dorsal or volar position
- Dorsal splint: two strips of tape, one in middle phalanx and other in distal phalanx; permits daily activities (is more effective to maintain full extension)
- Volar splint: five or six strips of tape, at the level of distal joint (is easy to apply but limits daily activities)
- Premolded plastic splints sometimes do not fit well and fail to maintain extension
- Splint should be followed closely with initial follow-up in 1 week
- After period of continuous immobilization, start weaning next 2 to 4 weeks (use at night and for high-risk activities)
- There is insufficient evidence to establish the preference of different type of splints

Exercises

- After immobilization light range of motion, grip exercises

Modalities

- Paraffin bath

Injection

- Not recommended

Surgical

- Surgery: indicated for fracture of more than 30% to 40% of articular surface involvement and volar subluxation of distal phalanx
- Joint is reduced, and transarticular Kirschner wire is inserted in the fractured fragment
- Complication of pressure sore can result if hyperextension occurs
- Comminuted fractures need internal fixation

Consults

- Orthopedic surgery or hand surgery

Complications/side effects

- Residual deformity, and weak grip

Prognosis

- Untreated mallet finger is not of serious functional consequences
- There are studies with surgery only in the presence of palmar subluxation with good results

Helpful Hints

- Early treatment gives best functional and cosmetic results

Suggested Readings

Cochrane Rev Abstract 2007. The Cochrane collaboration. Posted 07/01/2007.

Oetgen ME, Dodds SD. Non-operative treatment of common finger injuries. *Curr Rev Musculoskelet Med.* 2008;1(2): 97–102.

Medial Collateral Ligament Injury of the Knee

Lyle Micheli MD ■ Anne M. Chicorelli DO MPH

Description

The medial collateral ligament (MCL) consists of two layers: the superficial MCL and the deep MCL. The superficial MCL originates on the posterior aspect of the medial femoral condyle and inserts on the tibial metaphysis beneath the pes anserinus. It resists valgus loads, predominantly from 30° to 90° of flexion and also controls internal rotation in flexion. The deep MCL inserts onto the tibial plateau and medial meniscus and controls anterior tibial drawer of the flexed and externally rotated knee and is a secondary restraint to valgus stress.

Injury to this ligament is associated with valgus stress across the knee joint, can occur in isolation, or associated with injury to other structures.

Etiology/Types

- Contact injury (football, wrestling, judo)
- Noncontact injury (skiing)
- Partial or complete
- Isolated or combined with other structures
- More severe damage usually caused by contact injury
- Injuries to the collateral ligaments are graded in severity:
  - Grade I: less than 5 mm laxity (partial tear)
  - Grade II: 5 to 10 mm laxity
  - Grade III: more than 10 mm laxity indicating a complete tear

Epidemiology

- Sports involvement
- Most commonly injured knee ligament in sports
- Dependent upon severity of trauma and associated injuries

Pathogenesis

- Injury may occur due to valgus stress to knee

Risk Factors

- External force on limb
- Contact sport participation
- Biomechanical deficits: muscle weakness and poor balance

Clinical Features

- Pain
- Effusion/edema
- Decreased range of motion
- Subjective instability

Natural History

- First and second degree injuries heal without surgery
- Full thickness tears may require surgery
- May be part of combined injuries (anterior cruciate ligament [ACL], meniscus)

Diagnosis

Differential diagnosis

- Intra-articular ligament injury: ACL/posterior cruciate ligament (PCL)
- Fracture
- Muscle strain/sprain
- Meniscal pathology
- Knee dislocation

History

- Position of knee at time of injury
- Weight bearing status
- Force applied
- Immediate or delayed effusion
- Audible "pop"

Exam

- Visual inspection: ecchymosis, edema, knee effusion
- Palpation of structures surrounding knee: bony vs soft tissue tenderness
- Neurovascular examination
- Hip and ankle physical examination
- Range of motion: active and passive
- Varus stress test in 0° and 30° of flexio: assess LCL
- Valgus stress test in 0° and 30° of flexion: assess MCL

Testing

- X-ray
- Magnetic resonance imaging (MRI)
- Computed tomography (CT) scan
- Ultrasound of lower extremity

Pitfalls

- Failure to diagnose multiligamentous injury, knee dislocation, neurovascular injury

Red Flags

- Infection
- Fracture
- Neoplasm
- Dislocation
- Neurological dysfunction

Treatment

Medical

- Nonsteroidal anti-inflammatory medications
- Analgesics
- Knee immobilization

Exercises

- Rest/protected weight bearing
- Gradual motion (progress gradually into full extension)
- Isometrics/static exercises
- Strengthening as swelling decreases closed chain and open chain exercises
- Aquatic rehabilitation
- Plyometrics and balance training

Modalities

- Heat
- Ice
- Electrical stimulation

Surgical

- MCL Grade III isolated injury rehabilitation is preferred treatment
- Combined ligamentous injury with ACL tears; surgery may be considered

Consults

- Orthopedic surgery
- Physical medicine and rehabilitation
- Sports medicine

Complications/side effects

- Stiffness
- Instability
- Weakness

Prognosis

- Variable, dependent upon grade of ligamentous injury, and other structures injured

Helpful Hints

- Isolated MCL injuries are infrequent. A thorough physical examination of all ligamentous structures is imperative to rule out associated injuries

Suggested Readings

Indelicato PA. Isolated medial collateral ligament injuries in the knee. *J Am Acad Orthop Surg.* 1995;3:9–14.

Indelicato PA, Linton RC. Medial ligament injuries. In: DeLee JC, Drez D, eds. *De Lee & Drez's Orthopedic Sports Medicine Principles and Practice.* 2nd ed. Philadelphia, PA: Elsevier-Saunders; 2003:1937–1949.

Medial Tibial Stress Syndrome

Robert P. Wilder MD FASCM ▪ Eric Magrum PT

Description

Medial tibial stress syndrome (MTSS), also known as shin splints, is described as diffuse posteromedial leg pain located on the distal third of the tibia usually related with physical activity.

Etiology/Types

- Overuse injury related with running or jumping activities
- Mild forms occur only with exercise
- More severe cases can have pain at rest
- May precede stress fracture of the tibia

Epidemiology

- Sixty percent of cases of leg pain in runners
- Between 13% and 17% of all running injuries

Pathogenesis

- Precise pathogenesis of MTSS is unknown
- The most probable theory appears to be a traction periostitis due to excessive stress on the medial tibial fascia by the deep posterior compartment muscles including posterior tibialis, soleus, or flexor digitorum longus
- The eccentric contraction of the medial aspect of the soleus required to control pronation, from initial contact to mid stance with running, increases the stress of the fascial origin of the soleus, possibly disrupting Sharpey's fibers that traverse through the periosteum to insert in the fibrocartilaginous aspect of the tibia

Risk Factors

- Intrinsic risk factors:
  - Low bone mineral density
  - Hormonal imbalance
  - Decreased flexibility and strength (including decreased plantarflexion range of motion [ROM])
  - Lower quarter alignment dysfunction including rearfoot varum, forefoot varum, foot pronation, lower standing foot angle, increased navicular drop, increased pronation velocity and excursion
- Extrinsic factors:
  - Novice runners
  - Abrupt increase in training
  - Use of orthotics
  - Improper shoe wear
  - Uneven or harder surfaces
  - Female gender
  - Previous history of MTSS

Clinical Features

- Diffuse aching pain in the distal two-third of the posteromedial tibia
- Symptoms associated with activity
- Pain with palpation

Natural History

- Pain worsens with activity if not treated
- Resolves with management, including relative rest, appropriate shoes, orthotics, and rehabilitation
- Some individuals will present with pain at rest, and may develop stress fractures

Diagnosis

Differential diagnosis

- Tibial stress fracture
- Exertional compartment syndrome
- Posterior tibial tendinopathy
- Neurological claudication/lumbar radiculopathy
- Vascular claudication

History

- Leg pain with activity
- Novice runner, poor physical condition
- Female athletes with abnormal biomechanics
- Training on hard surfaces
- Improper shoes for running
- In the early stages, symptoms improve with rest

Exam

- Diffuse posteromedial leg tenderness
- Tight heel cords
- Pronated feet
- Weak posterior tibial, soleus, and gastrocnemius muscles
- Normal sensory examination
- Normal pulses
- Single-leg hopping may reproduce pain in patients with stress fracture

- A functional biomechanical screen including active pronation/supination, single-leg stance, single-leg squat, bilateral squat, step-down tests to document abnormal biomechanics
- Walking/running gait assessment

Testing
- X-rays should be normal and ordered to rule out anterior tibial stress fracture
- Bone scan will show linear uptake; can be used to rule out stress fractures that result in focal abnormalities
- Magnetic resonance imaging (MRI) can be ordered in individuals with pain at rest to rule out stress fracture
- Compartment pressure measurement if exertional compartment syndrome is considered

Pitfalls
- Missing biomechanical abnormalities that predispose the individual to MTSS
- Tibial stress fractures may be missed if not suspected

Red Flags
- Pain at rest
- Localized tenderness and swelling
- Worsening symptoms despite treatment

Treatment

Medical
- Relative rest
- Anti-inflammatory medications
- Shock reducing insoles/over-the-counter arch supports
- Custom-made orthoses

Exercises
- Flexibility exercises for gastrocnemius and soleus
- Concentric and eccentric strengthening of leg muscles
- Balance exercises/work on pronation control

Modalities
- Cryotherapy
- Superficial heat

- Ultrasound
- Soft tissue laser

Injection
- Not indicated

Surgical
- No surgical treatment for MTSS

Consults
- Physical medicine and rehabilitation
- Sports medicine
- Orthopedic surgery

Complications/side effects
- Inability to participate in sports
- Tibial stress fractures

Prognosis
- Good with prompt diagnosis and correction of causative factors

Helpful Hints
- Addressing lower quarter muscle imbalances and abnormal mechanics including gastroc soleus flexibility/myofascial mobility, plantarflexor weakness, eccentric pronation control and lower quarter kinetic chain alignment; improves treatment results
- In individuals with pain at rest not responsive to treatment suspect stress fracture

Suggested Readings

Hubbard TJ, Carpenter EM, Cordova ML. Contributing factors to medial tibia stress syndrome: a prospective investigation. *Med Sci Sports Exerc.* 2009;41(3):490–496.

Plinsky MS, Rauh MJ, Heiderscheit B, et al. Medial tibia stress syndrome in high school cross-country runners: incidence and risk factors. *J Orthop Sports Phys Ther.* 2007;37(2):40–47.

Thacker SB, Gilchrist J, Stroup DT, et al. The prevention of shin splints in sports: a systematic review of the literature. *Med Sci SportsExerc.* 2002;34(1):32–40.

Yates B, White S. The incidence and risk factors in the development of medial tibia stress syndrome among naval recruits. *Am J Sports Med.* 2004;32(3):772–780.

Meniscal Tears

Eduardo Amy MD

Description

The medial and lateral menisci are semicircular cartilaginous structures important for knee function. They are subject to stress and strain in sports and activities of daily living and are commonly injured.

Etiology/Types

- Acute traumatic tears
- Chronic degenerative tears
- Longitudinal, radial, flap, and complex tears based on location
- Associated with lateral discoid meniscus (anatomical variant, meniscus covers complete lateral tibial plateau, seen in young individuals)

Epidemiology

- Acute traumatic tears with incidence of 61/100,000
- In patients over 65 years, there is a 60% prevalence of degenerative tears
- Medial meniscus tears more common
- Lateral meniscus tears common in young patients, associated with anterior cruciate ligament (ACL) injury

Pathogenesis

- Meniscus functions as a shock absorber (elastohydrodynamic properties), and in load distribution
- Acts as a knee stabilizer, creating a concavity within the joint
- Promotes articular cartilage nutrition by distribution of synovial fluid
- Lateral meniscus fails to stresses most commonly in extension
- Medial meniscus fails to stresses most commonly in flexion
- Hyperextension produces tears of the anterior horn of the lateral meniscus
- Hyperflexion produces tears of the posterior horn of the medial meniscus
- Twisting of the knee on a planted foot produces tears of both menisci
- Total meniscectomy 235% force increase across the knee joint

Risk Factors

- Twisting and cutting sports
- Acute and chronic ACL tears
- Acute ACL-medial collateral ligament (MCL) tears
- Any ligamentous instability of the knee

Clinical Features

- Pain
- Swelling
- Locking
- Knee giving way/instability associated with activity

Natural History

- Small or peripheral tears may heal on their own
- Larger or complex tears lead to recurrent locking, giving way, and frequent effusions with activity
- Progression of tear with continued sports activity
- Loss of motion
- Activity limited by pain
- Increased incidence of degenerative arthritis

Diagnosis

Differential diagnosis

- Patellofemoral pain
- Osteoarthritis
- Loose bodies/chondral lesions
- Patellar instability

History

- Twisting injury to the knee, painful crack
- Knee may lock completely, severe pain with attempted motion
- Effusion usually develops the following day
- Pain and crepitus

Exam

- Presence of effusion
- Medial or lateral joint line tenderness, high clinical correlation for lateral and medial meniscus tear
- Positive McMurray's test (combines flexion, rotation, varus, and valgus to evaluate medial and lateral meniscus, reproduces pain, or results in a palpable click) may or may not be present
- Painful extension (positive bounce test) may or may not be seen

- Lachman's, valgus, and varus stress tests to rule out associated injury

Testing
- X-rays to rule out loose bodies, associated with osteoarthritis
- Magnetic resonance imaging (MRI) golden standard, high sensitivity and specificity; however, subject to interpretation. Common findings of meniscal tears in older patients with arthritis
- Diagnostic arthroscopy definitive diagnosis

Pitfalls
- Overinterpretation of diagnostic studies
- Early surgical referral for patients with osteoarthritis and findings of meniscal tear in MRI

Red Flags
- Persistent pain, effusions, and joint line tenderness
- Recurrent locking with negative studies

Treatment

Medical
- Protected weight bearing
- Anti-inflammatory/analgesic medications
- Stable tears <1 cm; not symptomatic; do not require surgery

Exercises
- Active range of motion (ROM)
- Static/dynamic strengthening exercises in pain-free ROM
- Closed chain exercises avoiding full flexion
- Bicycle, elliptical trainer, aquatic rehabilitation

Modalities
- Cryotherapy
- Superficial heat
- Electrical stimulation

Injection
- Aspiration of effusion, and injection may be considered for patients with associated osteoarthritis, degenerative tears, and absence of mechanical symptoms such as locking or giving way

Surgical
- Meniscal repair for peripheral tears, particularly in young patients and in patients with associated ACL injury, which requires reconstruction
- Partial meniscectomy for patients with complex tears, and tears away from the vascular zone of the meniscus
- Total meniscectomy (should be avoided)
- Meniscus transplant

Consults
- Orthopedic surgery
- Physical medicine and rehabilitation

Complications/side effects
- Infection
- Loss of motion and quadriceps weakness
- Pain following surgery

Prognosis
- Eighty five percent of meniscus repairs have good results if repairable
- Less than 40% of menisci are repairable
- Eighty percent to 95% good short-term results after partial meniscectomy
- Eighty percent good long-term results after partial meniscectomy
- Predictably poor results after total meniscectomy

Helpful Hints
- Small tears may be amenable to conservative treatment
- Surgical referral for patients with continued mechanical symptoms

Suggested Readings
Alatakis S, Naidoo P. MR imaging of meniscal and cartilage injuries of the knee. *Magn Reson Imaging Clin N Am.* 2009;17(4):741–756.
DeHaven KE, Black KP, Griffiths H. Open meniscus repair: technique and two to nine year results. *Am J Sports Med.* 1989;17:788–795.
Konan S, Rayan F, Haddad FS. Do physical diagnostic tests accurately detect meniscal tears? *Knee Surg Sports Traumatol Arthrosc.* 2009;17(7):806–811.

Meralgia Paresthetica

Steve Geringer MD

Description

Neuropathy of the lateral femoral cutaneous nerve (LFCN). Meralgia derives from *meros* (thigh) and *algo* (pain).

Etiology/Types

- Compression at the inguinal ligament
- Pregnancy
- Direct trauma
- Postsurgical
- External compression from tight clothing, equipment belts, etc
- Case reports relate meralgia to a bout of strenuous exercise and to body armor

Epidemiology

- Most common in middle age
- Equal incidence right to left

Pathogenesis

- From results of nerve conduction testing, one can infer the usual sequence arising from nerve compression: demyelination initially followed by axon loss.

Risk Factors

- Obesity—it is possible that obesity is itself a cause, but it does seem to be at least a predisposing factor
- Underlying polyneuropathy. Any such condition affecting sensory fibers (the vast majority do) will predispose to isolated, focal neuropathies

Clinical Features

- Symptoms in the anterior-lateral thigh
- Usually not frank pain
- Numbness/tingling
- Crawling sensations (formication)
- Hyperpathia
- Symptoms aggravated by prolonged standing/walking, relieved by sitting

Natural History

- Acute vs slow onset of symptoms depending on cause
- After acute onset, gradual reduction of symptoms
- Often a long-lasting residual degree of numbness

Diagnosis

Differential diagnosis

- Femoral neuropathy
- Lumbar plexopathy
- Mid-lumbar radiculopathy
- Hip joint osteoarthritis
- Trochanteric bursitis
- Iliotibial band syndrome

History

- Area of symptoms not as broad as the territory of the nerve itself
- Insidious vs rapid onset (depends on the cause)
- Possible contribution of tight clothing or equipment
- Possible distal, symmetric symptoms of polyneuropathy

Exam

- Territory of diminished pin sensation smaller than that for large-fiber modalities
- Typical territory in anterior-lateral thigh
- Possible Tinel sign over lateral aspect of inguinal ligament
- Normal strength of all thigh muscles
- Normal muscle stretch reflexes, with particular attention to quadriceps

Testing

- Electrodiagnostic (nerve conduction) testing of the LFCN can be performed antidromically or orthodromically
- Must do side-to-side comparison; perform unaffected side first
- Main criterion is absence of response only on the affected side
- Relative amplitude reduction is of questionable relevance, given the small amplitudes to begin with
- Somatosensory evoked potential (SSEP) testing usually yields satisfactory results from the LFCN
- Limited needle electromyography (EMG) of thigh muscles—will be normal
- Computed tomography (CT) scan of pelvis if symptoms persist to look for tumors, lymphadenopathy

Pitfalls
- Not feasible to perform or compare conduction velocities, meaning that the earliest conduction abnormality, slowing, cannot be detected
- Sensory nerve action potentials (SNAP) amplitudes are small even in normals, which may not allow detection of lesions that involve only mild conduction block. SSEP could be helpful in that circumstance
- LFCN testing is technically difficult in the obese, yet that population can be predisposed to meralgia

Red Flags
- Any abnormality of the physical examination beyond impaired sensation in the distribution of the LFCN. This could signal femoral neuropathy, lumbar plexopathy, lumbar radiculopathy, quadriceps injury, among other conditions.

Treatment

Medical
- Weight loss if obesity is a factor
- Modification of tight clothing, belts, or equipment
- Avoidance of squatting/extreme hip flexion
- Expectant approach to pregnancy
- Gabapentin or pregabalin trial, particularly for night symptoms

Exercises
- Aerobic exercise for weight loss
- Hip flexor and iliotibial band stretching in patients with tight hip muscles

Modalities
- Transcutaneous electrical nerve stimulation (TENS)

Injection
- Inject 20 to 30 mm medial to the ASIS along the course of the inguinal ligament
- Diagnostic and/or therapeutic injection with 5 to 10 mL of anesthetic with or without corticosteroid
- Ultrasound guidance may be beneficial

Surgical
- Currently rarely performed or indicated
- If done, decompression at the inguinal ligament

Consults
- Orthopedic or neurological surgery for decompression

Complications/side effects
- Femoral nerve injury from injection
- Any of the potential surgical complications

Prognosis
- Usually very good, if the predisposing or causative factor can be successfully addressed
- Guarded with a recalcitrant predisposing factor, for example obesity or polyneuropathy

Helpful Hints
- May be observed in patients who fluctuate in weight, not necessarily obese
- In acute presentation following activity, reassure patient of good recovery

Suggested Readings

Harney D, Patijn J. Meralgia paresthetica: diagnosis and management strategies. *Pain Med.* 2007;8(8):669–677.

Seror P, Seror R. Meralgia paresthetica: clinical and electrophysiological diagnosis in 120 cases. *Muscle Nerve.* 2006;33(5):650–654.

Metatarsalgia

Rebecca Rodriguez-Negrón MD DABFM

Description
Pain in metatarsophalangeal joints (MP joints) attributed to excessive pressure under metatarsal heads with weight bearing activities.

Etiology/Types
- Primary metatarsalgia: due to inherent anatomical deformities of patient's foot or toes
- Secondary metatarsalgia: due to systemic conditions
- Iatrogenic metatarsalgia: due to complications of foot surgery

Epidemiology
- Prevalence increases with age, reports of 83% in patients older than 65 years
- Male-to-female ratio 1:2

Pathogenesis
- Overloading of MP joint causing synovitis and irritation to adjacent tissues, including the skin, causing pain and callosities
- Unstable MP joints with extrinsic vs intrinsic muscle imbalance causing hyperextension of MP joint and distal displacement of its fat pad
- Floating ray with overload of adjacent metatarsals

Risk Factors
- Primary metatarsalgia: associated with excessively long second metatarsal, plantarflexed metatarsal head, hammer toes, claw toes, hallux valgus (bunion), pes cavus, gastroc-soleus contracture.
- Secondary metatarsalgia: inflammatory, metabolic, neurological, and infectious etiologies. Examples are: rheumatoid arthritis, gout, diabetes mellitus causing a Charcot-like arthropathy, muscular dystrophy, Charcot-Marie-Tooth disease, poliomyelitis, leprosy affecting peripheral nerves causing severe claw toes. Also in Freiberg's disease, infarction of dorsal part of a metatarsal head, usually the second metatarsal.
- Iatrogenic metatarsalgia: Short or floating metatarsal due to an osteotomy or a metatarsal head resection that causes overloading of adjacent metatarsals.

Clinical Features
- Pain in first metatarsal head, as in hallux valgus; on the four lateral metatarsal heads, as in hammer toes or claw toes; or generalized, which is usually bilateral in patients with pes cavus along with hammer toes or claw toes, as well as in systemic conditions
- Pain in different phases of gait or running cycle. During propulsion phase of gait as in excessively long second metatarsal, or at mid-stance as in plantarflexed metatarsal head

Natural History
- Progression of deformities with lateral subluxation of MP joints, overriding second toe, increase in pain and size of callosities

Diagnosis

Differential diagnosis
- Morton's neuroma
- Bone or soft tissue tumors (rare)
- Stress fracture
- Bursitis

History
- Insidious pain in metatarsal heads with weight bearing activities
- Aggravated with the use of high heels, high impact sports activities, walking barefoot

Exam
- Presence of foot and toe deformities with distally displaced metatarsal head fat pad
- Localized or diffuse callosities under metatarsal heads
- Pain upon direct palpation of metatarsal head, especially dorsally
- Laxity of the MP joint
- Absence of pain in interdigital spaces or a Mulder's click help to rule out Morton's neuroma

Testing
- Diagnosis is usually clinical
- CBC and differential, sedimentation rate, C-reactive protein (CRP), and serological tests if inflammatory or infectious etiologies are suspected
- Foot radiographs with patient standing (anteroposterior, lateral and internal oblique) looking

for plantarflexed metatarsals, metatarsal length, MP joint subluxation or widening (synovitis). Check for signs of a secondary pathology like joint erosion, Freiberg's disease. Check for stress fractures, old calluses
- Ultrasound or magnetic resonance imaging (MRI) when cause is not clear (soft tissue tumors, neuroma, bursitis)
- Foot pressure studies (rarely used)
- Intermetatarsal space steroid injection if history and physical examination cannot differentiate from a neuroma

Pitfalls
- Not correcting biomechanical abnormalities

Red Flags
- In pain that does not improve, consider stress fracture
- Numbness may be associated with peripheral neuropathy

Treatment
Medical
- Ice, rest, and analgesics; usually nonsteroidal anti-inflammatory drugs (NSAIDs)
- Treating the underlying condition, especially in secondary metatarsalgia
- Semi-rigid insoles, redistributing excessive load in affected areas with metatarsal pads or bars, arch support if needed
- Wide toe box shoes, rocker bottom shoes

Exercises
- Gastroc-soleus stretching
- Posterior tibial, and foot intrinsic muscle strengthening
- Proprioceptive and balance training

Modalities
- Ice
- Ultrasound

Injection
- Steroid injection to MP joint in its midline; dorsally and angled from proximal to distal

Surgical
- Metatarsal osteotomy to relocalize the metatarsal head
- Transfer of flexor digitorum longus tendon for correction of second MP joint subluxation
- Resection of metatarsal head (rarely used due to complications)

Consults
- In secondary metatarsalgia according to cause (inflammatory, infectious, neurological)
- Orthopedic Surgery if failure of conservative treatment

Complications/side effects
- Progression of deformities and worsening of pain
- Ulcer formation on pressure points, especially in patients with a neuropathy (diabetics)
- Surgery complications: infection, nonunion, iatrogenic metatarsalgia

Prognosis
- Usually good with conservative treatment

Helpful Hints
- Look for the cause and treat any secondary conditions
- Maximize conservative treatment

Suggested Readings
Espinosa N, Maceira E, Myerson MS. Current concept review: metatarsalgia. *Foot & Ankle Int.* 2008;29(8):871–879.
Miller SD. Technique tip: forefoot pain: diagnosing metatarsophalangeal joint synovitis from interdigital neuroma. *Foot & Ankle Int.* 2001;22(11):914–915.
Wu KK. Morton neuroma and metatarsalgia. *Curr Opin Rheumatol.* 2000;12(2):131–142.

Morton's Neuroma

Joseph A. Volpe MD MEd

Description

Morton's neuroma, also called interdigital or intermetatarsal neuroma, is not a true neuroma. The lesion actually results from injury to the interdigital nerve of the foot as it passes below the transverse ligament of the metatarsal heads.

Etiology/Types

- Due to repetitive trauma and fibrosis of the interdigital nerve
- Usually located between the third and fourth metatarsal heads
- Occur less commonly between the other digits

Epidemiology

- It is more common in women than in men at a ratio of 8:1
- Affects women between 30 and 50 years of age
- May affect young men active in sports

Pathogenesis

- Repetitive trauma leads to fibrosis of the interdigital nerve.
- Painful fusiform swelling of the nerve develops.
- During hyperpronation of the metatarsals, the interdigital nerve can be pinched in an area where the nerve is only covered by plantar skin.
- As a result, there is thickening of the tissues, perineural fibrosis, and a painful forefoot.

Risk Factors

- Running or walking with forefoot weight bearing
- Exercise on treadmills, steppers, and elliptical trainers
- High heels
- Narrow toe boxes in the shoe
- Rheumatoid or inflammatory arthritis
- Diabetes/diabetic neuropathy

Clinical Features

- Symptom onset is commonly insidious
- Complaint of progressively worsening forefoot pain and numbness in the area of the metatarsal heads
- Worse with activity
- Improves by removing the shoe and rubbing the forefoot
- Complaint of fullness and pain in the area of the metatarsals
- Frequently misdiagnosed as metatarsalgia

Natural History

- Worsens with continued activity and prolonged standing
- Response to conservative treatment if identified early
- May require surgery if patients have continued symptoms and fixed foot deformities

Diagnosis

Differential diagnosis

- Metatarsalgia
- Metatarsal stress fractures
- Peripheral neuropathy
- Tarsal tunnel syndrome
- Peripheral vascular disease

History

- The classic presentation involves forefoot pain that radiates into the toes with a sensation of pins and needles or numbness
- Pain with activity
- Feeling of fullness in the sole of foot
- Improves with rest

Exam

- Localized pain and tenderness is elicited by palpating or compressing between the metatarsal heads
- In severe cases, a click can be felt in this area
- Transverse compression of the forefoot can also reproduce similar pain
- Intact sensation
- Normal pulses
- Tight Achilles tendon and toe extensors
- Weak foot intrinsic muscles

Testing

- X-rays to document foot, ankle, bone anomalies
- Ultrasound to evaluate for interdigital nerve swelling
- Magnetic resonance imaging (MRI) may be used to evaluate the interdigital nerve and to rule out stress fractures
- Electrodiagnostic testing to evaluate for underlying peripheral neuropathy

- Vascular studies if peripheral vascular disease is suspected

Pitfalls

- Diagnosing metatarsalgia because of lack of suspicion
- Failure to identify biomechanical abnormalities or causative factors such as inappropriate shoe wear

Red Flags

- Worsening symptoms with activity
- Pain at rest

Treatment

Medical

- Anti-inflammatory medications
- Unloading of the forefoot using metatarsal bars, gel inserts, custom orthoses with premetatarsal padding, and proper shoe wear

Exercises

- Achilles tendon and foot muscle stretching
- Strengthening of the intrinsic foot muscles, posterior tibialis, and other leg muscles can help improve and maintain the transverse arch of the foot
- Cross training with stationary bicycle and aquatic exercises

Modalities

- Cryotherapy
- Hydrotherapy
- Iontophoresis/phonophoresis

Injection

- In cases where the aforementioned treatment does not work, local injection of anesthetics and corticosteroids can sometimes provide long-lasting relief.

Surgical

- If all conservative measures fail, surgical excision of the lesion is indicated.

- Dorsal resection of the neuroma proximal to the intermetatarsal ligament is usually the initial approach because of faster recovery; however, the plantar approach allows direct visualization of the nerve.
- Recurrence of symptoms may occur if the patient does not correct the mechanism of the injury.

Consults

- Orthopedics/foot-and-ankle surgeon
- Podiatry
- Physical medicine and rehabilitation

Complications/side effects

- Skin and fat pad atrophy
- Chronic foot pain
- Intolerance to exercise

Prognosis

- Good with early identification of the causative factors, correction of abnormal foot anatomy and biomechanics, and modification of activity and shoe wear

Helpful Hints

- Suspect Morton's neuroma in patients with complaints of burning feet
- Strengthen the foot intrinsic muscles in running athletes

Suggested Readings

Agosta J. Foot pain. In: Brukner P, Khan K, eds. *Clinical Sports Medicine*. Sydney: McGraw-Hill; 2001:599.

Dec KL. Foot and toes. In: McKeag DB, Moeller JL, eds. *ACSM's Primary Care Sports Medicine*. Philadelphia, PA: Lippincott Williams & Wilkins; 2007:524–525.

Hansen PA, Willick SE. Musculoskeletal disorders of the lower limb. In: Braddom RL, ed. *Physical Medicine & Rehabilitation*. Philadelphia: Saunders-Elsevier; 2007:874.

Neuralgic Amyotrophy

Jayson Takata MD

Description

Neuralgic amyotrophy is also known as acute brachial plexus neuropathy, Parsonage-Turner syndrome, brachial neuritis, shoulder girdle syndrome, idiopathic brachial plexus neuropathy, cryptogenic brachial neuropathy, and brachial radiculoplexopathy. It is an acute to subacute neuropathy involving the brachial plexus and/or upper extremity peripheral nerves.

Etiology/Types

- Unknown etiology
- Suspected to be caused by immune-mediated nerve damage with multiple possible triggering events (vaccines, infections)

Epidemiology

- Incidence: 1.6 per 100,000 population
- Right > left
- Range: 20 to 70 years of age
- More common in males

Pathogenesis

- Suspected immune-mediated microvasculitis

Risk Factors

- Upper respiratory infection
- Other bacterial or viral disease
- Systemic illness
- Vaccination
- Childbirth
- Trauma
- Surgery or invasive diagnostic procedure

Clinical Features

- Acute onset shoulder region pain
- Pain onset is frequently nocturnal
- Weakness develops as pain subsides over a few days to a week or two

Natural History

- Severe pain subsides in 7 to 10 days
- Persistent ache for several months
- Predominantly, the proximal upper extremity muscles in rapid onset of atrophy and weakness (occurs over a few weeks)
- Gradual recovery over several months

Diagnosis

Differential diagnosis

- Hereditary neuralgic amyotrophy
- Hereditary neuropathy with liability to pressure palsies
- Cervical radiculopathy
- Mononeuropathy multiplex
- Traumatic brachial plexopathy
- Neoplastic plexopathy
- Motor neuron disease

History

- Sudden onset of acute pain, usually in the superior scapula extending into the upper arm. Usually nonradicular pattern
- Chronic ache lasting for months
- Onset of weakness occurs often as pain is subsiding over first few weeks
- Flaccid weakness of shoulder girdle and often in the arm

Exam

- Weakness: often patchy, variable distribution, and severity
- Most commonly affected muscles: deltoid, serratus anterior, supraspinatous, infraspinatous, biceps, and triceps
- May affect muscles in a single nerve distribution: long thoracic, suprascapular, axillary, radial, anterior interosseous, phrenic, and musculocutaneous
- Mild sensory loss: usually lateral forearm, lateral deltoid region
- Prominent atrophy of affected muscles
- Deep tendon reflexes normal unless musculocutaneous nerve involved

Testing

- Spinal fluid: normal
- Nerve conduction studies
- Routine nerves (median and ulnar) often unremarkable
- Abnormal lateral antebrachial cutaneous in 50%
- Reduced compound muscle action potential recording from affected muscle (deltoid, biceps)

- Electromyogram: denervation
- Nerve distributions of the brachial plexus
- Phrenic, spinal accessory, and laryngeal nerve may also be involved
- Patchy distribution: differential fascicular involvement (eg, supraspinatus may be much more affected than the infraspinatus)

Pitfalls
- Often mistaken for acute shoulder joint disorder because pain is often worsened by shoulder movement
- May be confused with cervical radiculopathy in patients with abnormal cervical spine magnetic resonance imaging (MRI)

Red Flags
- Unremitting pain and lower trunk deficits may indicate neoplastic plexopathy

Treatment

Medical
- Analgesics, often requiring narcotic medication
- Corticosteroids may reduce acute pain

Exercises
- Range of motion of affected joints to prevent contractures
- Submaximal strengthening

Modalities
- Cryotherapy
- Heat
- Transcutaneous electrical nerve stimulation (TENS)
- Electrical stimulation

Injection
- Subacromial corticosteroid injection for secondary shoulder impingement syndrome
- Trigger point injection for secondary myofascial pain

Surgical
- No surgery indicated

Consults
- Neuromuscular neurology
- Physical medicine and rehabilitation

Complications/side effects
- Secondary shoulder adhesive capsulitis or myofascial pain of compensatory muscles

Prognosis
- Improvement after 1 or more months
- Thirty-six percent recover in 1 year
- Eighty percent functionally recover within 2 years
- Five percent recurrence
- Lower trunk lesions improve more slowly

Helpful Hints
- Important to clinically distinguish from iatrogenic nerve injury since onset can be seen following surgery or other medical procedures.

Suggested Readings

Stewart J. Brachial plexus. In: Stewart J, ed. *Focal Peripheral Neuropathies*. Philadelphia, PA: Lippincott Williams & Wilkins; 2000:141–145.

Wilbourn AJ. Plexopathies. In: Mendell JR, Kissel JT, Cornblath DR, eds. *Diagnosis and Management of Peripheral Nerve Disorders*. New York: Oxford; 2001:660–662.

Osgood Schlatter's Syndrome (Tibial Tubercle Apophysitis)

Fernando L. Zayas MD

Description

Osgood Schlatter's syndrome is a common sport lesion. This is an overuse syndrome that occurs more commonly in the active preteen or early teenage child. Its classical presentation is discomfort, swelling, and tenderness at the tibial tubercle related to sport activities that involve jumping, running, and direct trauma to the area.

Etiology/Types

- Traction apophysitis of the tibial tubercle is due to repetitive strain and chronic avulsion of the secondary ossification center of the tibial tuberosity.
- Repetitive strain is due to the strong pull of the quadriceps muscle during sport activity.
- Minor avulsion fractures occur, and tubercle enlargement is the result of repair and attempts and healing.

Epidemiology

- More common in those actively participating in sports (28%); only 4.5% nonparticipants
- More common in boys than in girls (3:1)
- Boys more symptomatic between ages 12 and 15 years; girls between ages of 8 and 12 years
- Bilateral in 20% of cases

Pathogenesis

- There are four stages of tibial tubercle development: cartilaginous stage (birth to 11 years), apophyseal stage (11 to 14 years), epiphyseal stage, the tibial epiphysis coalesces (14 to 18 years), and bony stage; epiphysis is fused (>18 years).
- Caused by submaximal repetitive tensile stresses on a developing secondary ossification center, which is unable to withstand the forces from the patellar tendon, resulting in avulsion of the center and later formation of extra bone between the fragments.

Risk Factors

- Sport activities that involve jumping (basketball, volleyball, running)
- Repetitive direct contact (eg, kneeling)

Clinical Features

- Usually present with gradual onset of pain and swelling in the region of the tibial tuberosity, which is exacerbated with sport activity
- On physical examination, there is tenderness, local swelling, and prominence in the area of tibial tuberosity
- Increased pain with knee extension against resistance

Natural History

- Majority are asymptomatic at adulthood. Some residual prominence of the tibial tubercle is common.
- Those with tubercle fragmentation can present with persistent symptoms while kneeling.

Diagnosis

Differential diagnosis

- Referred hip pain
- Sinding-Larsen-Johansson disease (analogous condition at inferior pole of the patella)
- Tibial tubercle avulsion fracture
- Patellar tendonitis (infrapatellar ligament)
- Infection
- Malignancy

History

- Gradually increasing upper anterior tibial pain with continuous sports activities
- Occasional acute episodes with strenuous activities or direct blow

Exam

- Tenderness, local swelling, and prominence in the area of tibial tuberosity (see Figure 1)
- Increased pain with knee extension against resistance
- Hamstring and quadriceps may be shortened
- Stable knee joint

Testing

- Usually not necessary (clinical diagnosis)

- Radiographs of the knee anteroposterior and lateral (leg internally rotated 10% to 20%) reveal soft tissue swelling anterior to the tibial tubercle (may be the only abnormality). Other signs include elevation of the tubercle away from the shaft; irregularity, fragmentation, or increased density of the tubercle (see Figure 2); a superficial ossicle in the patellar tendon; and calcification within or thickening of the patellar tendon (infrapatellar ligament)

Pitfalls

- Acute pain may be associated with an avulsion fracture of the tibial tubercle.

Red Flags

- Infection
- Fractures
- Malignancy

Treatment

Medical

- Conservative treatment is the mainstay of therapy; family members and athletes must be told that 12 to 18 months may be required for symptoms to resolve; this is the time required for physiological epiphysiodesis to occur.
- Acute treatment involves the use of modification of activities, oral nonsteroidal anti-inflammatory drugs (NSAIDs), and protective knee padding.
- Those with mild disease are allowed to continue with sports activities with the use a contoured knee pad (Osgood Schlatter's pad); this cushions the knee,

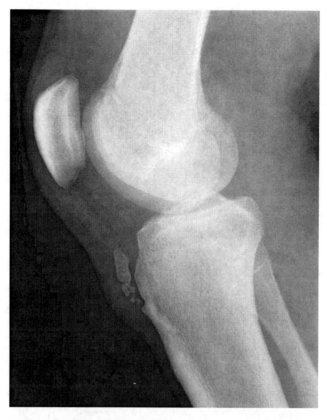

Figure 2. Fragmentation of anterior tibial tubercle.

decreases patellar mobility and forces on the tibial tubercle, and provides increased proprioception. Those with moderate to severe pain require rest from activity.

Exercises

- Flexibility exercises for the hamstrings, quadriceps, gastrocnemius, and soleus muscles
- Quadriceps, hamstring, and hip open chain muscle strengthening
- Closed chain lower extremity exercises
- Balance and proprioceptive training

Modalities

- Cryotherapy
- Superficial heat
- Transcutaneous electrical nerve stimulation (TENS)
- Electrical stimulation

Injection

- Not indicated

Surgical

- Uncommon
- Majority of surgical cases have an ossicle, which represents a nonunion

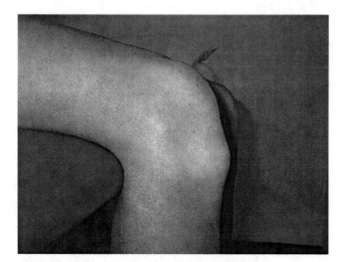

Figure 1. Prominent anterior tibial tuberosity.

- Ossicle and bursa removal may be performed prior to skeletal maturity
- In skeletal mature individuals, debulking of the prominent tubercle at the time of ossicle excision produces excellent results

Consults
- Physical medicine and rehabilitation
- Orthopedic surgery (severe cases)

Complications/side effects
- Tibial fractures
- Premature fusion of the anterior part upper tibial epiphyseal plate leading to genu recurvatum

Prognosis
- Very good

Helpful Hints
- Benign condition
- When identified early and treated, it has a very good prognosis

Suggested Readings

Bush MT. Sport injuries in young athletes. In: Morrissy RT, Weinstein SL, eds. *Lovell & Winter's Pediatric Orthopedics.* 5th ed. Philadelphia, PA: Lippincott Williams & Wilkins; 2000.

Frey S, Hosalkar H, Cameron DB, et al. Tibial tuberosity fractures in adolescents. *J Child Orthop.* 2008;2(6): 469–474.

Gholve PA, Scher DM, Khakharia S, et al. Osgood Schlatter syndrome. *Curr Opin Pediatr.* 2007;19(1):44–50.

Osteitis Pubis

Luis Baerga MD ■ Leonardo Pirillo MD

Description

Osteitis pubis is a noninfectious painful inflammatory condition of the pubic symphysis and surrounding fascia, caused by repetitive trauma or excessive stress across the joint and adjacent structures.

Etiology/Types

- Repetitive microtrauma
- Shear forces across the pubic symphysis
- Pregnancy and childbirth
- Pelvic surgeries
- Rheumatologic disease

Epidemiology

- Groin injuries account for 2% to 5% of all sport injuries
- Osteitis pubis and adductor strain are the two most common groin injuries and their incidence will depend on the type of athlete
- More common in sports that involve running, kicking, and rapid lateral movements, such as soccer
- Can be seen in sports that have frequent flexion and/ or adduction of hip, such as football, hurdlers, discus throwers, and weightlifters
- More common in men than in women

Pathogenesis

- Inflammation of the pubic symphysis characterized by sclerosis and bony changes

Risk Factors

- Leg length discrepancy
- Sacroiliac joint dysfunction
- Poor sports biomechanics

Clinical Features

- Pain and tenderness over the symphysis pubis
- Lower abdominal pain
- Groin or medial thigh pain, possible testicular pain
- Symptoms aggravated with running or with adduction of thigh
- Pain while walking, climbing stairs, coughing, or sneezing
- Onset can be abrupt but usually insidious
- Inability to stand or jump in one leg

Natural History

- Early in the disease the athlete can complain of groin or testicular pain
- Medial thigh or lower abdominal pain could be the chief complaint
- Poorly treated adductor strain or an adductor strain that will not heal
- Athlete is unable to compete
- Pain responds to appropriate treatment but biomechanical abnormalities need to be addressed for recovery

Diagnosis

Differential diagnosis

- Osteomyelitis pubis
- Adductor strain
- Rectus abdominus strain
- Inguinal hernia
- Sports hernia
- Stress fracture
- Other urologic and gynecologic diseases

History

- Pain at pubic symphysis and pubic bone
- Groin and testicular pain
- Lower abdominal and medial thigh pain
- Pain or weakness with running, flexing, or adducting the hip

Exam

- Exquisite tenderness at the symphysis, rectus abdominis insertion, and hip adductors origin
- Pain with passive abduction of hip
- Pain with active or resisted flexion, adduction, and internal rotation
- Pain or discomfort with sit-ups
- Pain or inability to perform single leg hop
- Pubic symphysis gap test with pain reproduction during isometric adduction contraction against the examiner fists with the hip and the knee flexed at 90°

Testing

- X-rays (pelvis anteroposterior) demonstrate widening of the symphysis pubis; acute injuries could show cortical outline asymmetry or irregularity with bony

resorption; chronic injuries will show subcortical bone sclerosis, cystic changes
- Bone scans or SPECT may be negative but usually will show increased uptake over the symphysis or unilaterally
- Magnetic resonance imaging (MRI) will show marrow edema at the pubic bone
- MRI with fat suppression will help visualize soft tissue edema at the rectus abdominis insertion and adductor origin, which could help with the etiology of the injury

Pitfalls
- Presentation could vary depending on chronicity of symptoms
- High incidence of recurrence

Red Flags
- Fevers, chills, or erythema

Treatment

Medical
- Nonsteroidal anti-inflammatory medications
- Analgesics

Modalities
- Ice
- Transcutaneous electrical nerve stimulation
- Ultrasound

Exercises
- Relative rest
- Stretching program for hip and abdominal musculature with emphasis on adductors and hip flexors
- Core strengthening, followed by closed chain hip exercises
- If patient has no pain with exercise, progression to open chain concentric and eccentric exercises
- Initiate sports-specific training if no symptoms arise
- Biomechanical evaluation to determine a cause for injury and subsequent correction of mechanics or muscular imbalance

Injection
- Fluoroscopy-guided symphysis pubis injection (Figure 1)

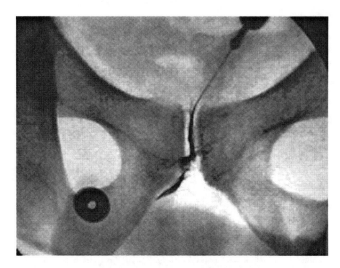

Figure 1. Fluoroscopy guided symphysis pubis injection.

Surgical
- Curettage
- Arthrodesis
- Wedge resection or wide resection

Consults
- Orthopedic surgery
- Infectious disease specialist

Complications
- Progressive pain and dysfunction, which requires surgical intervention
- Misdiagnosed osteomyelitis

Prognosis
- Five percent to 10% failure of conservative management
- Full recovery expected at 3 to 9 months but some cases may last for up to 12 months, depending on initial presentation

Helpful Hints
- High suspicion with athletes in kicking sports with the triad of groin, lower abdominal, and medial thigh pain

Suggested Readings
Johnson R. Osteitis pubis. *Curr Sports Med Rep.* 2003;2(2):98–102.
Macintyre J. Groin pain in athletes. *Curr Sports Med Rep.* 2006;5(6):293–299.

Osteoarthritis of the Hand

Maricarmen Cruz-Jimenez MD

Description

Hand osteoarthritis (HOA) is the progressive damage of joint cartilage, producing structural and functional changes around the joints. These changes can include fluid accumulation, bony overgrowth, and loosening and weakness of muscles and tendons, all of which may limit movement and cause pain and swelling.

Etiology/Types

- There is no definite mechanism, but any event that alters the environment of the chondrocyte has the potential to cause HOA
- There are two types
- Primary (idiopathic):
  - Localized: hands, feet, knee, hip, spine
  - Generalized: three or more joint sites
  - Erosive: more aggressive subset, rapidly progressive symptoms
- Secondary:
  - Trauma
  - Congenital
  - Calcium pyrophosphate crystal deposition (CPPD)
  - Other bone and joint disease, as well as other medical conditions (i.e., diabetes mellitus, hypothyroidism)

Epidemiology

- Prevalence increases with age, regardless of the definition used (clinical vs radiological)
- Joints more commonly involved in decreasing order of occurrence are distal interphalangeal (DIP), thumb base carpometacarpal (CMC), proximal interphalangeal (PIP), and metacarpophalangeal (MCP) joint
- Women are more frequently affected
- Unilateral involvement is more common on the dominant hand
- Cotton picking and other manual occupations raise the risk of HOA, mainly DIP and MCP

Pathogenesis

- Articular cartilage failure induced by a complex interplay of genetic, mechanical, metabolic, and biochemical factors with secondary components of inflammation creating an imbalance between the degradation and repair process of cartilage, bone, and synovium
- Contributing factors: monocyte-derived peptide, cartilage fragments, interleukin-I, growth factors

Risk Factors

- Age (being older than 40 years)
- Gender (female preference)
- Menopausal status (theory about estrogen deficiency role)
- Family history (susceptibility genes identified)
- Obesity (associated with CMC OA)
- Prior hand injury/trauma
- Joint laxity
- Higher bone mineral density
- Greater forearm muscle strength (increased mechanical forces)
- High grip strength
- Occupation or recreation-related usage

Clinical Features

- Hand pain, aching, or stiffness (<30 minutes in the morning) with functional limitations
- Hard tissue/bony enlargement
- Soft tissue swelling
- Deformities of the joint/joint instability
- Evidence recommends combining a series of defined joints in both hands to increase the sensitivity and specificity of the clinical diagnosis
- Second and third DIP
- Second and third PIP
- Thumb CMC

Natural History

- Typically, the initial presentation will be that of mild troublesome inflammatory pain, with variable duration
- Stiffness and joint deformity develops, subsequently leading to loss or limitation of hand function
- Rapid evolution of joint damage is observed in the erosive type OA. This appears to be a subtype of HOA with worse clinical and structural outcome

Diagnosis

Differential diagnosis

- CPPD
- Rheumatoid arthritis (RA)
- Infectious monoarticular disease
- Psoriathric arthritis
- Gout
- Hemochromatosis

History

- Joint pain is the typical presentation
- Morning joint stiffness <30 minutes
- Soft tissue swelling
- Hard or bony enlargement
- Deformity of the hand

Exam

Findings will vary on the stage of presentation:

- Synovial swelling
- Joint deformities
- Joint malalignment
- Bouchard's nodes if PIP involved
- Heberden's nodes if DIP involved
- Tenderness to joint palpation
- Limited range of motion
- Normal or weak hand grip

Testing

- X-rays may reveal cartilage loss, bone spurs, and joint damage that might *not* correlate with the amount of pain and disability
- Other findings could be bone erosions and alignment deviations
- Ultrasound shown to better evaluate synovitis
- Not that reliable defining joint space narrowing and cartilage defects
- Laboratory workup is used mostly to exclude other etiologies. Panel includes:
  - Acute phase reactants (C-reactive protein (CRP), sedimentation rate)
  - Rheumatoid factor titers
  - Evaluation of synovial fluid
  - Serum uric acid
  - Thyroid-stimulating hormone
  - Complete blood count

Pitfalls

- Cardiac and gastrointestinal (GI) toxicities associated with medication
- Postinjection infections
- Skin blanching after injections

Red Flags

- Constitutional symptoms
- Symmetric presentation
- Type of joints involved

Treatment

Medical

- Topical nonsteroidal anti-inflammatory drugs (NSAIDs) and capsaicin: safe and effective, particularly in mild to moderate pain or when a small number of joints is involved
- Oral medications
- Acetaminophen is the analgesic of choice, particularly for the long term and in mild to moderate pain
- Oral NSAIDs should be used at the lowest effective dose and for the shortest duration when there is a poor response to acetaminophen and in moderate to severe pain. Consideration should be given to on GI and cardiac risk
- Nutritional supplements (glucosamine, chondroitin sulfate, avocado soybean unsaponifiables, diacerhein), all may offer symptomatic relief with apparent low toxicity (questionable effect on disease progression)
- Mechanical and orthotic
- The goal is focused on promoting joint protection and prevention of deformities. This is achieved through:
  - Education on joint protection techniques and energy conservation
  - Evaluation of assistive devices
  - Splinting of the thumb base can prevent or correct lateral angulation and flexion deformity

Exercises

- The goal is to promote functional range of motion and strength
- Isotonic gripper, weights
- Isometric grip strengthening

Modalities

- Moist heat
- Paraffin baths
- Therapeutic ultrasound

Injection

- Steroid injections of long-acting corticosteroid are effective for flare-ups

- Intra-articular hyaluran has not shown clinically relevant structure modification or pharmacoeconomic benefits

Surgical

- Considered the last resort when conservative fails and the patient has marked pain and/or disability
- Interposition arthroplasty, osteotomy, or arthrodesis are effective for severe thumb base OA
- Includes removing cysts or excess bony growths

Consults

- Rheumatologist
- Hand/orthopedic surgery

Complications/side effects

- Sequelae are site-specific, such as interference with grip and fine precision pinch
- Dissatisfaction with cosmetic appearance

Prognosis

- Will depend on the joint involved and severity

Helpful Hints

- On examination, search for grinding on the thumb base
- In HOA, joint swelling is hard and bony
- Osteophytes are the most sensitive and specific of the radiographic features in individual joint groups
- Functional impairment in HOA may be similar in severity to that resulting from RA

Suggested Readings

Altman R, Alarcon G, Appelrouth D, et al. The American College of Rheumatology Criteria for the classification and reporting of osteoarthritis of the hand. *Arthritis Rheum.* 1990;33(11):1601–1610.

Zhang W, Doherty M, Leeb BF, et al. EULAR evidence-based recommendations for the diagnosis of hand osteoarthritis: report of a task force of ESCISIT. *Ann Rheum Dis.* 2009;68:8–17.

Osteoarthritis of the Hip

Antonio Otero-López MD ▪ Beatriz García-Cardona MD

Description
Noninflammatory degenerative disease of the hip joint, which usually appears in late middle or old age that leads to degenerative loss of articular cartilage of the acetabulum or the femoral head.

Etiology/Types
- Unknown
- Primary osteoarthritis (OA) is idiopathic
- Secondary OA is the most common type, due to congenital causes, developmental abnormalities (slipped capital femoral epiphysis, or Legg-Calvé-Perthes disease), avascular necrosis (AVN), or prior trauma, which creates a predisposing anatomic abnormality that leads to hip degeneration due to mechanical factors
- Developmental dislocation (dysplasia) of the hip is a risk factor for hip OA

Epidemiology
- Hip OA is one of the leading causes of disability worldwide
- One in four Americans can expect to develop OA of the hip during his/her lifetime
- More than 200,000 annual hip replacements have been done in the United States for OA

Pathogenesis
- Progressive erosion of articular cartilage
- In response to stress, chondrocytes release degradative proteolytic enzymes
- Inflammatory pathways are up-regulated, releasing inflammatory cytokines that further damage articular cartilage

Risk Factors
- Obesity
- Advancing age
- Hip trauma
- Genetic
- Occupation: heavy lifting and farming

Clinical Features
- Restricted internal rotation of the hip
- Groin pain most specific
- Lateral trunk lean toward the involved side (Trendelenburg gait) will decrease mechanical stress on joint and thereby lessen pain
- Leg length discrepancy
- May experience acute hip pain due to rupture of subchondral cyst into the joint

Natural History
- Variable clinical course due to the repair and remodeling reactions that occur after cartilage injury
- The course is usually slowly progressive but may be aggressive
- Deformities progress from passively correctable to fixed (ankylosis)
- Some patients have only mild symptoms controlled by nonsteroidal anti-inflammatory drugs (NSAIDs) and activity modification

Diagnosis

Differential diagnosis
- Inflammatory arthritis
- Infectious arthritis
- Gouty arthritis
- Hemorrhagic arthritis
- Hip labral tear
- Transient osteoporosis of the hip (TOI)
- AVN
- Spinal stenosis
- Herniated discs
- Lateral femoral nerve entrapment
- Vascular claudication

History
- Pain with ambulation, noticeable limp that increases with physical activity
- Gradual loss of hip motion
- Groin or gluteal pain, or referred pain to the knee

Exam
- Examine spine, abdomen, and neurovascular structures as they may be associated with hip pain
- Internal rotation of the hip reproduces the pain
- Flexion contractures: Thomas test
- Asymmetric hip abductor weakness
- Leg length

- Labral impingement signs (pain with hip flexion, internal rotation, and axial loading)
- Patrick's (pain over the groin region with hip flexion, abduction, and external rotation)
- Stinchfield tests (from a supine position with the knee extended, the patient is asked to actively elevate the leg against manual resistance, reproduction of pain in the groin, thigh, or buttock confirms a positive response)

Testing
- Plain films: low anteroposterior (AP) pelvis and frog views
- Femur AP/lateral in developmental dysplasia of the hip
- Magnetic resonance imaging: suspected AVN, TOI, or labral pathology
- Aspiration of the hip

Pitfalls
- Late diagnosis due to misleading symptoms of knee pain or back pain

Red flags
- Pain at rest
- Fever
- Groin pain following treatment with steroids

Treatment

Medical
- Weight loss
- Activity modification/limitation
- Anti-inflammatory medication (NSAIDs)
- Glucosamine
- Prescription of a cane to be used with the opposite upper extremity (unloads the hip joint with weight bearing)

Exercises
- First goal: stretching to improve the range of motion
- Second goal: strengthening the surrounding muscles, and then a plan for aerobic exercise, such as swimming or bicycling, to increase overall fitness and to control weight

Modalities
- Rest, ice, elevation, and activity modification are still called on to treat flare-ups
- Persistent pain can be addressed by transcutaneous electrical nerve stimulation and heat, which can be useful in opening circulation to alleviate swelling
- Cryotherapy and therapeutic ultrasound have proven to be effective components of pain-management strategies
- Hydrotherapy and hydrocollator packs improve myotendinous flexibility and allow enhanced stretching
- Pulsed electrical stimulation may relieve pain and improve function

Injection
- Intra-articular steroids
- Local anesthetics are most commonly used for diagnostic purposes than steroids
- Viscosupplementation (needs further studies but clinically used)

Surgical
- Corrective osteotomy for localized disease
- Total hip replacement: surface replacement vs traditional implants
- Newer bearings with promising results for young patients
- Hip arthroscopy: labral tears and loose bodies
- Hip arthrodesis: rarely used for young heavy laborers

Consults
- Orthopedic surgery
- Physical medicine and rehabilitation

Complications
- Progressive pain and dysfunction
- Inability to ambulate and therefore wheelchair-dependent

Prognosis
- Variable; with surgical reconstruction, there is high patient satisfaction

Helpful Hints
- Inflammation is not a major component of OA (despite the suffix -itis)
- Start your physical examination of the hip by examining the knee and back
- Stability of the hip replacement is a priority over leg length correction
- Watch for lateral trunk lean in patients with knee pain

Suggested Reading
O'Connor MI. Sex differences in osteoarthritis of the hip and knee. *J Am Acad Orthop Surg.* 2007;1(15):S22-S25.

Osteoarthritis of the Knee

Antonio Otero-López MD ■ Beatriz García-Cardona MD

Description

Osteoarthritis (OA) is the most common type of joint disease, resulting in degenerative changes of the joints. It is a noninflammatory arthritis. The classically involved joints are the hip and the knee; the latter being the most commonly involved joint in the body.

Etiology/Types

- Unknown; most likely a failed attempt of chondrocytes to repair cartilage
- Primary, or idiopathic OA, occurs with no apparent initiating cause, just aging
- Secondary OA can result from joint trauma, infections, or metabolic, neurological, or developmental disorders
- Meniscal tears and ligamentous injuries create an unstable joint that can predispose for the development of knee OA

Epidemiology

- OA is the most common cause of musculoskeletal pain and disability
- The knee is the most commonly affected joint
- OA is the number 1 cause of arthritis of the knee in the United States
- OA is more common in women than in men, which may be due to the fact that articular cartilage of the distal femur is less thick in women than in men
- African American women have a higher prevalence of knee OA
- In 2002, 350,000 knee replacements were done, tripling the number over 10 years

Pathogenesis

- Progressive erosion of articular cartilage
- Although inflammatory cells are present, the inflammatory response is mild
- Interleukin is increased and leads to production of degradative enzymes such as metalloproteinases
- Decreased content of proteoglycans due to increased rate of degradation
- Collagen becomes disordered and matrix framework breaks down
- Chondroitin sulfate concentration increases, whereas keratin sulfate concentration decreases
- Decreased modulus of elasticity
- Increased cellularity and bone deposition leading to bone eburnation

Risk Factors

- Obesity
- Occupation: squatting and heavy lifting
- Endocrine disorders (i.e., diabetes and acromegaly)
- Metabolic disorders (i.e., Paget's and gout)

Clinical Features

- Knee pain: deep, poorly localized, and chronic
- Symptoms related to activities and worst at the end of the day
- May experience morning stiffness for <30 minutes
- Genu varus is the most common deformity in the knee due to destruction and distortion of capsular ligaments
- Intermittent swelling and stiffness after period of inactivity
- Weather changes increase the pain
- Decreasing function and mobility
- Increasing weakness of periarticular muscle group

Natural History

- Variable clinical course due to the repair and remodeling reactions that occur after cartilage injury
- The course is usually slowly progressive but may be aggressive
- Deformities progress from passively correctable to fixed
- Some patients have only mild symptoms controlled by nonsteroidal anti-inflammatory drugs and activity modification
- Varus deformity can develop due to stress transmission to the medial compartment

150

Diagnosis

Differential diagnosis
- Inflammatory arthritis, such as rheumatoid arthritis and systemic lupus erythematous arthritis
- Infectious arthritis
- Hemorrhagic arthritis: hemophilia and sickle cell anemia
- Noninflammatory arthritis: osteonecrosis and neuropathic joint

History
- Knee pain with activity
- Swelling and loss of motion
- Difficulty with stairs

Exam
- Joint effusion
- Joint line tenderness
- Palpable crepitus
- Bony prominences: osteophytes
- Muscle atrophy
- Limitation of motion: mostly with terminal knee extension

Testing
- X-rays: anteroposterior/lateral views, sunrise views, standing knee films, 45° views
- Varus/valgus stress views to assess full cartilage loss vs asymmetric compartment involvement
- Magnetic resonance imaging (MRI): if joint space is preserved in x-rays and mechanical symptoms present
- Knee aspiration: Will show <200 white blood cells, 25% polymorphonuclear leukocytes (PMNs), glucose, and protein equal to serum

Pitfalls
- Ordering MRI studies before plain films

Red Flags
- Coronal plane deformities can lead to incompetence of medial collateral ligaments and severe bone loss, which make reconstruction harder

Treatment

Medical
- Nonsteroidal anti-inflammatory medications
- Analgesics
- Nutritional supplements: glucosamine sulfate (theorize to slow cartilage damage in OA, clinical studies shows mixed results, may be better for patients with moderate to severe pain)
- Topical treatments: capsaicin cream
- Bracing: unloading knee braces (single or double upright orthosis, which reduces the load on the affected compartment of the knee using a 3-point pressure system)

Exercises
- First goal: stretching to improve the range of motion
- Second goal: strengthening the surrounding muscles, and then a plan for aerobic exercise, such as swimming or bicycling, to increase overall fitness and control weight

Modalities
- Rest, ice, elevation, and activity modification on to treat flare-ups
- Persistent pain can be addressed by transcutaneous electrical nerve stimulation and heat
- Cryotherapy and therapeutic ultrasound have proven to be effective components of pain-management strategies
- Hydrotherapy and hydrocollator packs improve myotendinous flexibility and allow enhanced stretching
- Pulsed electrical stimulation relieves pain and improves function

Injection
- Intra-articular steroids
- Intra-articular hyaluronic acid

Surgical
- Arthroscopy: short-term mechanical symptoms with residual joint space
- Osteotomy: for young heavy patients with unicompartmental involvement
- Unicompartmental knee replacement: indications include symptoms in one compartment and correctable deformity in the coronal plane
- Total knee replacement: indicated for bicompartmental and tricompartmental knee arthritis

Consults
- Orthopedic surgery
- Physical medicine and rehabilitation

Complications
- Progressive pain and dysfunction

Prognosis

- Variable; with surgical reconstruction, there is high patient satisfaction

Helpful Hints

- Inflammation is not a major component of OA despite the suffix -itis
- Asymmetric wear pattern of knee compartments differentiates OA from inflammatory arthritides
- Osteophytes are attempts to increase contact area between joint surfaces with eroded cartilage

Suggested Readings

Englund M. The role of biomechanics in the initiation and progression of OA of the knee. *Best Pract Res Clin Rheumatol.* 2010;24(1):39–46.

Hoaglund FT, Steinbach LS. Primary osteoarthritis of the hip: etiology and epidemiology. *J Am Acad Orthop Surg.* 2001;9(5):320–327.

Zhang W, Kuki G, Moskowitz RW, et al. OARSI recommendations for the management of hip and knee osteoarthritis: part III: changes in evidence following systematic cumulative update of research published through January 2009. *Osteoarthritis Cartilage.* 2010;18(4): 476–479.

Osteochondritis Dissecans of the Elbow

Francisco M. López-González MD FAAOS

Description
Most common cause of lateral elbow pain in adolescent baseball players. Capitellar osteochondral lesion caused by high stress area.

Etiology/Types
Repetitive force applied to the capitellum is the main etiological factor in osteochondritis dissecans (OCD). Increased load at the radiocapitellar joint during valgus stress in late cocking and early acceleration phases of throwing.

Epidemiology
- Overuse injury
- High prevalence among individuals who have played baseball actively since childhood
- Dominant arm mostly involved
- Eleven to 15 years of age high prevalence

Pathogenesis
- During the acceleration phase of throwing, the elbow is stressed in a valgus direction and the capitellum is subjected to compression and shear forces

Risk Factors
- Baseball, gymnastics, wrestling, activities that increase valgus load on elbow

Clinical Features
- Age of presentation 11 to 15 years, mean age 15 years
- Decreased range of motion (mean 13° to 128°)
- Lateral elbow pain, catching, locking

Natural History
- Depends on stage of presentation
- Stable lesions heal with rest
- If athlete continues to play, loosening or fragmentation may occur, with progression to unstable lesion
- OCD with closed physes should be treated with surgery
- Fragment excision alone good option for lesions involving <50% of capitellar articular width

Diagnosis

Differential diagnosis
- Panner's disease (osteochondroses) >90% younger than age 10
- OCD of the radial head
- Angular deformity of radial neck

History
- Lateral elbow pain with throwing
- Lateral pain with valgus force, pushing with arms, handstands, tumbling
- Locking, catching, limited elbow motion
- Deep, dull ache
- Limited return to sports

Exam
- Restricted arc of motion common, around 20° extensor lag
- Tenderness over lateral elbow
- Catching with forearm rotation may be present
- Locking with active motion
- Deep, dull ache
- Weak forearm, shoulder muscles

Testing
- Anteroposterior/lateral elbow x-rays
- Computed tomography scan
- Magnetic resonance imaging best for cartilage and detachment of fragments
- Radiological classification:
  - Grade I: localized flattening or radiolucency
  - Grade II: nondisplaced fragment
  - Grade III: displaced or detached fragment
  - Stable lesion: immature capitellum with open growth plate, flattening of radiolucency of subchondral bone (Grade I), almost normal motion
  - Unstable lesion: mature capitellum with a closed growth plate, fragmentation (Grades II and III) or restricted elbow motion >20°

Pitfalls
- Might go undiagnosed in early stages

Red Flags
- Infection
- Fracture

■ Neoplasm

Treatment

Medical
■ Rest—no throwing or weight bearing on extremity for patients with open physes

Exercises
■ Gentle range of motion
■ Light upper extremity strengthening
■ Scapular stabilizer and core muscle strengthening

Modalities
■ Heat
■ Ice
■ Transcutaneous electrical nerve stimulation
■ Ultrasound

Injection
■ Not recommended

Surgical
■ Debridement
■ Fragment excision alone good option for lesions involving <50% of capitellar articular width
■ Fragment fixation with bone graft
■ Reconstruction with osteochondral graft from lateral femoral condyle

Consults
■ Orthopedic surgeon
■ Physical medicine and rehabilitation

Complications/side effects
■ Progression of pain and dysfunction
■ Elbow stiffness, loss of motion

Prognosis
The range of elbow motion at the time of presentation is associated with final outcome, with limited motion predictive of more pain, decreased ability to return to sports, and worse radiographical findings.

Helpful Hints
■ X-ray contralateral elbow and compare
■ Progression based on age of presentation, younger than 10 years consider Panner's disease-osteochondroses with benign prognosis

Suggested Readings

Kobayasbi K, Burton K, Rodner C, et al. Lateral compression injuries in the pediatric elbow: Panner's disease and osteochondritis dissecans of capitellum. *J Am Acad Orthop Surg.* 2004;12:246–254.

Takahara M, Mura N, Sasaki J, et al. Classification, treatment, and outcome of osteochondritis dissecans of the humeral capitellum. *J Bone Joint Surg Am.* 2007;89:1205–1214.

Osteochondritis Dissecans of the Knee

Francisco J. Otero-López MD ■ Omar Morales-Abella MD

Description

Osteochondritis dissecans (OCD) is a disorder of the ossification centers of the knee characterized by involvement of both cartilage and bone, degeneration, or aseptic necrosis and calcification. OCD of the knee classically affects the lateral aspect of the medial femoral condyle (Figures 1 and 2).

Etiology/Types

- Remains unclear
- Hereditary predisposition unproven
- Poor blood supply to affected area may decrease healing response
- Microtrauma vs macrotrauma
- Shear forces around the knee
- Juvenile and adult forms of the condition exist

Epidemiology

- Incidence 0.02% to 1.2% of the population
- Male-to-female ratio 2:1
- Prevalence 19/100,000 in females and 29/100,000 in males

Pathogenesis

- Impaired healing of subchondral bone lesion develops into a spectrum that begins with softening of the overlying articular cartilage followed by early cartilage separation
- Partial detachment of the lesion occurs and finally, osteochondral separation with articular loose bodies

Risk Factors

- Meniscectomy/discoid meniscus
- Genu recurvatum
- Condylar flattening
- Any condition that increases shear forces at the knee joint

Clinical Features

- Juvenile onset before epiphyseal plate closure; adult onset after epiphyseal plate closure
- Anterior knee pain with intermittent swelling (early)
- Persistent swelling with complains of catching or giving away occurs as the disease progresses

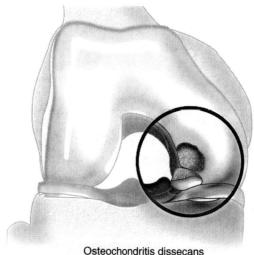

Osteochondritis dissecans

Figure 1. Knee osteochondritis dissecans.

- Late-stage disease correlates with complaints of a loose body in the knee
- Symptoms exacerbated with increased activity
- External rotation of the affected leg during gait alleviates symptoms

Natural History

- Juvenile onset OCD has better prognosis due to better healing potential
- Lesions at the classic location have a better prognosis
- Lesions <2 cm have a better prognosis
- OCD fragments that have not detached do better than dissected fragments
- Larger lesions may lead to articular surface irregularities and subsequent arthritis

Diagnosis

Differential diagnosis

- Patellofemoral pain/knee extensor mechanism disorders
- Fracture
- Rheumatoid arthritis
- Neoplasm
- Septic arthritis
- Osteoarthritis

History

- Anterior knee pain that is exacerbated by activity

- Intermittent swelling
- Catching, locking, and complaints of loose body in articulation

Exam
- Passive and active range of motion (ROM)
- Wilson's test (internal rotation of leg while extending knee from 90° to 30° will reproduce symptoms if classic OCD present)
- Ballotment/milking to assess for effusion
- Varus/valgus stress
- Lachman's test

Testing
- Weight bearing knee anteroposterior and lateral x-rays (Figure 2). Aids in classification of OCD lesion due to location and staging
- Notch view x-ray
- Bone scan Tc-99 for assessment of juvenile OCD
- Magnetic resonance imaging

Pitfalls
- May miss early diagnosis if not suspected

Red Flags
- Trauma
- Infection
- Neoplasm
- Inflammatory arthritis

Treatment

Medical
- Analgesic medications such as acetaminophen is recommended for juvenile OCD
- Nonsteroid anti-inflammatory drugs for adult OCD

Exercises
- Limit activity, especially sports participation, for up to 3 months
- Weight bearing is recommended
- Weight control
- ROM/gentle stretching

- Strengthening exercises for quadriceps, hamstrings, and hip muscles in older patients who commonly have concomitant pathology (osteoarthritis, instability, malalignment)

Modalities
- Cryotherapy
- Heat
- Electrical stimulation
- Ultrasound (adult individuals)

Injection
- Not commonly used

Surgical
- Arthroscopy
- Subchondral/transchondral drilling
- Osteochondral grafting
- Chondrocyte transplantation

Consult
- Orthopedics
- Sports medicine
- Physical medicine and rehabilitation

Complications/side effects
- Degenerative arthrosis

Prognosis
- Variable
- Better prognosis for juvenile OCD, stable OCD fragments, and for small lesions (<2 cm)

Helpful Hints
- Nonsurgical management is successful in 50% of patients. The main objective of both surgical and conservative management is to restore a normal joint surface

Suggested Readings
Cahill BM. Osteochondritis dissecans of the knee: treatment of juvenile and adult forms. *J Am Acad Orthop Surg.* 1995;3:237–247.

Crawford DC, Safran MR. Osteochondritis dissecans of the knee. *J Am Acad Orthop Surg.* 2006;14:90–100.

Osteolysis of the Clavicle

Efrain Deliz MD

Description
Distal clavicle osteolysis (DCO), also known as weight-lifter's clavicle, is an infrequent entity.

It is often bilateral and usually occurs in young adult males.

Etiology/Types
- Overuse injury associated with heavy weightlifting

Epidemiology
- Twenty-eight percent of elite weightlifters present with DCO
- Bilateral involvement in 79% of weightlifters at the time of presentation

Pathogenesis
- The acromioclavicular (AC) joint is a diarthrodial joint stabilized via the coracoclavicular ligaments (conoid and trapezoid-vertical stability) and the superior and inferior AC ligaments (horizontal stability)
- A fibrocartilaginous disc adds congruency to the joint
- Subchondral bone microfractures with a subsequent repair attempt, making it consistent with repetitive microtrauma
- Pathological specimens show articular degeneration, chronic inflammation, fibrosis, loss of trabecular structure, and osteoblastic activity

Risk Factors
- Repeated overhead activity
- Heavy weightlifting

Clinical Features
- Insidious pain
- Pain localized to the AC joint, may radiate to the trapezius muscle
- Associated with weightlifting activities

Natural History
- Symptoms improve with activity modification and cross training
- Worsening of symptoms with continued weightlifting

Diagnosis

Differential diagnosis
- AC joint osteoarthritis
- Rotator cuff tendinopathy
- Biceps tendinopathy
- Hyperparathyroidism
- Gout
- Scleroderma
- Rheumatoid arthritis
- Multiple myeloma
- Infection
- Gorham's disease (vanishing bone disease, associated with proliferation of vascular channels, and bone osteolysis)
- Referred cervical pain

History
- Insidious pain, exacerbated with exercise, especially weight training
- Symptoms may worsen over time hurting with any motion as well as during sleep
- Trauma is usually not recalled

Exam
- Pinpoint tenderness over the AC joint
- Occasional swelling
- Deformity
- Crepitance
- Cross arm adduction test (pain reproduction)
- O'Briens active compression test (arm forward flexed, adducted 10°, internally rotated while flexion is resisted, reproduces AC joint pain, and differentiates from labral tears)
- Paxinos test (patient seated, arm resting along chest, acromion compressed with examiner's thumb while clavicle is compressed with index and long fingers, pain reproduction)
- AC joint stability is assessed by placing anterior and posterior stress loading to the clavicle

Testing
- Radiographs of both AC joints using an anteroposterior (AP) view with 35° of cephalad orientation or a Zanca's AP view with 15° cephalad orientation help avoid overlapping of the scapular spine

- Findings include distal clavicle subchondral bone loss, AC joint fluid, microcysts and widening of the AC joint. The acromial medial facet is sparred of lytic changes
- Scintigraphy may help in the early diagnosis but is usually not necessary
- Magnetic resonance imaging shows increase in signal intensity with the T2-weighted images
- Bone marrow edema may be present, but not on the acromial side. Imaging may also help the surgeon decide on the amount of bone to be resected

Pitfalls
- Low level of suspicion, missed diagnosis
- Continued weight training

Red Flags
- Worse pain despite treatment
- Fever
- Night pain

Treatment

Medical
- Activity modification, reduction of weight lifting
- Modify the bench press, narrow grip and avoid full extension of the arms
- Nonsteroidal anti-inflammatory medications

Exercises
- Range of motion, posterior capsule shoulder flexibility training
- Light rotator cuff and scapular stabilizers strengthening

Modalities
- Cryotherapy
- Superficial heat
- Electrical stimulation

Injection
- Intra-articular steroid injections may provide short-term pain relief

- Local infiltration may be done using a small gauge needle and small volume of medications (local anesthetic 1 mL and steroid 1 to 2 mL)
- May repeat a second injection in 3 months (usually no more than two given)

Surgical
- Once conservative treatment fails, surgical treatment should be considered
- Successful open and arthroscopic distal clavicle excision (ADCE) techniques are available
- Recently, arthroscopic procedures have gained popularity, and in most cases, a minimal amount of bone resection is needed (4–6 mm). ADCE offers less morbidity and complications rates

Consults
- Orthopedic surgery
- Physical medicine and rehabilitation
- Sports medicine

Complications/side effects
- Chronic pain
- Inability to return to weightlifting

Prognosis
- Variable; symptoms may become chronic if activity not modified

Helpful Hints
- High level of suspicion leads to early diagnosis
- Order x-rays on any young active individual with AC joint insidious pain

Suggested Readings

Beals RK, Saucer DD. Nontraumatic disorders of the clavicle. *J Am Acad Orthop Surg.* 2006;14:205–214.

Schaffer SS. Painful conditions of the acromioclavicular joint. *J Am Acad Orthop Surg.* 1999;7:176–188.

Schwarzkopf R, Ishak C. Distal clavicular osteolysis. *Bull Hosp Jt Dis.* 2008;66(2):94–101.

Osteoporosis

Enrique Vázquez MD MBA

Description
Osteoporosis is currently defined as a skeletal disorder characterized by low bone density and compromised bone strength, which predisposes to increased risk for fractures. Common and typical locations of osteoporotic fractures include the spine, hip, and wrist (Figure 1).

Etiology/Types
- Type I: involutional (postmenopausal); associated with reduction in estrogen, consequent osteoclast activation, and bone resorption
- Type II: related to aging and characterized by increase in parathyroid hormone (PTH) levels, increase in bone turnover, and decrease in osteoblastic activity
- Male osteoporosis is related to secondary factors of bone loss such as hypogonadism

Epidemiology
- Over 10 million females in the United States have established osteoporosis, an additional 34 million with osteopenia (bone mineral density [BMD] that is lower than normal peak but not low enough to be classified as osteoporosis)
- The annual incidence is more than heart attack, stroke, and breast cancer combined
- Five percent of males in the medicare population in 2001 diagnosed with osteoporosis
- A female left untreated has a 50% chance of suffering an osteoporosis-related fracture
- Fracture prevalence is estimated to be 1.5 million a year (over 700,000 spine and over 350,000 hip fractures) with excess mortality of up to 26% (hip fractures)
- Hip fracture morbidity is high, close to 30% to 50% of patients cannot assume prefracture function and 20% of these require nursing home placement
- The economic impact of fractures in the United States is $14 billion per year in direct expenditures with a cost of $21,000 per hip fracture

Pathogenesis
- Bone is in a state of constant turnover with a tight coupling of bone resorption (osteoclasts) and formation (osteoblasts) functions

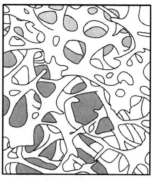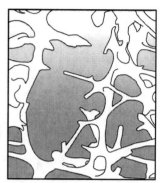

Normal bone   Bone with ospteoporosis

Figure 1. Comparison of normal and osteoporotic bone.

- Multiple factors (genetics, nutrition, lifestyle and habits, gender, race, menopause and aging, medications, and disease) can cause an "uncoupling" of these cell units with a potential net effect of decreased bone mass, microarchitectural deterioration, osteoporosis, and fractures
- The roles of cytokines (TNF, IL-1, IL-6), RANKL, transforming growth factor β, PTH, and 1,25-hydroxyvitamin D (among others) continue to emerge
- Menopause is characterized as a period of rapid bone loss (2% to 3% per year in the spine for up to 8 years). Aging (seventh decade of life) shows a slower decline in bone loss of 0.5% per year

Risk Factors
- Age
- Asian or white race
- Malabsorption disorders
- Postmenopausal status
- Low calcium intake and vitamin D deficiency
- Solid organ or bone marrow transplantation
- Alcoholism
- Hypogonadism, hyperparathyroidism
- Parental hip fracture, personal history of fragility fracture >40 years of age
- Chronic liver or kidney disease
- Sedentary lifestyle, inability to rise from a chair
- Body mass index (BMI) <19 or weight <127 pounds
- Long-term use of steroids or other medications (i.e., anticonvulsants, heparin, GnRH therapy for

prostate cancer, others), excessive consumption of caffeine

Clinical Features
- Fractures from minimal trauma (defined as falling from standing or sitting position) and after bending, stooping, or carrying a load
- Fractures located in the wrist, spine, and hip
- Chronic pain
- Dyspnea (related to changes in the thoracic spine, pain, and muscle weakness)
- Possibly restrictive lung disease

Natural History
- Unrecognized fractures of the spine may lead to kyphosis
- Chronic pain and loss of height
- Early identification of patients at risk improves results of treatment

Diagnosis

Differential diagnosis
- Osteomalacia
- Metastatic disease
- Hypogonadism
- Medications (glucocorticoids, immunosuppresants, heparin, anticonvulsants)
- Vitamin D deficiency
- Primary hyperparathyroidism, idiopathic hypercalciuria
- Alcoholism
- Gastrointestinal disorders (celiac sprue, inflammatory bowel disease)
- Endocrine disorders (hyperthyroidism, Cushing's syndrome)
- Hematologic disorders (multiple myeloma, monoclonal gammopathy of undetermined significance, mast cell disorders)

History
- Pain associated with falling, or lifting, and resultant fractures
- Progressive deformity of the spine
- Loss of height

Exam
- Thoracolumbar kyphosis
- Tenderness to palpation over the thoracolumbar spinous processes
- Pain with back motion, particularly flexion
- Deformity or limitation of motion associated with hip or wrist fractures

- Neurological deficits in patients with compression fractures of the spine, retropulsion, and nerve injury

Testing
- Laboratory studies
  - First Tier: complete blood count (CBC), renal profile, hepatic profile, alkaline phosphatase, phosphorus, 24-hour calcium, PTH levels, thyroid-stimulating hormone (TSH) levels, and 25-OH vitamin D
  - Second Tier: if indicated, testosterone in men, estradiol in women, tissue transglutaminase, 24-hour free cortisol or dexamethasone suppression, serum and urine protein electrophoresis
- The gold standard for diagnosis continues to be the central dual energy x-ray absorptiometry (DXA)
- WHO classification: BMD *T*-score (comparison with BMD of young normal patients)
  - Normal: BMD <1 SD of the young adult reference mean
  - Osteopenia: BMD values >1 SD below the young adult mean but <2.5 SDs below this value
  - Osteoporosis: BMD value 2.5 SD or more below the young adult mean
  - Severe osteoporosis: BMD value 2.5 SD or more below the young adult mean in the presence of one or more osteoporotic fractures
  - Since the WHO criteria for diagnosis of osteoporosis was based largely on postmenopausal white females, the International Society of Clinical Densitometry (ISCD) recommends that in other groups, the diagnosis should not be based on densitometric criteria alone and that the age match normal patient (*Z*-score) rather than the *T*-score be used:
  - Men < 50 years of age, premenopausal women, and children: use ethnic or race adjusted *Z*-score

Pitfalls
- Osteoporosis is "silent disease" only becoming manifest when fractures and their complications develop
- Spine fractures may go undetected for prolonged periods of time and only manifest by progressive loss of height (over 2 cm over 3 years) and dorsal kyphosis ("Dowager's hump")

Red Flags
- The occurrence of low trauma pelvic fractures should prompt the search for osteomalacia and metastatic bone disease
- Progressive spine deformity
- Severe night pain

Treatment

Medical
- Avoidance of excess alcohol
- Not smoking
- Calcium and vitamin D
- Clinical trials have shown that particularly in elderly, institutionalized patients with low levels of 25-OH vitamin D, supplementation with cholecalciferol (vitamin D3 800 IU/day) and calcium (1200 mg/day) increased proximal femur bone density and reduced hip fractures and other peripheral fractures by 25%
- Hip protectors decrease fracture risk but the compliance rate is low due to discomfort
- Pharmacological therapy
- Bisphosphonates side effects include gastrointestinal with swallowing difficulty, esophagitis, and gastric ulcer. Osteonecrosis of the jaw is a concern, however, mostly seen in patients with cancer. Reduces spine and hip fractures occurrence 36% to 50%
  - Alendronate (Fosamax)
  - Risendronate (Actonel)
  - Ibandronate (Boniva)
- Estrogen/estrogen progestin combination used to be considered first-line therapy, caution with used due to increased incidence of myocardial infarction (MI), stroke, invasive breast cancer, pulmonary emboli, deep vein phlebitis; reduces vertebral fractures by 34% and other osteoporotic fractures by 23%
- Raloxifene (Evista) has been shown to reduce the risk of estrogen receptor positive breast cancer. Increases the risk of deep vein thrombosis as well as hot flashes; reduces spine fractures by 30% in patients with and by 55% in patients without prior spine fracture
- Calcitonin (Miacalcin, Calcimar, or Fortical) has mild analgesic effect with reported (questionable) benefit in acute vertebral fractures; reduces vertebral fractures by 33%
- Parathyroid hormone (Forteo) is approved in postmenopausal women at high risk for fracture. The safety and efficacy has not been demonstrated beyond 2 years of treatment; reduces spine fractures by 65% and nonspine fractures by 53%

Exercises
- Back extension exercises
- Back and core-strengthening exercises
- Dynamic weight training for upper and lower extremities
- Weight bearing aerobic exercise (walking, running, low-impact aerobics)

Modalities
- Cryotherapy
- Superficial heat
- Transcutaneous electrical nerve stimulation

Injection
- Epidural blocks for root compression
- Vertebral augmentation with vertebroplasty or kyphoplasty is a treatment option with intractable pain caused by osteoporotic vertebral compression fracture (mixed results in the medical literature, limited change in vertebral height)

Surgical
- Rarely indicated for osteoporotic compression fracture

Consults
- Endocrinology
- Obstetrics and gynecology
- Physical medicine and rehabilitation
- Rheumatology

Complication/side effects
- Chronic pain
- Spine deformity
- Limitation in activity tolerance

Prognosis
- Osteoporosis progression can be controlled with early identification and appropriate treatment
- Complications from fractures include high excess mortality and disability as in the case of hip fractures and loss of height

Helpful Hints
- Suspect osteoporosis in females at risk
- Early diagnosis with DXA important for adequate treatment

Suggested Readings
Prather H, Hunt D, Watson JO, et al. Conservative care for patients with osteoporotic vertebral compression fractures. *Phys Med Rehabil Clin N Am.* 2007;18:577–591.

Wei GS, Jackson JL, Hatzigeorgiou C, et al. Osteoporosis management in the new millennium. *Prim Care.* 2003;30(4):711–741.

Patellar Extensor Mechanism Disorders

Margarita Tolentino MD ■ Sheila A. Dugan MD

Description

Extensor mechanism disorders are common sources of anterior and peripatellar knee pain.

Multiple causative factors are implicated, including repetitive use, musculoskeletal imbalances, trauma, and bony abnormalities.

Etiology/Types

- Patella/patellofemoral abnormalities: chondromalacia patella, patellar bursitis, osteochondritis dissecans (OCD), stress fracture of the patella, patellar fracture, symptomatic bipartite patella, and synovial plica inflammation
- Patellar tendon abnormalities: including patellar tendinopathy and tendinitis (Jumper's knee), Osgood-Schlatters syndrome (inflammation at the tibial tuberosity), Sinding-Larson-Johansson syndrome (apophysitis at inferior pole of patella), and patellar tendon avulsion
- Quadriceps/femoral dysfunction, including quadriceps tendinopathy and rupture, and vastus medialis oblique (VMO) weakness causing lateral patellar tracking
- Anatomical variants/factors: miserable malalignment syndrome, a combination of femoral anteversion, external tibial torsion, increased quadriceps (Q) angle, and patella alta, associated with genu valgum and foot pronation, which contribute to abnormal tracking of the patella and increased stresses on the patellofemoral joint

Epidemiology

- A reported 25% of patients with knee complaints, who present to sports medicine clinics, have anterior knee pain
- Women are more likely to be affected than men (wider pelvis, weak hip, and gluteal muscles, increased quadriceps angle) (Figure 1)
- Predominantly affects patients in 20 to 30 years of age

Pathogenesis

- Overuse with repetitive flexion/extension (as in running) or excessive jumping activities results

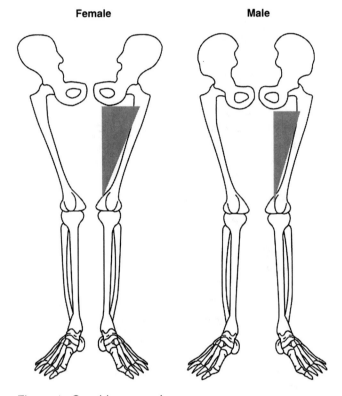

Female **Male**

Figure 1. Quadriceps angle.

in Osgood-Schlatters syndrome, Sinding-Larson-Johansson syndrome, and patellar and quadriceps tendinopathies
- Acute injury or direct trauma lead to symptomatic bipartite patella, synovial plica inflammation, patellar stress fracture, quadriceps rupture, OCD, and patellar bursitis

Risk Factors

- Lack of conditioning
- Previous trauma
- Degenerative arthritis/cartilage lesion
- Overtraining, incorrect training techniques, running on hard or irregular surfaces
- Improper foot wear

Clinical Features

- Pain with activity, stairs, and prolonged sitting

- Intermittent locking, and occasional giving way of the knee
- Mild effusion may be evident in plica inflammation, symptomatic bipartite patella, miserable malalignment syndrome, or in any injury due to trauma
- Tenderness at the tibial tuberosity, patellar tendon insertion, and quadriceps tendon is reproduced with palpation.

Natural History
- Persistent quadriceps inhibition/weakness associated to pain
- Tracking abnormalities
- Pain with activity if not treated
- Chronic degenerative changes, possibly associated with osteoarthritis, cartilage lesions/ chondromalacia may progress and lead to limitation of activity

Diagnosis
Differential diagnosis
- Ligamentous injury
- Meniscal injury
- Bony tumor
- Referred pain from hip
- L4 radiculopathy

History
- Pain may be acute or chronic in onset, indicating either trauma or overuse etiologies
- Patients may give history of pain, instability, and difficulty weight bearing during and after activity, specifically running, jumping, and going upstairs and downstairs; pain may also worsen with prolonged sitting (movie sign)
- Patients may complain of pain at the anterior knee, "behind the patella," or peripatellar region

Exam
- Gait assessment for excessive foot pronation and signs of lower extremity malalignment
- Skin inspection assessing for inflammation, acute signs of trauma, or obvious inflammation at the tibial tubercle
- Observe tracking of the patella on the trochlea during knee flexion and palpate along the peripatellar margins
- Patellar compression test may reproduce pain (compression of the patella against the femur)
- Assess for quadriceps tightness in the prone position; iliotibial band tightness/Ober's sign in the side-lying position, and hamstring flexibility when supine
- Quadriceps, hamstrings, and hip muscle strength testing sitting, supine, and prone
- Standing evaluation of single leg balance, step-down or single leg squat to assess hip and quadriceps muscle strength, as well as control of knee valgus and femoral internal rotation
- Apprehension test to assess patellar laxity

Testing
- X-rays remain the gold standard for evaluation
  - Axial views at 30° or 45° of knee flexion should be done for the evaluation of patellar alignment
  - Posterior/anterior, sunrise, and weight bearing films are standard in assessing any early degenerative changes or alignment issues
- Magnetic resonance imaging is beneficial for assessment of soft tissue injuries and patellar tendon abnormalities
- Ultrasound could be used to evaluate the quadriceps and patellar tendons

Pitfalls
- May be confused with meniscal injury or intra-articular pathology

Red Flags
- Continued pain may be due to OCD
- Suspect fracture if pain worsens despite treatment or insignificant trauma

Treatment
Medical
- Relative rest, ice, and nonsteroidal anti-inflammatory medications in acute trauma
- Knee sleeve with patellar opening for patellofemoral pain
- Infrapatellar strap for patellar tendinitis (Cho-Pat or equivalent orthotic device)
- Foot orthosis to correct pronation

Exercises
- Quadriceps, hamstrings, and iliotibial band stretching
- Quadriceps/VMO strengthening including straight leg raising, short arc, and terminal extension exercises
- Hip muscle strengthening
- Kinetic chain balancing/closed chain exercises including mini-squats, lunges, and step-down exercises

- Bicycle (high seat to reduce knee flexion, patellofemoral joint forces), elliptical trainer, aquatic exercises

Modalities
- Cryotherapy
- Electrical stimulation to facilitate muscle recruitment and reduce inhibition
- Ultrasound followed by quadriceps, iliotibial band, or hamstring stretching
- McConnell taping may be used to assist in modifying abnormal patellar tracking during activity

Surgical
- Lateral retinacular release and arthroscopy are reserved for patients who fail conservative treatment and have persistent, chronic pain associated with lateral patellar tilt
- Patients with medial peripatellar pain associated with thickened synovial plica may benefit from arthroscopic removal

Complications/side effect
- Prolonged symptoms lead to quadriceps inhibition and muscle atrophy
- Inability to participate in running and jumping sports

Prognosis
- With relative rest, cross training and rehabilitation that addresses the etiology of the pain, prognosis is good for return to sport and functional activity

Helpful Hints
- Address the whole kinetic chain in treatment
- Proximal lower extremity weakness
- Distal extremity abnormalities such as overpronation

Suggested Readings

Lowry CD, Cleland JA, Dyke K. Management of patients with patellofemoral pain syndrome using a multimodal approach: a case series. *J Orthop Sports Phys Ther.* 2008;38(11):691–702.

Prins MR, van der Wurff P. Females with patellofemoral pain syndrome have weak hip muscles: a systematic review. *Aust J Physiother.* 2009;55(1):9–15.

Patellar Instability

Margarita Tolentino MD ▪ Sheila A. Dugan MD

Description
Patellar instability is characterized by partial or total displacement of the patella from the femoral trochlea and is commonly associated with knee pain. It can be caused by direct trauma, anatomical variants, or biomechanical imbalances.

Etiology/Types
- Patellar subluxation
- Patellar dislocation
- Lateral unless iatrogenic factors (surgery) lead to medial instability

Epidemiology
- Female-to-male ratio of 2:1
- Fifteen percent of patients may have recurrent dislocation after an initial dislocation

Pathogenesis
- Traumatic dislocation typically occurs with twisting maneuvers, in conjunction with strong quadriceps contraction and knee positioned in valgus. Dislocation occurs laterally
- Associated with anatomical variants such as patella alta and hypoplastic femoral trochlea
- Increased quadriceps angle, muscle imbalances

Risk Factors
- Previous history of patellar dislocation and instability
- Abnormal patellar configurations including patella alta, patellar tilt, and hypoplastic trochlea
- Patellofemoral malalignment from disruption of the static stabilizers of the patella, which include weakened medial patellofemoral ligament (MPFL), medial patellomeniscal ligament, medial patellotibial ligament, and hypertonic iliotibial band, concomitant with imbalanced dynamic stabilizers of the patella, which include the vastus medialis (VMO) and adductor magnus
- Overuse
- Family history of patellar dislocation/subluxation

Clinical Features
- Swelling and hemarthrosis in acute patellar dislocation

- Mild recurrent swelling in patellar subluxation

Natural History
- Patellofemoral arthritis
- Development of crepitus beneath the patella
- Increased frequency of patellar dislocation or subluxation
- Chronic abnormal tracking of the patella
- Potential atrophy of the quadriceps

Diagnosis

Differential diagnosis
- Ligamentous injury
- Meniscal injury
- Osteochondritis dissecans of the patella

History
- Patient gives history of trauma during activity with knee in flexion and valgus
- Severe swelling and pain with initial dislocation
- Individuals may feel like the knee is slipping or unstable with any "cutting" or twisting movements

Exam
- There may be evidence of patella alta, genu valgus, knee recurvatum, and knee crepitus when examining the uninjured knee
- An acute dislocated patella can be seen over the lateral femoral condyle.
- After reduction, hemarthrosis will be present
- Subluxed patella may show mild effusion and will have hypermobility
- Positive apprehension test may be present
- Lachman's test; valgus stress tests are carried out to rule out associated injury

Testing
- Plain films, including anterior, posterior, and lateral views, are cost-effective but are limited in assessment of the surrounding soft tissue
- Merchant or sunrise views (tangential views with the knee in flexion) may show severity of subluxation and/or the presence of a maintained dislocation
- Computed tomography (CT) scan is more sensitive when compared with plain films in evaluating the degree of patellar subluxation

- Magnetic resonance imaging (MRI) may reveal lesions of the static stabilizers/dynamic stabilizers, MPFL

Pitfalls
- Missing associated osteochondral fracture or anterior cruciate ligament injury
- Missing instability in a dislocation that spontaneously reduced

Red Flags
- In severe swelling needs to rule out combined injuries

Treatment

Medical
- Acute dislocation can be reduced by extending the knee and applying pressure along the lateral aspect of patellar edge
- In acute subluxation, temporary immobilization until pain and swelling subside followed by rehabilitation and patellar bracing may be utilized. Extension immobilization can be considered, as needed for short term only to help reduce symptoms

Exercises
- Strengthening of the quadriceps, glutei, and hip external rotators combining static, straight leg raising, short arc, and full arc dynamic exercises
- Closed chain exercises starting with calf raises, mini-squats, lunges, and progressing from two legs to one leg
- Proprioceptive training
- Bicycle, elliptical training, and aquatic rehabilitation

Modalities
- Cryotherapy
- Electrical stimulation (for reduction of swelling, facilitation of quadriceps contraction)

- Patellar taping to control pain and assist in realigning the patella

Injection
- Aspiration of hemarthrosis may help to reduce symptoms
- Injection not indicated

Surgical
- Surgery should be considered if VMO or MPFL is disrupted
- Arthroscopic lateral release, repair of MPFL
- Open extensor mechanism reconstruction is reserved for patients with persistent, symptomatic subluxation

Consults
- Orthopedic surgery

Complications/side effects
- Recurrent symptoms results in muscle inhibition and inability to participate in sports
- Osteoarthritis associated with muscle inhibition, recurrent injury

Prognosis
- Functional recovery and return to activity is generally good after injury if rehabilitation addresses muscle imbalances, weakness, and proprioceptive deficits
- Variable recovery of function following surgery

Helpful Hints
- Following initial injury address proximal lower weakness, and muscle control of the gluteus and external rotators

Suggested Readings
Arendt EA, Fithian DC, Cohen E. Current concepts of lateral patella dislocation. *Clin Sports Med.* 2002;21(3):499–519.
Colvin AC, West RV. Patellar instability. *J Bone Joint Surg Am.* 2008;90(12):2751–2762.

Pelvic Pain Syndrome

Ignacio Echenique MD ■ Gerald Isenberg MD FACS FACRS ■ William Alemany MD

Description

Pelvic pain syndrome (PPS) is defined as lower genitourinary and pelvic symptoms in the pudendal region, perineum or genitalia, voiding symptoms, such as dysuria or frequency, and sexual difficulties. It is more common in women; it can be a set of symptoms of a disease; or it can represent a clinical condition by itself. Chronic PPS is diagnosed when the pelvic region pain persists longer than 6 months.

Etiology/Types

- Gastrointestinal: nonrelaxing puborectalis muscle, and levator ani syndrome
- Neuromuscular: pudendal neuralgia, and lumbosacral radiculopathy
- Musculoskeletal: myofascial pain syndrome, and coccygodynia
- Gynecological: vulvodynia, and pelvic floor dysfunction
- Genitourinary: chronic prostatitis (CP), and interstitial cystitis
- The large number of possible diagnoses suggests multiple etiologies with a large range of symptoms of mixed origins
- Patients with PPS will usually present with more than one condition/diagnosis and a confusing crossover representing medical and surgical conditions

Epidemiology

- Estimated prevalence in the United States: 15% to 25% in women and 15% in men (all diagnoses combined)
- More than 50% of women with age 55 and older suffer one or more of the problems caused by pelvic floor dysfunction
- PPS affects one in every seven women
- Men and women underreport chronic PPS due to embarrassment (the Latin word "pudendus" means shame)
- Nonbacterial CP or prostatodynia is the most common urological diagnosis in men over 50 years and third in those younger than 50 years
- In women, the most common etiologies are endometriosis, and interstitial cystitis
- Prevalence approaches that of migraine, asthma, or low back pain

Pathogenesis

- Varies, depending on specific cause; often indeterminate
- The "pelvic floor" is a combination of muscles, ligaments, and other tissues that support the pelvic organs
- When this system weakens, the organs may move, protrude, bulge, and push outward, or cause pressure on each other
- The high prevalence in both sexes suggests the possibility of a common underlying cause
- Women have wider pelvis, greater range of motion, and muscle imbalances
- Biomechanical alterations follow pregnancy and childbirth

Risk Factors

- Musculoskeletal disorders of the low back and pelvic region
- Neurological disorders (radiculopathy, peripheral neuropathy)
- Pregnancy/deliveries
- Physical inactivity
- Irritable bowel syndrome (IBS)
- Constipation
- Lower urinary tract symptoms
- History of sexual abuse

Clinical Features

- Most patients experience somatic or visceral symptoms
- Presentation dependent upon the primary etiology of the patient's condition
- The pain can be moderate to severe, soft or dull, intermittent or constant, and present
- Evaluated by multiple physicians and multiple diagnostic tests
- Emotional overlay

Natural History

- Progressive symptoms if not properly diagnosed
- Pain becomes diffuse and poorly localized
- Depends on the primary cause of symptoms

Diagnosis

Differential diagnosis

- Gastrointestinal: levator ani syndrome, proctalgia fugax, paradoxical puborectalis, anismus, nonrelaxing puborectalis, IBS, concealed or true rectal prolapse, proctitis, gastrointestinal tumors, retrorectal tumors, abscesses, anal fissures, anal fistulas
- Neuromuscular: high tone pelvic floor dysfunction, pelvic floor tension myalgia, coccygodynia, pudendal neuralgia (Alcock's syndrome, cyclist's syndrome, pudendal canal syndrome), anorectal neuralgia, piriformis syndrome, lumbosacral discogenic disease, neuropathy, sacroiliac joint dysfunction, arthritis
- Gynecological: endometriosis, chronic pelvic inflammatory disease (PID), interstitial cystitis, bladder pain syndrome, uterine descend-prolapse, vulvodynia, vestibulitis, pelvic contracture syndrome, pelvic congestion, pelvic floor hernias, pelvic floor dysfunction, cystocele, tumors, abscesses, pelvic adhesions
- Genitourinary: chronic or nonbacterial prostatitis, prostatodynia, interstitial cystitis bladder pain, kidney or bladder stones, cystocele, urinary tract infection (UTI), epidymitis
- Others: pelvic floor hernias, depression-psychogenic, history of sexual abuse, trauma, postpelvic surgery, idiopathic

History

- Low back pelvic, vaginal, testicular pain
- Painful defecation
- Dyspareunia
- Pain associated with erection, ejaculation
- Constipation
- Fecal and urinary incontinence
- Sensation of a foreign body
- Decreased urinary flow
- Urinary frequency and urgency
- Previous trauma, sexual abuse

Exam

- Palpation for lumbar, hip, coccygeal, and pelvic tender or trigger points
- Evaluation of hip range of motion, and back, hip, and hamstrings muscle flexibility
- Neurological examination
- Straight leg raising and Patrick's test
- Digital rectal examination
- Pelvic examination

Testing

- Intravesical potassium sensitivity test
- Analysis and cultures of urine, prostatic secretions, valginal secretions, and stool
- Manometry
- Flexible sigmoidoscopy/colonoscopy
- Cystoscopy evaluation under anesthesia and evaluation of bladder capacity without anesthesia
- Electrodiagnosis (electromyography [EMG]), pudendal nerve latency test
- Ultrasound: transvaginal, rectal, pelvis
- Defecography
- Cystography
- X-rays: lumbosacral, coccyx
- Magnetic resonance imaging (MRI): lumbosacral spine and pelvis

Pitfalls

- Low level of suspicion
- Delay in diagnosis
- Psychogenic cause/history of abuse

Red Flags

- Infection
- Neoplasm
- Rule out psychosomatic etiology

Treatment

Medical

- Multidisciplinary approach
- Pharmacological
- Nonsteroidal anti-inflammatory drugs for inflammatory and nociceptive pain
- Analgesics
- Gabapentin, pregabalin for neuropathic pain, burning sensation
- Amitriptyline for neuropathic pain, sleep dysfunction
- Tizanidine, cyclobenzaprine for painful muscle spasm, nonrelaxing puborectalis muscle
- Antibiotics for UTI, prostatitis, epididymitis
- Stool softener, dietary supplements (glucosamine, melatonin for sleep dysfunction)
- Psychotherapy, cognitive behavioral therapy

Exercises

- Hip, hamstrings, and low back flexibility exercises
- Pelvic floor muscle relaxation techniques
- Pelvic floor and core muscle strengthening exercises
- Aerobic exercises

Modalities

- Back, and hip massage and myofascial release
- Rectal and transvaginal (Thiele's) massage
- Whirlpool, sitz baths

- Pelvic toners, vaginal cones
- Electrical stimulation
- EMG biofeedback

Injection
- Trigger point injections
- Botulism toxin injection
- Lidocaine/methylprednisolone injections into the puborectalis
- Epidural blocks
- Sacral nerve stimulation
- Intrathecal pump

Surgical
- The rationale for surgery is the restoration of normal pelvic support, removal of abnormal structures, decompression of impinged nerves
- Laparoscopic surgery for endometriosis, adhesions
- Pelvic floor reconstruction
- Repair of rectal prolapse
- Hysterectomy
- Removal of stones, tumors
- Cystoscopy with irrigation (dimethyl sulfoxide, heparin, hyaluronic acid)
- Drainage of collections
- Decompressive nerve surgery
- Hernia repair
- Symphodesis (dislocated pubis symphysis repair)

Consults
- Obstetrics and gynecology
- Urology
- Gastroenterology
- Colorectal surgery
- Physical medicine and rehabilitation
- Neurology
- Psychiatry
- Pain medicine

Complications/side effects
- Urinary/fecal incontinence
- Chronic pain
- Poor activity tolerance
- Anxiety/depression

Prognosis
- Variable, depends on the primary diagnosis
- Early diagnosis and patient education improve outcome

Helpful Hints
- Meticulous history and physical examination required
- Multidisciplinary approach
- Early use of MRI and appropriate diagnostic tests important to make in reaching an accurate diagnosis

Suggested Readings
Butrick CW. Pelvic floor hypertonic disorders: identification and management. *Obstet Gynecol Clin N Am.* 2009;36(3):707–722.
Prather H, Monaco T, Dugan SA. Recognizing and treating pelvic pain and pelvic floor dysfunction. *Phys Med Rehab Clin N Am.* 2007;18:477–496.

Peroneal Tendon Subluxation

Jonathan S. Halperin MD

Description
Peroneal tendon subluxation is an uncommon form of lateral ankle pain and dysfunction. It was first described in ballet dancers in 1803.

Etiology/Types
- Peroneal tendon subluxation occurs when the superior peroneal retinaculum (SPR) is torn, allowing resultant subluxation/dislocation of the peroneus brevis and longus tendons
- It is more commonly encountered in downhill skiing, ice skating, football, basketball, soccer, and gymnastics
- A surgical classification system had been used but has shown to have no effect on prognosis

Epidemiology
- Estimated to occur in <1% of acute ankle injuries
- More than 90% are due to acute ankle trauma

Pathogenesis
- The peroneous longus and brevis tendons sublux or dislocate from the lateral retromalleolar groove. This results from a tear, or significant laxity of the SPR
- The injury can occur with a sudden reflex contraction of the peroneal muscles during an ankle sprain with inversion and dorsiflexion or forced dorsiflexion of an everted foot (ski boot)

Risk Factors
- Pre-existing lateral ankle instability
- Inadequate or shallow retromalleolar groove
- Laxity of the SPR
- Calcaneovalgus rearfoot

Clinical Features
- Acute: pain, swelling, and bruising over the lateral ankle
- Chronic: painful snapping or popping felt over the posterior/lateral ankle with activity

Natural History
- Initial pain and swelling subside in a similar fashion to a typical ankle inversion sprain
- Pain and instability persist until surgical fixation is performed

Diagnosis
Differential diagnosis
- Lateral ankle instability due to ankle inversion sprain
- Peroneal tendon tear
- Osteochondral lesions of the talar dome
- Tarsal coalition
- Stress fracture of the base of the fifth metatarsal, cuboid, or fibula

History
- Pain and swelling noted behind the lateral malleolus (distal fibula)
- Over time, the patient can develop a painful popping sensation on the lateral ankle with active dorsiflexion and eversion

Exam
- Palpable clicking, snapping, or crepitus is noted over the posterior/lateral ankle with active dorsiflexion, eversion, and circumduction of the ankle
- Acute injuries present with swelling, tenderness, and ecchymosis posterior to the lateral malleolus

Testing
- Weight bearing anteroposterior and lateral radiographs are needed to rule out an acute fracture, or chronic conditions (arthrosis, exostoses, or spuring of the retromalleolar groove). A fracture of the base of the fifth metatarsal can indicate an avulsion of the peroneous brevis tendon
- Magnetic resonance imaging (MRI) is the standard method for evaluating this condition. Multiplanar images provide essential information about the morphology of the retromalleolar groove and the integrity of the SPR and peroneal tendons
- Ultrasonography is gaining popularity in the evaluation of this condition. The positive predictive value approaches 100% in detecting peroneal tendon subluxation

Pitfalls
- This condition is commonly missed on initial injury
- Early surgical treatment is associated with the best long-term outcomes

Red Flags

- Fluoroquinolone use and local steroid injection can lead to tendon rupture
- Rheumatoid arthritis and diabetic neuropathy are associated with tendinopathy and tear

Treatment

Medical

- Initially: rest, ice, compression, elevation, and nonsteroidal anti-inflammatory drugs (NSAIDs)
- Orthopedic Surgery consult is required for persistent symptoms

Exercises

- Similar to those prescribed for acute ankle sprain: gentle motion (avoid forced inversion), isometrics, proprioception, and balance training

Modalities

- Cryotherapy
- Electrical stimulation
- Ultrasound
- Similar to those prescribed for acute ankle sprain

Injection

- Not usually indicated

Surgical

- Repair of the SPR with or without deepening of the fibular groove

Consults

- Orthopedic surgery
- Podiatry

Complications/side effects

- Pain, swelling, and instability if surgical treatment is not pursued

Prognosis

- Excellent if recognized early and surgical repair is considered

Helpful Hints

- Peroneal tendon subluxation should be suspected in any acute ankle sprain
- Early recognition and definitive treatment (surgery) are needed to prevent long-term symptoms

Suggested Readings

Heckman DS, Reddy D, Pedowitiz D, et al. Operative treatment for peroneal tendon disorders. *J Bone Joint Surg Am.* 2008;90(2):404–418.

Rosenfeld P. Acute and chronic peroneal tendon dislocations. *Foot Ankle Clin.* 2007;12(4):643–657.

Pes Anserine Bursitis

Carmen E. López-Acevedo MD ▪ Roxanna Amill MD

Description
Pes anserine bursitis is an inflammatory condition of the medial knee. The anserine bursa lies beneath the pes anserinus, name given to the conjoined tendon of the sartorius, gracilis, and semitendinosus muscle. Actually, the clinical syndrome of anserine bursitis may be a tendinitis or a fasciitis involving the insertion of the tendons. The tendon's name, which literally means "goose's foot," was inspired by the pes anserinus's webbed, foot-like structure.

Etiology/Types
- Overuse, due to abnormal biomechanics
- Trauma

Epidemiology
- Pes anserine bursitis can occur at any age but is common in overweight middle-aged women
- Due to anatomical differences, it is more common in females than in males
- May be associated with osteoarthritis of the knee
- It also occurs in athletes engaged in activities such as running, basketball, and racquet sports
- Pes anserinus syndrome (tendonitis and bursitis) is frequent in long distance runners
- It has been also seen in patients with Type II diabetes mellitus

Pathogenesis
- The pathogenesis of anserine bursitis is unclear, but stress on the bursa aggravated by obesity or osteoarthritic deformity of the knee produces thickening of the synovial lining and subsequent excessive fluid formation, thereby leading to localized swelling and pain

Risk Factors
- Osteoarthritis of the knee
- Obesity
- Genu valgum, flat foot, or pronated foot
- Incorrect training techniques
- Lack of flexibility of hamstrings muscles
- Overuse, repetitive trauma or constant friction on the bursa
- Lack of knee extension
- Patellar malalignment

Clinical Features
- Pain, tenderness, and swelling over the anteromedial aspect of the knee, 2 to 5 cm below the joint line
- Pain increases with knee flexion, exercise, and stairs
- Swelling over the anterior medial tibia, which can be mistaken for a cyst or a mass

Natural History
- Onset of symptoms may be acute or insidious, resulting from overuse

Diagnosis

Differential diagnosis
- Extra-articular cystic lesions or tumors such as synovial cysts, ganglion cysts, parameniscal cysts, pigmented villonodular synovitis, and synovial sarcoma
- Degenerative joint disease
- Proximal tibial stress fracture
- Medial meniscal tear
- Medial collateral ligament injury
- Crystal-induced bursitis
- Inflammatory arthritides
- Knee osteochondritis dissecans
- Saphenous nerve entrapment

History
- Patients may have a history of worsening pain when arising from a seated position or at night
- Patients typically deny pain with walking on level surfaces
- Local swelling may be noted
- History of athletic activity

Exam
- Pain to palpation over the proximal medial tibia at the insertion of the conjoined tendons of the pes anserinus approximately 2 to 5 cm below the anteromedial joint margin of the knee
- The bursa usually is not palpable unless effusion and thickening are present
- Palpable crepitus occasionally is observed

- With the chronic variant in older adults, usually no pain is experienced with flexion or extension of the knee
- Medial joint line tenderness may mimic a meniscal tear
- In the sports-related variant, symptoms may be reproduced with resisted internal rotation and resisted flexion of the knee
- Valgus stress may reproduce the symptoms in athletic individuals, making it hard to distinguish from medial collateral ligament (MCL) injuries. Typically, painful tenderness in association with MCL injuries is superior and posterior to the pes anserine bursa
- If swelling can be traced more proximally along the pes anserinus tendons, a formal tendonitis may be present, and a snapping of the pes anserinus tendons can occur
- An exostosis of the tibia has been described in athletes
- Disuse atrophy and weakness
- Compression of the saphenous nerve and its infrapatellar branch by swelling of the pes anserinus bursa may cause numbness below the patella

Testing
- Complete blood count, erythrocyte sedimentation rate, C-reactive protein
- X-rays anterposterior, lateral, standing
- Ultrasound
- Computed tomography scan
- Magnetic resonance imaging
- Arthrogram
- Aspiration of the bursa

Pitfalls
- Pes anserine bursitis is a clinical diagnosis but high level of suspicion is required for other causes of knee pain, such as medial compartment arthritis, stress fractures, infection, or crystal-induced bursitis and to avoid unnecessary arthroscopy

Red Flags
- Infection
- Fracture
- Neoplasm
- Neurological dysfunction

Treatment
Medical
- Nonsteroidal anti-inflammatory medications
- Analgesics
- Antibiotics if infectious origin

Exercises
- Pes anserine bursitis rehabilitation exercises include:
  - Hamstrings, quadriceps, and calf muscle stretching
  - Quadriceps and hamstrings isometrics
  - Dynamic strengthening
  - Heel slides

Modalities
- Rest, ice, compression, elevation
- Ultrasound
- Transcutaneous electrical nerve stimulation

Injection
- Corticosteroid

Surgical
- Incision and drainage
- Decompression

Consults
- Physical medicine and rehabilitation
- Orthopedic surgeon
- Rheumatologist

Complications
- Chronic bursitis leads to continued pain and antalgic gait
- Weakening of underlying ligaments and/or tendons that can lead to partial tearing and spontaneous rupture

Prognosis
- Good to excellent with compliance to prescribed medical and rehabilitation management
- Pes anserine bursitis is usually a self-limited condition and has few long-term sequelae. In most patients, a 6- to 8-week stretching and exercise program alleviates the symptoms

Helpful Hints
- Pes anserine bursitis is best prevented by a proper warm-up that includes stretching of the hip and thigh muscles and a strengthening program. Gradually increasing the activity level will also help prevent the development of pes anserine bursitis

Suggested Readings
Gnanadesigan N, Smith RL. Knee pain: osteoarthritis or anserine bursitis? *J Am Med Dir Assoc.* 2003;4(3):164–166.
Rennie WJ, Saifuddin A. Pes anserine bursitis: incidence in symptomatic knees and clinical presentation. *Skeletal Radiol.* 2005;34:395.

Piriformis Syndrome

Julio A. Martínez-Silvestrini MD

Description
Piriformis syndrome is an uncommon cause of buttock and hip pain. It is a controversial diagnosis that involves pain in the gluteal region, irritation or inflammation of the sciatic nerve, and leg symptoms.

Etiology/Types
- Intrinsic piriformis muscle (PM) pathology such as myofascial pain
- Anatomical variations
- Muscle hypertrophy
- Trauma
- Associated with sacroiliac joint (SIJ) dysfunction

Epidemiology
- Incidence of 6% to 8% of cases with low back pain
- Female-to-male ratio 6:1

Pathogenesis
- Overuse PM musculotendinous injury
- Rarely, the PM may compress the sciatic nerve (in some persons, the sciatic nerve completely or partially pierces the muscle)

Risk Factors
- SIJ dysfunction
- Lumbar disc disease
- Hip muscle weakness and inflexibility
- Anatomic variants

Clinical Features
- History of local trauma
- Pain localized to SIJ, greater sciatic notch, and PM
- Pain worsened by lifting or bending and relieved by traction
- Palpable sausage-shaped mass in the PM distribution
- Positive Lasegue test
- Atrophy of gluteal muscles

Diagnosis

Differential diagnosis
- Lumbar radiculopathy
- Spinal stenosis
- Facet syndrome
- SIJ dysfunction
- Trochanteric bursitis
- Pelvic floor dysfunction

History
- History of acute trauma or muscle overuse
- Buttock pain that can radiate down the ipsilateral leg

Exam
- Tenderness, or spindle-shaped mass along the course of the PM
- Palpable band with rectal and pelvic examination
- Pain aggravated by hip flexion, adduction, internal rotation (FAIR)
- Most patients will have normal strength and sensation
- Abnormal neurological examination, in cases with sciatic nerve compression
- Special tests
- Pace's maneuver: pain and weakness on resisted hip abduction with flexed hips in the sitting position
- Freiberg's maneuver: pain on forced internal rotation of the extended hip

Testing
- Musculoskeletal ultrasound
- Magnetic resonance imaging
- Electrodiagnostic studies may show prolonged H-reflex or denervation in sciatic nerve-innervated muscles

Pitfalls
- Repetitive nerve compression injuries may result in irreversible muscle atrophy and loss of mobility

Red Flags
- Progressive weakness
- Muscular atrophy

Treatment

Medical
- Nonsteroidal anti-inflammatory drugs
- Muscle relaxants
- Analgesics
- Anticonvulsants
- Antidepressants

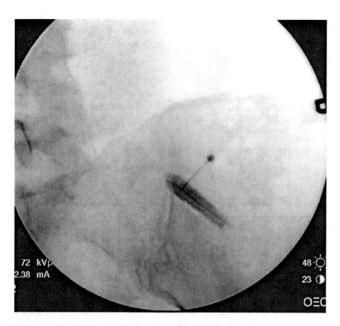

Figure 1. Fluoroscopy guided injection.

Exercises
- Stretching of PM muscle with hip flexion, adduction, and rotation (FAIR position)
- Strengthening of hip abductors, external rotators, and other core muscles
- Back stabilization program

Modalities
- Superficial heat
- Ultrasound
- Vapocoolant spray followed by deep tissue massage

Injection
- Local injections guided by computer tomography, electromyography, fluoroscopy (Figure 1), or ultrasound

- Local anesthetics, steroids, or botulinum toxin can be injected

Surgical
- In recalcitrant cases or with documented anatomic abnormalities
- To reduce the substance of the muscle, dissect or excise part of the muscle

Consults
- Physical medicine and rehabilitation
- Pain medicine
- Orthopedic surgery

Complications
- Leg atrophy
- Sciatic nerve injury
- Chronic pain syndrome

Prognosis
- Good with adequate treatment

Helpful Hints
- Radicular pain originating from the middle of the buttock is very common in patients with this condition
- Males with this syndrome may give a history of carrying their wallet in their back pocket

Suggested Readings
Kirschner JS, Foye PM, Cole JL. Piriformis syndrome, diagnosis and treatment. *Muscle Nerve.* 2009; 40(1):10–18.

Windish G, Braun EM, Anderhuber F. Piriformins muscle: clinical anatomy and consideration of the piriformis syndrome. *Surg Radiol Anat.* 2007;29:37–45.

Plantar Fasciitis

John C. Cianca MD

Description
A common rear foot problem that affects the plantar surface of the foot at the calcaneal origin of the plantar fascia, causing pain and intolerance to running, walking, and jumping

Etiology/Types
- Biomechanical inefficiency or error will cause excessive stretch (stiff feet) or loading (excessive pronation, limited ankle dorsiflexion) on the plantar fascia at its origin on the calcaneus
- Degenerative changes at origin

Epidemiology
- Most common cause of rear foot pain
- Prevalent in obese people
- More prevalent in women

Pathogenesis
- The plantar fascia stabilizes the longitudinal arch of the foot during normal motion of the foot
- During propulsion, the toes dorsiflex creates tension at the distal plantar insertion. The stiff plantar fascia passively pulls on the calcaneus, elevating and shortening the longitudinal arch
- In overpronating feet or with ankles that have limited dorsiflexion, the plantar fascia undergoes excessive weight-bearing force due to increased eversion and abduction
- In stiff feet, the plantar fascia has higher than usual tension placed on it during push off phase of gait
- Poor proximal and distal eccentric control causes further exacerbation

Risk Factors
- Obesity
- Overpronation, particularly when coupled with proximal weakness
- Stiff, cavus feet
- Tight Achilles tendons, limited ankle dorsiflexion

Clinical Features
- Tenderness at the medial plantar calcaneus
- Pain with transitional weight bearing, particularly in the morning and with prolonged standing or walking
- Pain when walking in bare feet or on tip toes

Natural History
- Insidious onset of plantar heel pain during weight bearing
- Associated with rapid increase in running or walking, particularly when hills and speed work are included
- Pain will worsen as weight bearing continues throughout the day or if unusual weight-bearing stress arises
- Chronic symptoms if mechanical or training issues are not corrected
- Tendinopathy changes in chronic cases

Diagnosis

Differential diagnosis
- Calcaneal or talar stress fractures
- Tarsal tunnel syndrome
- Nerve entrapment or S1 radiculopathy
- Plantar fascia avulsion
- Posterior tibialis tendinopathy
- Enthesopathy associated with spondyloarthropathies

History
- Plantar heel pain upon arising in the morning and later in the day
- Worse after running or walking

Exam
- Pain at the medial border of the plantar surface of the calcaneus
- Tenderness along the plantar fascia
- Passive dorsiflexion of the toes and foot causes pain
- Achilles tendons inflexibility, stiff feet, or excessively mobile feet
- Proximal weakness of the hip muscles

Testing
- X-rays to rule out fractures or avulsion, calcaneal spurs can be visualized, often not the cause of the pain
- Diagnostic ultrasound allows visualization of swelling and tissue changes, particularly when compared with the asymptomatic side
- Magnetic resonance imaging (MRI) and bone scan can be helpful if stress fracture is suspected

Pitfalls

- Do not forget to consider S1 radiculopathy particularly in people with a history of back problems
- Negative x-rays can be misleading; MRIs may highlight nonclinical changes
- Overaggressive treatment of bone spurs

Red Flags

- Bruising and swelling are indicative of plantar fascia rupture

Treatment

Medical

- Conservative treatment effective as much as 80% to 90% of the time
- May require weeks of treatment
- Reduce mileage and offending activities such as hill and speed work
- Symptomatic treatment includes ice, massage, and judicious use of pain relievers
- Provide arch support with orthotics, taping, and appropriate shoes
- Night splints may be effective in improving pain (Achilles tendon and plantar fascia flexibility improve, effective in reduction of symptoms)

Exercises

- Eccentric strengthening for proximal and distal muscles
- Correct mechanical deficits
- Functional exercise to improve landing and impact control

Modalities

- Shock wave therapy has been shown to be effective

Injection

- Steroid injections may provide pain relief for a month or so
- Injection of platelet rich plasma may prove effective

Surgical

- Release of the medial one-third of the plantar fascia with release of lateral plantar nerve and removal of spurs indicated for refractory cases

Consults

- Podiatry for orthotic fabrication

Complications/side effects

- Plantar fascia rupture or fat pad atrophy following steroid injections or surgery

Prognosis

- Most cases resolve with conservative treatment and time
- Identifying and correcting mechanical factors and training errors are critical to resolution and to prevention of recurrence

Helpful Hints

- Do not overlook S1 radiculopathy
- Treat the entire kinetic chain as it relates to the activities involved in causing symptoms

Suggested Readings

Barr KP, Harrast MA. Evidence-based treatment of foot and ankle injuries in runners. *Phys Med Rehabil Clin N Am.* 2005;16(3):779–800.

Simmons SM. Foot injuries in the runner. In: O'Connor FG, Wilder RP, eds. *Textbook of Running Medicine.* New York: McGraw-Hill; 2001:213–226.

Posterior Cruciate Ligament Injury

Antonio Soler MD

Description
The posterior cruciate ligament (PCL) is an important stabilizer of the knee joint being the primary restraint to posterior translation of the tibia on the femur, and a secondary restraint to knee external rotation. The understanding of PCL injuries is evolving, yet it lags behind that of anterior cruciate ligament (ACL) injuries. A PCL tear can result in varying degrees of disability, from minimal to severe impairment.

Etiology/Types
- Most commonly injured with a direct blow and posterior-directed force applied to the proximal tibia when the knee is flexed, as in a dashboard injury or striking the ground landing on the knee, with the foot plantar flexed
- Injury can also result from hyperextension, hyperflexion, and rotational stress
- Injury may be isolated or combined with other structures including the posterolateral corner (PLC; lateral collateral ligament, joint capsule, lateral meniscus)

Epidemiology
- Injuries to the PCL are less common than ACL injuries and frequently missed
- Injuries to the PCL have been historically under diagnosed because they are frequently asymptomatic
- The true incidence of PCL injuries remains unknown, but in general comprise between 3% and 20% of all knee ligament injuries

Pathogenesis
- The PCL is the primary restraint to posterior translation of the tibia on the femur and is also a secondary restraint to valgus, varus, and external rotation stress to the knee joint
- Broader and stronger than the ACL and has a tensile strength of 2000 N
- The PCL originates from the lateral border of the medial femoral condyle, and inserts approximately 1 cm below the joint line in a depression between the posterior aspects of the medial and lateral tibial plateaus

- The anatomic complex architecture of the PCL consists of two major reciprocal bundles. The thicker and stronger anterolateral band that becomes tight in flexion and the posteromedial band that conversely tightens in extension. Together, they act as the primary restraint to posterior translation of the tibia, with the collateral ligaments and the PLC acting as secondary restraints

Risk Factors
- Participation in contact sports, cycling, and motor sports
- Motor vehicle accidents

Clinical Features
- Initial presentation of pain with minimal swelling
- Recurrent instability
- Posttraumatic arthritis

Natural History
- Isolated injuries have good functional level
- Secondary meniscal, and patellofemoral injury (associated with abnormal patellofemoral and tibiofemoral joint forces because of posteriorly subluxed tibia)
- Surgical outcomes improving but not as good as ACL reconstruction

Diagnosis

Differential diagnosis
- PCL isolated vs combined lesion
- ACL injury
- Knee dislocation
- Patellar or tibial contusion

History
- Direct impact to proximal anterior tibia
- Contact sports
- Motor vehicle accidents (dashboard injuries)
- Minimal initial swelling
- Recurrent pain

Exam
- Proximal tibia contusion, abrasion
- Tenderness to palpation at the patella or anterior tibia

- Positive posterior drawer test (may be interpreted as a false positive anterior drawer test because of anterior migration of the posteriorly located tibia)
- Sag sign (observe position of the involved tibia and compare with the opposite side, knees and hips should be flexed to 90°)
- Collateral ligament varus valgus stress testing

Testing

- X-rays usually negative but look for avulsion fractures of PCL on posterior tibia and proximal fibula
- Magnetic resonance imaging essential for tear location and associated injuries

Pitfalls

- Diagnosed as ACL tear with false positive anterior drawer test

Red Flags

- Neurovascular injuries may be present and should not be missed

Treatment

Medical

- Nonsteroidal anti-inflammatory medications and analgesics
- Initial immobilization and splinting
- Limited success with functional bracing

Exercises

- Early range of motion and quadriceps strengthening are started as soon as pain permits
- Open-chain hamstring exercises in flexion angles higher than 60° are avoided to prevent any exacerbation of posterior subluxation

Modalities

- Heat
- Ice
- Ultrasound
- Trancutaneous electrical stimulation

Injection

- Rarely indicated

Surgical

- Surgical management is indicated for displaced avulsion fractures and combined ligament injuries
- Differences in surgical techniques, graft choices, single- or double-bundle reconstructions, and fixation methods create a nonuniform approach that causes difficulties in outcome studies

Consults

- Orthopedic surgeon
- Vascular surgery in the case of complications such as vascular injury
- Physical medicine and rehabilitation

Prognosis

- A PCL tear can result in varying degrees of disability, from minimal to severe impairment

Helpful Hints

- Suspect PCL injury in patients, which present with anterior knee trauma with knee in flexion
- Repeat examination after initial pain and swelling subside to document posterior tibial translation in the posterior drawer test

Suggested Readings

McAllister DR, Petrigliano FA. Diagnosis and treatment of posterior cruciate ligament injuries. *Curr Sports Med Rep.* 2007;6(5):293–299.

Schulz MS, Russe K, Weiler A, et al. Epidemiology of posterior cruciate ligament injuries. *Arch Orthop Trauma Surg.* 2003;123(4):186–191.

Wind WM, Bergfeld JA, Parker RD. Evaluation and treatment of posterior cruciate ligament injuries: revisited. *Am J Sports Med.* 2004;32(7):1765–1775.

Posterior Tibial Tendon Dysfunction

Kenneth Cintrón MD

Description

The spectrum of posterior tibial tendon dysfunction (PTTD) is broad, ranging from tenosynovitis to a complete tendon rupture. In the adult, PTTD is the most common cause of acquired flat foot deformity.

Etiology/Types

- Inflammatory synovitis, degenerative rupture, and acute traumatic injury are the most common causes
- Most ruptures are caused by an intrinsic abnormality of the tendon
- Frequently, ruptures occur in a degenerated tendon segment distal to the medial malleolus and corresponding to a zone of hypovascularity
- Classification:
  - Stage I: swelling, tenderness, mild weakness, minimal or no deformity present
  - Stage II: flexible planovalgus foot. The tendon is lengthened or ruptured
  - Stage III: rigid, flat foot deformity is present. Complete tendon degeneration
  - Stage IV: lateral tibiotalar degeneration and valgus ankle angulation

Epidemiology

- Common cause of acquired flatfoot deformity
- Typically affects women in the fourth to sixth decade
- Associated with prolonged standing, walking, and running
- 2.3% to 3.6% of runners seen in sports medicine clinics

Pathogenesis

- Tenosynovitis occurs with chronic, recurrent inflammation
- Fibrous adhesions make the tendon adherent to the inner surface of the tendon sheath
- Later, attenuation, insufficiency, and sometimes complete rupture may be seen

Risk Factors

- Hypertension
- Obesity
- Diabetes mellitus
- Exposure to steroids, local steroid injections
- Previous surgery or trauma about the medial aspect of the foot has been linked to PTTD

Clinical Features

- Swelling, erythema, and tenderness along the course of the tendon
- Pain with prolonged standing and walking
- Progressive deformity of hind foot

Natural History

- Patients with flexible deformity may respond to conservative treatment
- Progressive pain, deformity, and functional deficits if not treated adequately

Diagnosis

Differential diagnosis

- Spring ligament rupture
- Degenerative joint disease of the ankle, talonavicular, or tarsometatarsal joint
- Inflammatory arthritis of the hind foot
- Charcot's joint and neuromuscular injuries

History

- Insidious onset of pain on the medial aspect of the ankle
- Patients may notice swelling and pain along the course of the tendon
- Change in the shape of the foot (hyperpronation) may be identified
- Some describe a sensation of weakness or instability with ambulation

Exam

- Swelling at the medial ankle
- Tight Achilles tendon
- Weak ankle invertors, plantarflexors, and evertors
- "Single-heel rise test"; patient is unable to lift the heel of the ground on the metatarsal heads due to pain along the PTT
- "Double-heel rise test"; the affected heel will not swing into varus when the patient rises on the metatarsal heads
- "Too many toes sign"; more toes are seen lateral to the outer border of the leg on the involved foot when viewing the patient from behind

Testing
- X-rays: anteroposterior and lateral weight-bearing radiographs of foot and ankle
- Ultrasound can identify tendinopathy and peritendinitis
- Magnetic resonance imaging (MRI) provides clear details of abnormalities of the PTT, allows identification of partial and full thickness tears; however, it is used too frequently in clinical practice

Pitfalls
- Not treating the symptoms early
- Allowing progressive deformity of the foot

Red Flags
- Severe symptoms despite treatment
- Rigid deformity

Treatment

Medical
- Anti-inflammatory medication
- Orthoses such as the University of California at Berkley brace
- Short leg walking cast, or cast boot—short term for acute exacerbation or in early treatment

Exercises
- Achilles tendon stretching
- Ankle muscle strengthening (invertors, evertors, dorsiflexors, and plantarflexors)
- Foot intrinsic muscle strengthening (toe-curling exercises)
- Proprioception training
- Bicycle, aquatic exercises

Modalities
- Cryotherapy
- Superficial heat
- Ultrasound
- Electrical stimulation
- Soft tissue laser

Injection
- Local steroid injections can be used in the initial stages of tenosynovitis, pain, and swelling
- Repeated injections may weaken the tendon

Surgical
- Operative treatment is indicated after failed conservative measures
- Consists of rebalancing the foot by means of tendon transfers or lengthening, osteotomies, or joint fusions

Consults
- Orthopedic/foot-ankle surgery
- Physical medicine and rehabilitation

Complications/side effects
- Progressive flatfoot deformity
- Chronic ankle and foot pain

Prognosis
- Variable
- Flexible deformities diagnosed early may improve with nonsurgical treatment

Helpful Hints
- Evaluate patient for flexible deformities of the hindfoot
- These may respond to flexibility and strengthening programs, combined with orthoses

Suggested Readings

Mann RA. Flat foot in adults. In: Coughlin MJ, Mann RA, eds. *Surgery of the Foot and Ankle*. 7th ed. Vol. 1. St. Louis: Mosby Inc.; 1999:733–767.

Meehan RE, Brage M. Adult acquired flat foot deformity: clinical and radiographic examination. *Foot Ankle Clin N Am*. 2003;8:431–452.

Wilder RP, Sethi S. Overuse injuries: tendinopathies, stress fractures, compartment syndrome, and shin splits. *Clin Sports Med*. 2004;23:55–81.

Proximal Interphalangeal Joint Dislocation

Juan A. González MD ■ Carmen J. Martínez-Martínez MD

Description

Finger anatomy is very complex since many anatomical structures are localized in a small area. Fingers are composed of proximal, middle, and distal phalanges and three hinged joints: distal interphalangeal (DIP), proximal interphalangeal (PIP), and metacarpophalangeal (MCP). The thumb has a distal and proximal phalanx as well as an interphalangeal and MCP joint. Also, fingers have associated neurovascular structures, tendons, and lateral bands, which may be injured due to trauma (Figure 1).

Etiology/Types

- Usually sports-related
- Associated with a blow to the finger
- PIP dislocations are classified by the position of the distal phalanx
- There are three types of PIP dislocations:
  - Dorsal dislocation is associated with forced hyperextension of the finger. This kind of dislocation represents a major ligament injury
  - Volar dislocation (palmar dislocation) occurs when there is forced hyperflexion of the finger. Is a rare form of dislocation and usually irreducible
  - Lateral dislocation happens when there is a blow in either ulnar or radial direction

Epidemiology

- PIP joint dislocations are the most common hand dislocations
- Dorsal dislocations the most frequent

Pathogenesis

- PIP dislocations result after forced hyperextension or hyperflexion combined with axial loading of the finger
- Associated fractures can be seen

Risk Factors

- Contact and ball sports

Clinical Features

- Swelling and tenderness over PIP joint
- Inability to extend the joint

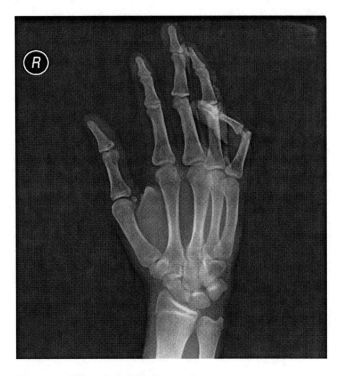

Figure 1. Fifth digit PIP dislocation.

Natural History

- Long-term prognosis after reduction is good
- Stiffness, swelling, and pain can persist for months
- Does not recur unless the finger is hyperextended or hyperflexed again

Diagnosis

Differential diagnosis

- Phalangeal fracture
- Collateral ligament injury

History

- Direct blow to finger, "jamming injury" during sports-related activity or due to a fall

Exam

- Gross deformity of the joint associated with swelling and tenderness
- Decreased range of motion of the joint
- Thorough neurovascular examination of the finger and complete hand

Testing

- Adequate examination is composed of three x-ray views of the hand: anteroposterior, true lateral, and oblique
- X-rays show displacement of the middle phalanx on the proximal phalanx
- Assess for any associated fractures

Pitfalls

- Undiagnosed neurovascular compromise
- Missing dorsal hood injury

Treatment

Medical

- Closed reduction of the dislocation after digital block anesthesia
- For dorsal dislocation, closed reduction can be performed by hyperextension, traction, and then gentle flexion of the joint
- Volar dislocation can be reduced by traction and manipulation of the middle phalanx while the metacarpophalangeal joint is held in flexion (which relaxes lateral bands)
- In the case of lateral dislocation, simple longitudinal traction will reduce the dislocation
- Evaluate active and passive movement after reduction
- Assess neurovascular function after reduction
- Immobilization by buddy taping, or splinting with PIP in slight flexion (20° to 30°) can be used
- Postreduction radiographs must be obtained
- Nonsteroidal anti-inflammatory drugs and analgesics should be given to treat the pain

Exercises

- Early mobilization/active motion

Modalities

- Cryotherapy
- Paraffin bath

Injection

- Digital block anesthesia for closed reduction

Surgical

- In cases where closed reduction is not possible, open reduction is required

Consults

- Orthopedic/hand surgeon evaluation maybe required if:
  - Avulsion fracture is present in dorsal dislocations
  - Neurovascular compromise after reduction is present
  - Joint instability present
  - Unsuccessful closed reduction

Complications

- Development of boutonniere and swan neck deformities in volar and dorsal dislocations, respectively
- Redislocation if inadequate immobilization is used
- Loss of joint mobility or instability

Prognosis

- Excellent prognosis if adequate reduction/ immobilization and orthopedic evaluation is performed

Suggested Readings

Chinchalkar SJ, Siang GB. Management of proximal interphalangeal joint fractures and dislocations. *J Hand Ther.* 2003;16(2):117–128.

Graham TJ, Mullen DJ. Athletic injuries of the adult hand section B. In: DeLee JC, Drez's D, eds. *Orthopaedic Sports Medicine: Principles and Practice.* 2nd ed. Philadelphia: Elsevier Science; 2003:1381–1431.

Kiefhaber TR, Stern PJ. Fracture dislocations of the proximal interphalangeal joint. *J Hand Surg.* 1998;23(3):368–380.

Quadriceps Contusion

David J. Kennedy MD ■ Joshua D. Rittenberg MD

Description

A frequent injury that is the result of a traumatic impact to the anterior, lateral, or medial thigh resulting in deep muscular bleeding and bruising.

Etiology/Types

- Results from a direct blow to the anterior, medial, or lateral thigh
- Rectus femoris is the most common injured muscle due to its anterior location
- Injury severity graded based on knee flexion range of motion
  - Mild: >120°
  - Moderate: between 90° and 120°
  - Severe: <90°

Epidemiology

- Contusion, second most common sports injury next to sprains/stains
- Exact prevalence is unknown as majority of injured persons do not seek medical care
- Highest prevalence in football, although higher per year incidence in other contact sports such as: rugby 4.7%, judo 2.3%, football 1.6%, all other sports <1%

Pathogenesis

- Quadriceps is in contact with the femur throughout its length, making it susceptible to compression forces
- Impact causes muscle fiber and connective tissue rupture
- Capillary disruption occurs leading to localized hemorrhage with hematoma formation and associated edema of the muscle
- Inflammatory cells and macrophages enter the site of injury and begin clearing necrotic muscle cells over 2 to 3 days after injury, followed by muscle cell regeneration and scar tissue formation

Risk Factors

- Contact sports
- Muscle fatigue

Clinical Features

- History of trauma
- Painful anterior thigh, especially with weight bearing and knee flexion
- Tense anterior compartment
- Swelling, stiffness, bruising, and impaired function and range of motion delayed 24 to 48 hours

Natural History

- Gradually worsens over first 24 to 48 hours
- Most are asymptomatic within few weeks and able to return to sports
- May develop into myositis ossificans, a form of heterotopic ossifications

Diagnosis

Differential diagnosis

- Quadriceps strain, overuse, or rupture
- Femoral/hip fracture
- Compartment syndrome
- Fascial rupture with muscle hernia
- Slipped capital femoral epiphysis
- Spine referred pain
- Myositis ossificans
- Deep vein thrombosis
- Soft tissue tumors

History

- Trauma
- Gradual worsening of symptoms over the following 24 to 48 hours

Exam

- Physical examination shows normal medial and posterior thigh with tender, tensely edematous anterior thigh and possible increased circumference of affected thigh
- Lower extremity neurovascular examination

Testing

- Laboratories generally not indicated, in severe cases in patients on anticoagulation order creatine kinase, hematocrit, and coagulation studies

- If patient develops spontaneous edema or is on anticoagulants, consider coagulation studies
- Compartment pressure measurements
- Imaging not indicated in mild injuries with clear history
- At 3 to 4 weeks if not painless full range of motion, consider plain films to rule out fracture or tissue calcification
- Magnetic resonance imaging (MRI) more useful than computed tomography scan, however, neither usually indicated; and if obtained imaging findings lag behind functional recovery
- Ultrasound shows some utility, although no clear indications at this time

Pitfalls
- Delay in diagnosis
- Development of myositis ossificans 2 to 3 months postinjury
- Missing a rupture

Red Flags
- Disproportionately high level of pain triggers suspicion of compartment syndrome
- Abnormal sensation in distal lower extremity, must consider nerve injury
- Failure to heal or sudden loss of range of motion, consider myositis ossificans
- Lower extremity extensor lag may indicate quadriceps tear
- Inability to perform active straight-leg raise or knee extension may indicate disruption of the extensor mechanism

Treatment

Medical
- Compression, ice, rest to prevent hemorrhage in first 24 to 48 hours
- Immobilize knee in 120° of flexion for 24 hours with non-weight-bearing status
- Avoid nonsteroidal anti-inflammatory drugs (NSAIDs) in first 72 hours due to potential of increased bleeding
- Early use of NSAIDs for muscular injuries may interfere with the inflammatory response and thus delay healing; however, with a loss of range of motion, a short course of NSAIDs may be warranted in later stages to prevent myositis ossificans
- Corticosteroids not indicated

- Anabolic steroids may be helpful in muscle healing but not currently used

Exercises
- Discontinue 120° of flexion at 24 hours and begin active pain-free quadriceps motion with a focus on achieving knee flexion
- Gradual return to strengthening and weight bearing as tolerated
- Return to sports only when pain-free full range of motion is obtained

Modalities
- Ice to affected area for 20 minutes every 2 to 3 hours for first 24 to 48 hours
- No ultrasound or heat therapy
- A hard shell protective pad larger than the injury site should be worn over the contused area for the duration of the season

Injections
- None indicated

Surgical
- Operative findings for compartment syndrome of the thigh are usually benign, suggesting most cases can be handled nonoperatively
- Myositis ossificans: surgery indicated as symptoms persist but should wait 6 to 12 months prior to surgical excision to allow bone to fully mature
- Partial intrasubstance tear of the rectus femoris that do not improve with a rehabilitation program, may be candidates for surgical repair of the tear
- Quadriceps muscle hernias do not usually meet the criteria for surgery

Consults
- Orthopedic surgery when a concern for compartment syndrome exists

Complications/side effects
- Acute compartment syndrome
- Myositis ossificans occurs an a rate of approximately 9% and increases with injury severity
- Initial factors that lead to increased risk of development of myositis ossificans includes: initial range of motion <120°, repeat injury to quadriceps, knee effusion, football injury, and treatment delayed >3 days

Prognosis

- If treated properly, a full recovery is expected, although recovery times vary with injury severity
- Treatment may require excision of heterotrophic bone formation, although most people return to full activity without special treatment
- Average return to play of 13 days for mild injury, 19 days for moderate injury, and 21 days for severe injury

Helpful Hints

- If not progressing consider myositis ossificans
- MRI findings lag behind functional outcomes

- Compartment syndrome in thigh is rare, and can usually be managed nonoperatively

Suggested Readings

Almekinders LC. Anti-inflammatory treatment of muscular injuries in sport. An update of recent studies. *Sports Med.* 1999;28(6):383–388.

Alonso A, Hekeik P, Adams R. Predicting a recovery time from the initial assessment of a quadriceps contusion injury. *Aust J Physiother.* 2000;46(3):167–177.

Aronen JG, Garrick JG, Chronister RD, McDevitt ER. Quadriceps contusions: clinical results of immediate immobilization in 120 degrees of knee flexion. *Clin J Sport Med.* 2006;16(5):383–387.

Radial Epiphyseal Injury

William Micheo MD ■ Harry Alverio Rodriguez MD

Description

Physeal injuries of the distal radius occur most frequently in the growing child or adolescent, as a result of excessive forces applied to the upper extremity. This type of injury can be seen in athletes who participate in gymnastics, cheerleading, diving, ice skating, roller skating, hockey, skateboarding, and weightlifting.

Etiology/Types

- Acute injuries: mechanical overload to the physeal plate, such as a fall on an outstretched hand
- Overuse injuries: repetitive dorsiflexion and axial loading result in distal radius physeal injuries

Epidemiology

- Incidence of physeal injury in boys is twice than that in girls and most likely secondary to trauma
- Peak incidence during early adolescence
- Bilateral in one-third of the cases
- Fifteen percent to 30% of long bone injuries involve the physeal plate
- Ten percent to 30% have been reported to be sports-related
- Distal radial physis is the most common site of physeal injury
- Seen in athletes that have heavier training schedules (35 hours/week)
- Chronic wrist pain in 79% of young gymnasts
- Injuries in 2.7 per 100 participants per year in gymnastics
- Female gymnasts are more affected between 12 and 14 years of age
- Prevalence in gymnastics between 8% and 42%

Pathogenesis

- Acute trauma
- Falling with an outstretched hand causes mechanical overload to the wrist with separation of the hypertrophic zone and the metaphyseal bone
- Chronic trauma
- Repetitive dorsiflexion and axial loading induces temporary metaphyseal ischemia that may prevent cartilage calcification, causing physis to widen

- As the growth plate widens, the distal radial physis develops microfracture, which may result in growth impairment
- Physeal fractures typically occur through the zone of provisional calcification but may traverse several zones
- Compressive forces affect the normal endochondral process of ossification on the metaphyseal side of the physis
- Tension forces affect the proliferative zone

Risk Factors

- Age: children and adolescents
- Immature physeal plate
- High repetitive wrist dorsiflexion
- Axial loading to upper extremities
- Increased training intensity
- Sports with high mechanical load to wrist joints
- Acute traumatic event is more in boys than in girls

Clinical Features

- Acute trauma
- Progressive wrist pain after trauma to the wrist
- Swelling, erythema, and pain to touch around the circumference of the wrist
- Decreased range of motion of the wrist
- Chronic trauma
- Pain on the dorsal side of the wrist that worsens with workout
- Pain decreases with suspension of the offending activities
- Radial wrist pain that occurs with passive and active wrist hyperextension activities

Natural History

- In acute injuries, there is development of acute pain in the wrist associated with swelling and/or wrist deformity after a fall
- In chronic injuries, the growth plate widens under repeated stress; prolonged exposure to mechanical loads leads to distal radial physeal fracture; finally, bone growth is affected resulting in positive ulnar variance

Diagnosis

Differential diagnosis
- Distal fracture of the ulna or radius
- Soft tissue contusion
- Wrist impingement
- Metacarpal fractures
- Scaphoid fracture
- De Quervain's tenosynovitis

History
- Trauma to the long bones, joint dislocation, or ligament injury
- Landing on outstretched arm resulting in pain, swelling, and wrist deformity
- Chronic lesions usually present with pain of the wrist during activity, which may persist after activity and affect activities of daily living
- Change to more intense activity, change in sport technique or equipment
- Isolated involvement of the wrists and no other joints, which may require evaluation for malignancy, juvenile rheumatoid arthritis, or infectious process

Exam
- Tenderness or focal pain around the circumference of the distal radius
- In chronic injury, tenderness involves the dorsal, radial, and volar aspect of the physis
- Painful limitation of wrist range of motion
- Pain with axial loading

Testing
- X-rays of the wrist with comparative views of the contralateral extremity
- If suspected and initial negative x-rays, stress radiographs should be considered
- Radiographs show with widening of the growth plate, haziness of the physis, cystic changes on the metaphyseal side of the growth plate, and a beaked effect of the distal aspect of the epiphysis on the radial and volar sides pointing toward the physeal plate
- Salter-Harris classification of fractures
  - Type I: involves the hypertrophic zone of the physis
  - Type II: involves the physis and the metaphysis, but the epiphysis is not involved
  - Type III: affects the physis and the epiphysis
  - Type IV: affects the intra-articular region
  - Type V: is a compression or crush injury of the epiphyseal plate with no associated epiphyseal or metaphyseal fracture
  - Type VI: damage to the perichondral ring
- Staging system for chronic trauma
  - Stage I: clinical diagnosis
  - Stage II: physeal widening, irregular and cystic changes involving the metaphyseal, beaked distal epiphysis, and indistinct physeal appearance
  - Stage III: positive ulnar variance
- Bone scan to assess for stress fractures
- Magnetic resonance imaging (MRI) to assess for bone edema, stress reaction, and stress fracture

Pitfalls
- May be confused with soft tissue injury

Red Flags
- Infection
- Fracture
- Neoplasm
- Neurological dysfunction

Treatment

Medical
- Non-narcotic pain management
- Rest from causative activity
- Salter-Harris Types I and II fractures can be treated with closed reduction and immobilization

Exercises
- Gentle assisted range of motion and stretching
- Static wrist extensor strengthening
- Progressive strengthening as pain decreases, avoidance of axial loading until pain free

Modalities
- Heat
- Ice
- Transcutaneous electrical nerve stimulation

Injection
- Not indicated

Surgical
- Salter-Harris Types III and IV physeal injuries require anatomic reduction. Type IV injuries require accurate alignment to prevent bony bridges
- Salter-Harris Types V and VI: early diagnosis can be delayed, diagnosed mostly when bony bridge is seen across the physis
- In chronic stress injuries, if conservative measures fail, orthopedic evaluation is recommended for wrist arthroscopy in order to debride or repair the triangular fibrocartilage complex lesions

- Ulnar shortening osteotomy may be the procedure of choice if the young athlete exhibits ulnar positive variance

Consults
- Orthopedic surgery
- Physical medicine and rehabilitation

Complications/side effects
- Wrist deformities
- Progressive pain and dysfunction
- Growth arrest (may be seen in those with more severe injury; gymnasts may present with premature closure of the radius physis)
- Ulnar positive variance
- Ulnocarpal impingement

Prognosis
- Salter-Harris Types I, II, and III have an excellent prognosis

- Salter-Harris Types IV and V have poor prognosis

Helpful Hints
- In traumatic injury in a growing child, a physeal injury must be ruled out
- Repetitive dorsiflexion and axial loading of the wrist in sports in which the upper extremity is weight-bearing results in injury to the distal radial physis

Suggested Readings
Cannata G, De Maio F, Mancini F, Ippolito E. Physeal fractures of the distal radius and ulna: long-term prognosis. *J Orthop Trauma.* 2003;17(3):172–179.

DiFiori JP, Caine DJ, Malina RM. Wrist pain, distal radial physeal injury, and ulnar variance in the young gymnast. *Am J Sports Med.* 2006;34(5):840–849.

Shanmugam C, Maffulli N. Sports injuries in children. *Br Med Bull.* 2008;86:33–57.

Radial Head Fractures

Francisco M. López-González MD FAAOS

Description
The radial head is fractured in approximately 20% of elbow trauma cases.

Etiology/Types
- Usually result from fall into the outstretched hand
- May be isolated or associated with complex injuries around the elbow, fractures of the coronoid process of the ulna, ulnar collateral ligament tears, interosseous membrane disruption (Essex Lopresti) lesion
- Type I: minimally displaced fracture, no mechanical block to forearm rotation, intra-articular displacement <2 mm
- Type II: fracture displaced >2 mm or angulated, possible mechanical block to forearm rotation
- Type III: severely comminuted fracture, mechanical block to motion
- Type IV: radial fracture with associated elbow dislocation

Epidemiology
- All fractures from 1.5% to 4%
- Thirty-three percent of all elbow fractures
- Involved in 20% of elbow trauma cases
- Present in 5% to 10% of elbow dislocations
- Eighty-five percent occur in adults 20 to 60 years of age
- Male-to-female ratio 2:3, as the age increases about 50, the number of female patients becomes significantly higher than males

Pathogenesis
- Fall with abducted arm between 0° and 80° of flexion
- Valgus—pronation force transmitted around proximal radius to the elbow—radial head is pushed against the capitellum
- Capitellum articular cartilage may be damaged as well

Risk Factors
- Female predominance 3:2
- Stair climbing (falls)
- Working or standing over unstable objects (falls)

Clinical Features
- Elbow can rarely be extended in acute phase (hemarthrosis)
- Pain limits arc of motion flexion/extension/pronation/supination
- Elbow locking or catching can be present
- Wrist pain can be present due to interosseous membrane damage

Natural History
- Good long-term results for uncomplicated radial head fractures
- Radiographic arthritis on displaced fractures/articular cartilage damage
- Variable degrees of loss of motion can be expected with increasing fracture severity
- Associated injuries can lead to instability and/or stiffness

Diagnosis

Differential diagnosis
- Elbow muscle strain or ligament tear
- Synovitis
- Congenital dislocation of the radial head

History
- Fall on outstretched hand
- Elbow pain and swelling after fall

Exam
- Limited motion of elbow
- Elbow swelling
- Tenderness over radiocapitellar joint
- "Click" with rotation can be present

Testing
- Anteroposterior (AP)/lateral (LAT) x-ray of elbow
- AP projection perpendicular to radial head
- AP/LAT x-rays of wrist to evaluate distal radioulnar joint
- Computed tomography scan may be helpful in defining comminution and degree of displacement

Pitfalls
- Contracture, occasional pain, and inflammation are common

- Osteochondral fractures of capitellum may cause poor result for otherwise benign appearing radial head fracture
- Missed associated ligament or bone injuries

Red Flags

- Wrist pain with proximal fragment migration on x-rays associated with interosseous membrane injury and longitudinal instability of forearm

Treatment

- Principal goal: maintain good elbow function and thus retain adequate motion and stability
- Based on fracture type and the presence of any associated injury

Medical

- Type I: undisplaced fractures: brief period of immobilization 7 to 10 days followed by active range of motion (ROM) as swelling and pain decrease
- Static adjustable orthoses for contractures

Exercises

- Early active assistive ROM (AAROM) of elbow with endpoint stretching
- Stretch pronation, supination, flexion, and extension
- Avoid loading of joint—pushing or pulling with arm or lifting more than 10 lbs, in first 3 months

Modalities

- Cryotherapy
- Heat
- Transcutaneous electrical nerve stimulation
- Ultrasound

Injection

- Xylocaine injection after hematoma aspiration decrease pain and help examination

Surgical

- Type II: (controversial). Evaluation of mechanical block important in final treatment decision. If mechanical block present with <70° pronation/70° supination, then repair with small screws and/or plates
- Type III: comminuted fractures. Radial head excision for isolated injuries, contraindicated if concomitant

ulnar collateral ligament injury, or interosseous membrane injury, in these repair with small plates and screws. Radial head replacement may be needed if not able to reconstruct the radial head
- Type IV: fracture dislocation. Associated with ulnar collateral, lateral ulnar collateral or coronoid fractures. Radial head should be preserved or replaced

Consults

- Orthopedic surgeon
- Physical medicine and rehabilitation

Complications/side effects

- Pain
- Loss of motion
- Instability or non union of fracture
- Arthritis (posttraumatic)
- Complex regional pain syndrome

Prognosis

Variable, depending on fracture type:
- Good results expected in 86% to 100% of patients
- Type II good. Satisfactory results in 90% of cases. Loss of motion 10° to 15° usually seen
- Type IV fair. Loss of elbow flexion and rotation on average of 20° usually seen. Seventy-five percent satisfactory results. Higher incidence of heterotopic bone

Helpful Hints

- Serial x-rays are needed to confirm elbow reduction
- Associated coronoid and ligament injuries are very common
- Isolated radial head fracture "rare"

Suggested Readings

Kaas L, van Riet RP, Vroemen JP, et al. The epidemiology of radial head fractures. *J Shoulder Elbow Surg.* 2010;19(4):520–523.

Roidis N, Papdakis S, Rigopoulus N, et al. Current concepts and controversies in the management of radial head fractures. *Orthopedics.* 2006;29(10):904–916.

Tejwani N, Mehta H. Fractures of the radial head and neck: current concepts in management. *J Am Acad Orthop Surg.* 2007;15:380–387.

Radial Neuropathy

Jayson Takata MD

Description

The radial nerve is derived from the C5 to C8 nerve roots and includes contributions from all three trunks of the brachial plexus before merging into the posterior cord. Less common entrapment neuropathy compared with median and ulnar nerves.

Etiology/Types

- Axilla: pressure palsy, missile injury
- Upper arm: pressure palsy, tourniquet, humerus fracture, injections, scar/fracture callus, neoplasm, hereditary neuropathy with liability to pressure palsies, multifocal motor neuropathy
- Posterior interosseous: radius fracture/dislocation, soft tissue mass, iatrogenic, idiopathic, elbow deformity, rheumatoid synovitis, ganglion cyst, radial tunnel syndrome, supinator syndrome
- Superficial radial: compression (handcuffs, casts, wristwatch band), trauma, de Quervain's surgery, intravenous needles, nerve tumors (also known as Wartenberg syndrome or Cheiralgia paresthetica)

Epidemiology

- More often involved in traumatic injuries to the arm compared with the median and ulnar nerves

Pathogenesis

- Compression, traction, or laceration of the nerve causing focal demyelination and axonal degeneration

Risk Factors

- Extreme fatigue, alcohol, excessive sedation, and general anesthesia increase risk of compression neuropathy
- Bone callus following fracture may cause nerve compression or entrapment

Clinical Features

- Upper arm lesion: usually painless weakness of wrist and digit extensors with numbness in the superficial radial nerve distribution
- Posterior interosseous lesion: weakness of wrist and digit extensors without numbness. Pain in extensor region of the forearm with radial tunnel syndrome
- Superficial radial lesion: numbness or pain in the dorsoradial surface of the wrist, hand, thumb, index, middle and ring fingers. Strength normal

Natural History

- Pressure palsies that occur during sleep, coma, or anesthesia usually recover in 6 to 8 weeks
- Tourniquet injuries usually recover in several months
- Closed fractures of the humerus: 75% recover spontaneously
- Complex fractures of the humerus: nerve is frequently entrapped and may require early surgical exploration

Diagnosis

Differential diagnosis

- C7 radiculopathy
- Posterior cord brachial plexopathy
- Rupture of the tendons of the thumb and finger extensors
- Focal lesions of the precentral motor cortex

History

- Usually painless onset of wrist and finger drop with or without numbness and paresthesias in the superficial radial nerve distribution
- Posterior interosseous neuropathy may be painful without numbness

Exam

- Proximal radial neuropathy: weakness of triceps, brachioradialis, extensor muscles of the wrist/thumb/fingers and numbness in the dorsolateral region of the hand and first three digits
- Posterior interosseous neuropathy: weakness of the finger and thumb extensors at the metacarpophalangeal joint, radial deviation with wrist extension (weakness of extensor carpi ulnaris), and normal sensation
- Superficial radial neuropathy: sensory disturbance in dorsolateral region of the hand and first three digits, normal strength, positive Tinel's sign

Testing

- Electrodiagnosis

- Radial sensory nerve action potential amplitude reduced with some proximal radial neuropathies and most superficial radial neuropathies
- Radial sensory distal latency may be prolonged with superficial radial neuropathies
- Radial motor conduction studies may reveal reduced compound muscle action potential amplitude and/or conduction block
- Electromyography reveals denervation in radial innervated muscles distal to the lesion
- Radiographs to evaluate for elbow joint abnormalities
- Magnetic resonance imaging to evaluate nerve at the arcade of Frohse and possible cysts/tumors

Pitfalls
- Radial nerve lesions may cause a false sense of grip weakness, which may lead to incorrect suspicion of median nerve injury

Red Flags
- Delayed onset of neuropathy following fracture may indicate nerve entrapment in fracture callus or scar tissue

Treatment

Medical
- Dynamic wrist-hand-finger orthosis with stabilization of the wrist and extension of the fingers
- Occupational/hand therapist for activities of daily living, equipment evaluation, and fine motor skills
- Educate patient to avoid constricting clothing or accessories (eg, tight watchband), forceful elbow movements

Exercises
- Range of motion of wrist and fingers to prevent contractures
- Gentle stretches and submaximal strengthening of affected muscles

Modalities
- Cryotherapy
- Heat
- Electrical stimulation

Injection
- Corticosteroid and anesthetic injections for entrapment of superficial radial nerve
- Intra-articular steroid injections for nerve lesions affected by the joint

Surgical
- Surgical exploration if no recovery in 8 to 10 weeks following fracture or dislocation
- Surgical excision if mass is compressing the nerve
- Suture or grafting of nerve if lacerated
- Tendon transfer procedures to provide digit extension if suture or grafting fails

Consults
- Neurosurgery
- Hand surgery
- Occupational/hand therapist

Complications/side effects
- Radial nerve laceration may develop painful neuroma

Prognosis
- Majority of lesions resolve spontaneously
- Lesions that are a result of complex fractures, dislocations, and orthopedic procedures have a guarded prognosis and may require surgical exploration
- Slower recovery with significant axonal degeneration on electromyography

Helpful Hints
- Triceps muscle is spared with lesions at the spiral groove of the humerus

Suggested Readings
Freimer M, Brushart TM, Cornblath DR, et al. Entrapment neuropathies. In: Mendell JR, Kissel JT, Cornblath DR, eds. *Diagnosis and Management of Peripheral Nerve Disorders.* New York: Oxford; 2001:614–621.
Stewart JD. Radial nerve. In: Stewart J, ed. *Focal Peripheral Neuropathies.* Philadelphia: Lippincott Williams & Wilkins; 2000:281–305.

Rotator Cuff Tendinopathy

Brian J. Krabak MD MBA ■ Maureen Noh, MD

Description

Rotator cuff tendinopathy describes a degenerative overuse injury of the muscles about the shoulder joint that can lead to pain and dysfunction.

Etiology/Types

- Repetitive use causes microtears in the tendons of the rotator cuff (supraspinatus, infraspinatus, teres minor, and subscapularis). This leads to a decrease in local blood flow to the tendons, resulting in decreased tensile strength, increased risk of tears, and shoulder dysfunction
- There may be higher risk of injury if there is initial glenohumeral laxity, imbalanced strength or range of motion of the shoulder and scapula, or bony abnormalities

Epidemiology

- Most common cause of nontraumatic shoulder pain
- Prevalence of shoulder pain is approximately 20% in the general population
- Sixty percent to 75% of shoulder pain is attributed to rotator cuff disease
- Incidence increases with aging and repetitive overhead activities
- Evidence of degeneration increases after 40 years of age with peak incidence between 40 and 60 years of age
- Specific athletes at risk include swimmers, baseball pitchers, and tennis players

Pathogenesis

- Rotator cuff muscles originate on the scapula and insert on the humeral head; they are at risk for impingement as they pass underneath the coracromial arch and subacromial bursa, and over the glenohumeral joint
- Repetitive overuse (submaximal loading) leads to local decreased blood flow to the tendons, making them more susceptible to degeneration
- Chronic changes occur within tendons, including angiofibrotic hyperplasia

- Continued use of the degenerative tendon can lead to subsequent tearing
- In evaluation of tissue histology, inflammation is not seen; thus described as "tendinopathy" instead of "tendonitis"

Risk Factors

- Increasing age
- Repetitive overhead activities in sports or occupation
- Bony abnormalities including hooked acromion, spurs at the acromion, clavicle, or AC joint
- Shoulder trauma
- Glenohumeral instability
- Imbalance in strength or flexibility at the shoulder
- Poor lower body mechanics in a closed kinetic chain, leading to increased stresses at the shoulder

Clinical Features

- Anterolateral shoulder pain with movement, especially overhead activities
- Weakness
- Stiffness

Natural History

- Degeneration leads to pain and shoulder dysfunction, placing increased stresses on the shoulder
- Continued overuse can lead to tear of the tendon

Diagnosis

Differential diagnosis

- Bursitis, especially of the subacromial bursa
- Rotator cuff tear
- Arthritis of the acromioclavicular (AC) joint
- Adhesive capsulitis (frozen shoulder)
- Bicipital tendonitis
- Cervical radiculopathy
- Cardiac referred pain
- Infection
- Fracture
- Neoplasm

History

- Anterolateral shoulder pain, worse with movement, overhead activities, and at night (relative area of ischemia seen in the rotator cuff with the arm at the side)
- Weakness and stiffness
- Crepitus
- Usually insidious onset, although may have history of trauma

Exam

- May have atrophy of deltoid, supraspinatus, and infraspinatus, if severe
- Painful arc between 60° and 120° of shoulder abduction
- Passive range of motion usually normal; active range of motion limited in flexion, abduction, internal and/or external rotation
- Weakness particularly of the supraspinatus ("empty can" test) and external rotators
- Positive impingement: Hawkins-Kennedy (pain with flexion of the shoulder to 90° and internal rotation), and Neer (reproduction of symptoms with forward flexion with the forearm in supination)
- Scapular instability with winging

Testing

- Plain films may show osteoarthritis or calcific changes of the supraspinatus tendon or subacromial bursa

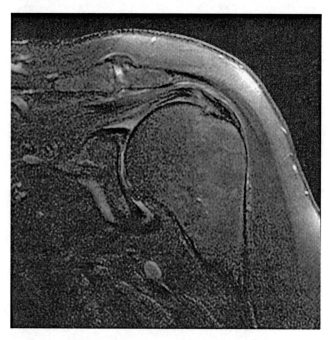

Figure 1. T2 fat saturated image shows increased signal on the undersurface of the supraspinatus tendon suggesting a tendonopathy.

- Magnetic resonance imaging (MRI) (Figure 1) better defines the capsular anatomy, tendons, bursae, and areas of impingement (sensitivity 98%, specificity 36%), especially if concern for tear (sensitivity and specificity for tear nearly 100% with the addition of intra-articular gadolinium)
- Diagnostic ultrasound by an experienced technician has a diagnostic accuracy of 77% to 95% in diagnosis of rotator cuff tear
- Complete blood count and sedimentation rate if concern for infection

Pitfalls

- Consider further imaging of neck and electrodiagnostics if concern for cervical disease
- Corticosteroid injections inhibit collagen biosynthesis and may be detrimental to tendons

Red Flags

- Constitutional symptoms concerning for neoplasm or infection
- Neurological deficits
- Red, warm, swollen joint
- Fracture

Treatment

Medical

- Nonsteroidal anti-inflammatories for pain; consider a 2-week course

Exercises

- Shoulder stretching, especially of the posterior capsule
- Pain-free range of motion
- Scapular stabilizers muscle recruitment, strengthening (closed chain initially, followed by open-chain exercises)
- Rotator cuff strengthening (initially below 90°, rotation at side) with gradual progression to functional upper extremity movements
- Hip and trunk stretching and strengthening

Modalities

- Ice
- Ultrasound
- Transcutaneous electrical nerve stimulation
- Extracorporeal shock wave (ECW) in calcific tendinitis

Injection

- Corticosteroid injection to the subacromial space may decrease pain and improve function at 4 weeks when compared with physical therapy, but has not been shown to have a benefit at 6 months

Surgical

■ Consider tendon debridement or repair, with decompression of the subacromial space for rotator cuff tears, and AC joint arthritis with osteophyte formation in patients not responding to conservative therapies
■ Surgical intervention should be followed by rehabilitation

Consults

■ Orthopedic surgeon
■ Sports medicine physician
■ Physical medicine and rehabilitation

Complications

■ Progressive pain and dysfunction
■ Adhesive capsulitis from prolonged immobility

Prognosis

■ Consider surgical treatment early if evidence of full thickness tear or failure of conservative therapy greater than 6 months

Helpful Hints

■ Shoulder dysfunction can be caused by faulty lower body biomechanics in a closed kinetic chain and should be addressed in treatment

Suggested Readings

Bushbinder R, Green S, Youd JM. Corticosteroid injections for shoulder pain. *Cochrane Database Syst Rev.* 2003;(1):CD004016.

Kibler WB. Rehabilitation of rotator cuff tendinopathy. *Clin Sports Med.* 2003;22:837–847.

Krabak BJ, Sugar R, McFarland EG. Practical nonoperative management of rotator cuff injuries. *Clin J Sport Med.* 2003;13:102–105.

Sacroiliac Joint Dysfunction

Heidi Prather DO

Description

Sacroiliac joint (SIJ) dysfunction and pain describes a subset of posterior pelvic (low back) pain. It stems from a wide variety of disorders and is typically multifactorial in etiology.

Etiology/Types

- Referred pain from multiple sites including the lumbar spine, pelvis, and hip
- Idiopathic, which may be associated with repetitive asymmetric stress, and biomechanical abnormalities not easily diagnosed
- Traumatic injury affecting the spine, hips, and lower extremities
- Inflammatory/metabolic associated with connective tissue disease
- Iatrogenic seen following spine, or hip surgery

Epidemiology

- Occurs in both men and women, though women predominant
- Forty-four percent to 58% of patients report a history of trauma
- Twenty-one percent of patients have a history of repetitive overload injury
- Fifty percent to 80% of women experience posterior pelvic pain during pregnancy

Pathogenesis

- SIJ dysfunction can occur in association with a traumatic event
- Insidious in onset without trauma, may be associated with repetitive motion in rotation, jumping or landing on one lower extremity
- Associated with pregnancy, hormones promote ligamentous laxity
- This in turn reduces force closure across the joint, allowing increased motion at the joint and therefore the potential for pain and dysfunction
- Disorders involving the lumbar spine, pubic symphysis, and hip may allow for dysfunctional loading across the SIJ, which in turn may cause a secondary adaptive disorder that manifests as pain related to the SIJ
- Some evidence to suggest pain may be periarticular

Risk Factors

- Trauma
- Repetitive pivoting, hip flexion and rotation, bending and twisting
- Conditions resulting in ligamentous laxity
- Spondyloarthropathy
- Sacral or iliac fracture
- Some evidence to suggest pain may also be periarticular

Clinical Features

- Pain in the posterior pelvis at the sacral sulci or posterior superior iliac spine (PSIS) and distally into the gluteal region and sometimes into the lower extremity
- Some will have pain that travels from the PSIS region laterally around the hip and into the groin
- Mechanical symptoms such as clicking or catching along the posterior pelvis or hip with lower extremity movement
- Pain worsened with walking, transitional motion, pivoting, and impact activities (running and jumping)
- SIJ pain can vary from self-limiting to chronic

Natural History

- Gender differences in anatomy and biomechanics predispose to SIJ dysfunction
- Common in young women and individuals with pathology of the lumbar spine
- Adaptive patterns due to disorders of the lower extremities or upper trunk and changes associated with pregnancy may result in shear or torsional forces through the SIJ and chronic symptoms
- Symptoms may progress if not appropriately diagnosed and the causative factors addresses

Diagnosis

Differential diagnosis

- Lumbar spine pathology

- Radiculopathy
- Facet-mediated pain
- Hip deformity
- Hip labral tear
- Hip chondrosis
- Hip osteoarthritis
- Spondyloarthropathy
- Piriformis syndrome
- Sacral fracture
- Pelvic floor dysfunction
- Infection
- Tumor
- Pregnancy
- Iatrogenic instability

History
- Pain localization to posterior pelvis, thigh, groin, and sacral sulci
- Often unilateral
- Provocative activities, usually single leg loading
- Sitting
- Transitional activities, supine to sit, sit to stand
- Increases with faster walking pace
- Popping or clicking in posterior pelvis

Exam
- Antalgic to normal gait
- Normal neurological examination
- Muscle imbalance across the hip, spine, and pelvis
- Positive active straight leg raise test
- Provocative tests (no test used in isolation has shown to be definitive in detecting SIJ pain, tests used together is of benefit in detecting SIJ pain)
- FABER/Patrick's test
- Sacral compression
- Distraction
- Thigh trust
- Gaenslen's test

Testing
- X-rays
  - Changes do not indicate source of pain
  - Best view 30° angle to anteroposterior
- Bone scan
  - Assess tumor, fracture, inflammatory joint changes
- Computed tomography (CT)
  - Best to show bony abnormalities
  - Can show early joint narrowing
  - Can show healing fracture

- Magnetic resonance imaging (MRI)
  - Most specific to assess bony edema and fracture
- Color Doppler ultrasound
  - Demonstrates stiffness across the SIJ

Pitfalls
- No single test diagnostic, may miss diagnosis

Red Flags
- Nighttime pain
- Pain unresponsive to treatment
- Fractures
- Neoplasm
- Infection

Treatment
Medical
- Relative rest with avoidance of aggravating activities such as pivoting and high impact activities
- Nonsteroidal anti-inflammatory medications
- Analgesics as indicated

Exercises
- A focused, specific physical therapy program
- Physical therapy goals include improvement of lumbopelvic quality of motion, reduced anterior femoral glide, and improved pelvic floor and core muscle strength
- Back stabilization, core muscle recruitment (abdominal hollowing), and dynamic flexibility (exercises in sagittal, frontal, and transverse planes) should be combined
- Taping and bracing in combination with exercise may facilitate pain reduction and muscle reeducation
- Joint mobilization can be useful for early on patients with SIJ hypomobility

Modalities
- Heat
- Ice
- Ultrasound

Injections
- Fluoroscopically guided SIJ injections can be used
- Diagnostic tool to confirm or rule out the diagnosis
- Therapeutically benefits patients with idiopathic pain and benefits patients with spondyloarthropathies

- Some evidence suggests prolotherapy can be helpful for SIJ pain (still controversial, needs more scientific evidence, may be beneficial if ligamentous abnormalities are part of the problem)

Surgical
- Extremely rare cases progress to SIJ fusion

Consults
- Physical therapist with expertise in hip, pelvis, and spine care

Complications/side effects
- Chronic pain
- Secondary dysfunction in the spine due to compensatory mechanisms

Prognosis
- Good

- Improved prognosis when recognized and treated early

Helpful Hints
- Pain not responding to comprehensive treatment should be reevaluated to determine the etiology
- Treat coexisting disorders (spine, hip)

Suggested Readings

Dreyfuss P, Michaelsen M, Pauza K, McLarty J, Bogduk N. The value of medical history and physical examination in diagnosing sacroiliac joint pain. *Spine.* 1996;21(22):2594–25602.

Prather H. Sacroiliac joint pain: practical management. *Clin J Sports Med.* 2003;13(4):252–255.

Slipman CW, Sterenfeld EB, Chou LH, Herzog R, Vresilovic E. The predictive value of provocative sacroiliac joint stress maneuvers in the diagnosis of sacroiliac joint syndrome. *Arch Phys Med Rehabil.* 1998;79(3):288–292.

Scaphoid Fractures

Gerardo E. Miranda MD ▪ William Micheo MD

Description

The scaphoid (carpal navicular) is the most commonly fractured carpal bone. It serves as a bridge between the proximal and distal carpal rows, transfers compression loads from the hand to the forearm, maintains normal wrist joint stability, and assists in wrist motion. The scaphoid bone is located distal to the radius and is stabilized by the radioscaphoid and scapholunate ligaments. It articulates with the radius, lunate, capitate, and trapezium.

Etiology/Types (Figure 1)

■ Fracture location
  – Distal 1/3 (distal pole)—10% of scaphoid fractures (heal readily)
  – Central 1/3 (waist)—65% of scaphoid fractures. May be subclassified as transverse, vertical oblique, horizontal oblique (heal without surgery if not displaced)
  – Proximal 1/3 (proximal pole)—15% of scaphoid fractures (will not heal if displaced, requires surgery)
  – Tuberosity—8% scaphoid fractures
■ Fracture timeframe
  – Acute: <3 weeks
  – Delayed union: 4 to 6 months
  – Nonunion fracture: >6 months
■ Fracture instability
  – Displacement >1 mm in any direction
  – Lateral intrascaphoid angulation >35°, scapholunate angle >60°, radiolunate angle >15°
  – Substantial bone loss or comminution
  – Associated with dorsal intercalated segment instability

Epidemiology

■ Account for approximately 10% of all hand fractures
■ Account for 60% to 70% of all carpal fractures
■ Annual incidence of 46/100,000 people
■ Most common in young active males
■ Four times more common in males than in females

Pathogenesis

■ Fall on an outstretched hand with the wrist extended and radially deviated

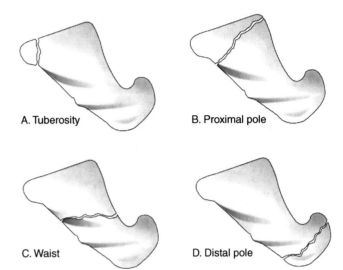

Figure 1. Fractures. Modified from Boles CA. Wrist, Scaphoid Fractures and Complications: Multimedia.

■ Forced palmar flexion of the wrist
■ Direct axial compression on a closed fist
■ Vascular flow enters the scaphoid from distal to proximal; fractures, particularly displaced and comminuted ones will affect the proximal scaphoid pole arterial circulation, and lead to nonunion and avascular necrosis
■ Abnormal force transmission across the wrist will result in arthritis

Risk Factors

■ Participation in contact sports
■ Skiing, snowboarding, and skateboarding

Clinical Features

■ Fall on the outstretched hand, wrist in extension
■ Pain, limited motion, and swelling
■ Tenderness over the anatomic snuffbox (distal to the radial styloid, bordered by the extensor pollicis longus ulnarly and extensor pollicis brevis radially)

Natural History

■ Non-displaced distal pole and waist fractures heal with cast immobilization

- Proximal scaphoid fractures may progress to nonunion
- Undiagnosed scaphoid fracture may be associated with arthritis of the wrist

Diagnosis

Differential diagnosis
- Wrist ligamentous injury
- Scapholunate dissociation
- Distal radial fractures
- Osteoarthritis/synovitis of the wrist

History
- Typically the patient reports some type of axial load to the wrist, or fall onto an outstretched hand
- Pain is localized to the radial aspect of the wrist and classically in the anatomical snuff box

Physical exam
- Swelling may be present on the dorsoradial aspect of the wrist
- Tenderness to palpation over the anatomical snuff box, volar prominence at the distal wrist crease, and just distal to Lister's tubercle
- Pain with wrist extension, and radial deviation

Testing
- Plain radiographs—wrist x-rays posteroanterior (PA), true lateral, scaphoid view (PA with the wrist at 45° of oblique pronation, and 45° of ulnar deviation)
- Bone scan—very sensitive, but not specific, and may be positive at 3 to 5 days after initial injury
- Computed tomography (CT scan)—accurately diagnose and delineate the fracture line, more readily available, and less costly than MRI
- Magnetic resonance imaging (MRI)—test of choice in symptomatic patients and athletes with negative or inconclusive x-rays
  - Helps to diagnose concomitant injuries (other carpal or radial fractures, ligamentous injury)
  - Helps to evaluate scaphoid vascularity to assess avascular necrosis

Pitfalls
- May miss the fracture if plain x-rays are negative and index of suspicion is low

Red Flags
- Continued pain despite negative x-rays
- Progressive wrist stiffness

Treatment

Medical
- Immobilization in a thumb-spica splint or preferably a thumb-spica cast, even if radiographs are negative, then repeat plain radiographs in 7 to 10 days
- Non-displaced distal scaphoid fracture (<1 mm)—immobilization in a short-arm thumb spica cast with the thumb IP joint-free and wrist in slight extension for 4 to 6 weeks
- Non-displaced waist and proximal pole—immobilization in a long arm thumb-spica cast for 10 to 20 weeks
- Follow-up x-rays every 2 weeks
- Bone stimulator or surgical referral if 3 to 4 months radiographical healing is not evident

Exercises
- Physical or occupational therapy to decrease muscle atrophy and maintain range of motion (ROM) following casting or surgery
- After cast removal (non-displaced fractures) gentle ROM, static wrist exercises, and dynamic strengthening
- Following surgical treatment, and cast immobilization (displaced fractures, usually after 6 weeks) start ROM, static and dynamic strengthening
- Athletes may be allowed participation in their sport with a soft cast (non-displaced fractures after 3 to 6 weeks, following surgery after 1 to 2 weeks for noncontact sports and after 3 to 6 weeks for contact sports)

Modalities
- To reduce inflammation, pain, and to facilitate rehabilitation following cast immobilization or surgery
- Cryotherapy
- Paraffin baths
- Transcutaneous electrical nerve stimulation (TENS)/electrical stimulation

Injection
- Not indicated

Surgical
Surgical referral if:
- Fracture displaced by ≥1 mm
- Increased tilt of the lunate
- Nonunion develops during follow-up
- Osteonecrosis of the scaphoid

- Suspected scapholunate dissociation
- Patient unwilling or unable to be immobilized for at least 3 months
- Percutaneous internal fixation non-displaced fractures
  - Arthroscopically assisted reduction—may also allow diagnosis of associated injuries (TFCC tears, lunotriquetal or scapholunate ligament injuries, chondral injuries)
  - Less postsurgical complications than ORIF
- Open reduction and internal fixation (ORIF) for displaced fractures using compression screws
  - More rapid return to work or sports than with conservative treatment
- Vascularized bone grafts are an alternative for patients with nonunion and avascularity of the proximal pole

Consults
- Orthopedic surgery/Sports medicine
- Hand surgery
- Physical medicine and rehabilitation

Complications/side effects
- Nonunion, chronic wrist pain
- Osteoarthritis of the wrist
- Postoperative infection, collapse of fracture segments

Prognosis
- Variable
- Good for distal pole fractures
- Proximal pole fractures may progress to nonunion, avascular necrosis

Helpful Hints
- Suspect scaphoid fracture in any patient with localized wrist pain and swelling after falling on an outstretched hand
- Normal x-rays do not rule out scaphoid fracture; need to repeat in 7 to 10 days
- MRI highly sensitive for scaphoid fractures; use early in athletes

Suggested Readings

Brotzman SB, Meyers SJ, Lee ML. Hand and wrist injuries. In: *Clinical Orthopaedic Rehabilitation*. Philadelphia, PA: Mosby; 2003:50–55.

Rizzo M, Shin AY. Treatment of acute scaphoid fracture in the athlete. *Curr Sports Med Rep.* 2006;5:242–248.

Yin Z, Zhang J, Kan S, Wang P. Treatment of acute scaphoid fracture, systemic review and meta-analysis. *Clin Orthop Rel Res.* 2007;480:142–151.

Scapholunate Dissociation

José A. Báez MD FAAPMR

Description
The most commonly injured ligament in the wrist is the scapholunate ligament (SLL). It is located between the scaphoid and the lunate at the proximal carpal row (Figure 1). The SLL maintains the proximal pole of the scaphoid adjacent to the lunate (scapholunate gap), stabilizes the palmar rotation force of the scaphoid against the dorsal rotation force of the lunate (scapholunate angle), and is crucial to wrist stability.

Etiology/Types
- Traumatic: fall on an outstretched extended and ulnar deviated wrist is the most common etiology
- Nontraumatic: chronic damage of supporting ligaments due to an underlying disease process (eg, rheumatoid arthritis)

Epidemiology
- Wrist injuries (the majority of which are sprains and strains) account for <3% of emergency room visits in the United States each year

Pathogenesis
- A fall on an outstretched hand will produce an impact load to the base of the thenar region of the hand with the wrist in extension, ulnar deviation, and supination
- The trauma may cause a partial SLL tear with pain but no instability
- A more extensive SLL tear may result in normal plain x-rays, pain with use, but increase in the scapholunate gap on a clenched fist stress x-ray (dynamic scapholunate instability)
- Complete disruption of the SLL results in an instability pattern visible on plain x-rays (static scapholunate instability)

Risk Factors
- Occupational
  - Athletes and individuals who participate in recreational sports
  - Workers who experience lifting or twisting stresses with their hands
- Anatomical
  - Ulnar minus variance

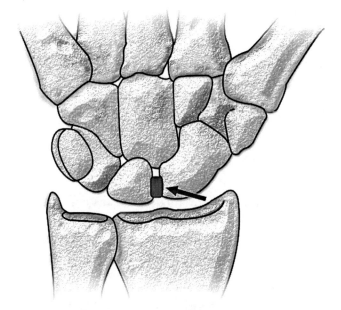

Figure 1. The scapholunate ligament.

  - Slope of radial articular surface
  - Lunotriquetral coalition
- Disease
  - Degenerative joint diseases (eg, rheumatoid arthritis, pseudogout)

Clinical Features
- Tenderness over the radial aspect of the dorsal wrist
- Pain
- Swelling
- Weakness
- Giving way
- Click, snap, and clunk with use

Natural History
- If not properly treated, this injury can lead to:
  - Chronic wrist pain
  - Weakness
  - Stiffness
  - Locking of the wrist
  - Unstable degenerative wrist arthritis (scapholunate advanced collapse pattern [SLAC])

Diagnosis

Differential diagnosis
- Scaphoid fracture
- Distal radial fracture
- De Quervain's tenosynovitis
- Dorsal ganglion cyst
- Radial wrist arthritis
- Kienböck's disease
- Other carpal bone fractures

History
- Fall on outstretched hand developing pain, swelling, and tenderness on the radial aspect of the wrist

Exam
- Bilateral wrist/hand examination recommended for comparison
- Inspection: swelling over the scapholunate region
- Range of motion (ROM): usually normal initially, but may be associated with pain or clicks with extremes of wrist flexion, extension, ulnar and radial deviation
- Palpation: tenderness over the dorsal aspect of a flexed wrist distal to Lister's tubercle
- Provocative maneuver: Watson's scaphoid shift test may produce pain or audible clunk (low specificity) (Figure 2)

Testing
- Plain x-ray
  - Anterior posterior (AP) view: widening of the scapholunate gap >2 mm ("frontal tooth gap sign") suggests static instability
  - Lateral view: increased scapholunate angle suggests dorsal intercalated segmental instability (DISI)
- Stress x-ray
  - Posterior anterior view: ulnar and radial deviation with clenched-fist
  - Widening of the scapholunate gap >2 mm suggests dynamic instability
- Bone scan: may be positive in 24 hours but low specificity
- Arthrogram: low sensitivity when compared with arthroscopy
- Magnetic resonance imaging: not as useful in small joints due to difficulties in interpretation
- Arthroscopy: gold standard for identifying and grading SLL injuries

Pitfalls
- Surgical repair will most likely result in some degree of permanent loss of wrist motion
- Diagnosis is frequently delayed due to:

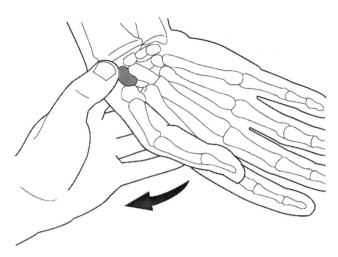

Figure 2. Scaphoid shift test (Watson test).

- Patient not seeking initial care due to mild symptoms
- Initially dismissed as a "wrist sprain"
- Normal plain x-rays
- Overlooked injury due to concomitant distal radius fracture

Red Flags
- SLL injury is highly associated with scaphoid, lunate, and distal radius fractures

Treatment

Medical
- Immobilization until imaging studies performed

Exercises
- Active ROM
- Static strengthening in the acute phase
- Dynamic strengthening as symptoms improve

Modalities
- Aimed at reducing pain, swelling, and increasing ROM
  - Ultrasound
  - Heat/cold therapy
  - Electrical stimulation

Injection
- Not indicated

Surgical
- Various orthopedic approaches depending upon the extent of ligament/bone injury, instability, and degenerative changes found
- Arthroscopy and ligament repair if diagnosed early

- Wrist fusion may be required in chronic injury

Consult
- Orthopedic surgery
- Physical medicine and rehabilitation

Complications/side effects
- Chronic wrist pain
- Wrist instability
- Degenerative changes
- Arthritis
- Loss of ROM
- Loss of function

Prognosis
- Early diagnosis and surgical treatment offers the best chance for long-term stability and function

Helpful Hints
- High degree of suspicion is necessary for a timely diagnosis and treatment
- Order clenched fist AP x-rays if diagnosis is suspected

Suggested Readings

Jaworski CA, Krause M, Brown J. Rehabilitation of the wrist and hand following sports injury. *Clin Sports Med.* 2010;29(1):61–80.

Kuo CE, Wolfe SW. Scapholunate instability: current concepts in diagnosis and management. *J Hand Surg Am.* 2008;33(6):998–1013.

Manuel J, Moran SL. The diagnosis and treatment of scapholunate instability. *Orthop Clin N Am.* 2007; 38:261–277.

Scheuermann's Disease

Edwardo Ramos-Cortes MD

Description
Initially described by Scheuermann as a rigid kyphosis of the thoracic or thoracolumbar spine occurring in adolescents

Etiology
- Unknown

Epidemiology
- Overall prevalence 2.8%; 2.1% among women, 3.6% men

Pathogenesis
- Biological factors
  - Disorganized endochondral ossification
  - A reduction in collagen and an increase in mucopolysaccharide in the vertebral endplates
  - Degeneration of the disc
- Mechanical factors
  - Thickening of the anterior longitudinal ligament
  - Partial wedging of the vertebral body

Risk Factors
- Increased familiar incidence

Clinical Features
- Rigid spine kyphosis; thoracic or thoracolumbar
- Back pain
- Fatigue

Natural History
- Lack of literature regarding the natural history of Scheuermann's kyphosis
- Rigid kyphosis that appears in the adolescent
- If resultant deformity is <75°, no long-term difficulties
- Patients with deformities of >75°, who have untreated disease, may seek medical attention as adults due to progressive curve and chronic back pain
- Studies have found that subjects with Scheuermann's kyphosis work in lighter jobs than controls
- More severe back pain and interference with activities of daily living
- More concern with their appearance

- Neurological complications in some subjects with untreated condition include dural cyst and thoracic disc herniation

Diagnosis

Differential diagnosis
- Postural kyphosis
- Associated with medical conditions
  - Neurofibromatosis (NF-1)
  - Congenital kyphosis
  - Kyphosis associated with Marfan syndrome

History
- Kyphosis in the thoracic or thoracolumbar area in the adolescent
- Occasional back pain

Exam
- Rigid kyphosis in the thoracic or thoracolumbar area
- Hyperlordosis of the lumbar spine that is flexible
- Forward protrusion of the head that is flexible
- Tight anterior shoulder girdle and hamstring muscles

Testing
- Routine x-ray; 36-inch posterior anterior and lateral, supine hyperextension lateral radiograph
- The normal range of thoracic kyphosis is from 20° to 40°, as measured by Cobb method
- Radiological criteria for Scheuermann's: the thoracic curve must be greater than 40°
- A 20° kyphosis in the area of T10 to L2 may be indicative of thoracolumbar Scheuermann's kyphosis
- Wedging of greater than 5° of more than three consecutive vertebrae
- Associated radiographical findings include Schmorl's nodes, irregularity and flattening of the intervertebral disc spaces
- MRI may be required in patients with neurologic symptoms to rule out thoracic disc herniation

Pitfalls
- Not doing an magnetic resonance imaging (MRI) prior to performing surgery and missing cord compression

Red Flags
- Presence of upper motor neuron signs in the lower extremities

Treatment

Medical
- Depends on the severity and location of the deformity, presence of pain, and age of the patient
- Analgesics
- Brace

Exercises
- Kyphosis <50°, needs only an exercise program with emphasis on increasing flexibility of the lower extremities, hip and spine, and postural muscles endurance training
- Kyphosis >55° thoracic, or 40° thoracolumbar bracing should be considered (23 hours/day) along with a back extension exercise program

Modalities
- Heat
- Ice
- Transcutaneous electrical stimulation

Injection
- Normally not used

Surgical
- Indications for surgical treatment are not clear. In general, adolescent with a symptomatic kyphotic deformity of 80° in the thoracic spine or 65° in the thoracolumbar spine

- A thoracic MRI should be obtained before surgery, because a thoracic disc herniation is occasionally present in Scheuermann's disease and may result in cord compression
- Posterior or anterior/posterior approach using pedicle screws and/or hooks

Consults
- Neurosurgeon or orthopedic-spine surgery

Complications/side effects
- Pain
- Neurological complications associated with cord compression

Prognosis
- Highly variable

Helpful Hints
- Scheuermann's kyphosis is a spinal deformity of the adolescent, which has a major impact in appearance and may require treatment depending on the magnitude of the curve

Suggested Readings

Betz RR. Kyphosis of the thoracic and thoracolumbar spine in the pediatric patient: normal sagittal parameters and scope of the problem. *Instr Course Lect.* 2004;53:479–484.

Lowe TG. Scheuermann's kyphosis. *Neurosurg Clin N Am.* 2007;18:303–315.

Lowe TG, Line BG. Evidence based medicine analysis of Scheuermann's kyphosis. *Spine.* 2007;32:S115-S119.

Pizzutillo PD. Non surgical treatment of kyphosis. *Instr Course Lect.* 2004;53:485–491.

Scoliosis

Manuel Garcia-Ariz MD

Description
Scoliosis is a multifactorial condition characterized by spinal deformity, mostly in the frontal (coronal) plane. Significant curves exceed 10°, and may have an associated rotatory component (Figure 1).

Etiology/Types
- Idiopathic
  - Infantile (<3 years of age)
  - Juvenile (3–10 years of age)
  - Adolescent (10–14 years of age)
- Congenital (vertebral defect)
- Neuromuscular (cerebral palsy, myelodysplasia, muscle dystrophy, anterior horn cell disease, polio spinal muscular atrophy [SMA])
- Functional
- Associated with spine tumors
- Hysterical
- Traumatic

Epidemiology
- Overall prevalence 0.3% to 2% of the population
- Incidence 3 to 5 per 1000
- Usually affects adolescents, girls twice as often as boys
- Eighty-five percent of cases are idiopathic scoliosis

Pathogenesis
- The cause of idiopathic scoliosis is unknown
- Congenital scoliosis is associated with intrinsic spine factors such as bony anomalies
- Acquired scoliosis is associated with trauma, infection, tumors, or degenerative changes
- Neuromuscular disease leads to scoliosis because of abnormalities in tone, muscle strength, and balance

Risk Factors
- Family history
- Connective tissue disorders
- Trauma
- Degenerative spine disease

Clinical Features
- Asymmetric shoulders and hips
- Dorsolateral rib hump
- Short trunk
- Breast asymmetry

Natural History
- Small curves usually do not progress and may be asymptomatic
- Larger curves may progress even into adulthood and require surgery

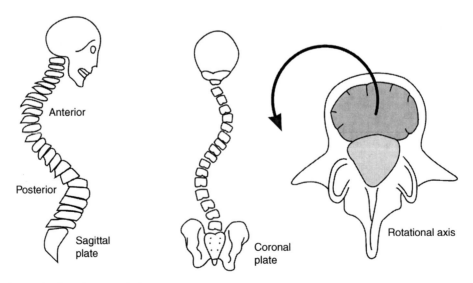

Figure 1. Scoliosis sagittal and coronal views.

Diagnosis

Differential diagnosis

- Idiopathic
- Congenital
- Neuromuscular
- Traumatic
- Tumors of the spine
- Functional

History

- Usually in an adolescent, presents with scapular asymmetry and rib hump
- Family history of spinal deformity; presents to clinic with a body image complaint
- Usually no complaints of pain; if present may be of musculoskeletal origin
- Severe pain, particularly at night, which awakens the patient may be a sign of intraspinal pathology

Exam

- Forward bending to identify fixed vs flexible deformity
  - Structural
  - Nonstructural
- Range of motion of hip, knee, and spine
- Flexibility testing of hip, hamstrings, and spine muscles
- Muscle strength of abdominal, back, and lower extremity muscles
- Reflexes
  - Abdominal
  - Knee
  - Ankle
- Measurement of leg length
- Visual gait analysis

Testing

- Simple 36″ thoracolumbar standing radiographs
- Measure the curves with Cobb method (note the upper and lower borders of the curve, measure the angle between lines drawn parallel to the endplates of the upper and lower vertebrae of the curve; if the lines do not intersect in the film, draw lines perpendicular to each of the above lines and measure)
- Determine the degree of rotation by looking at the pedicles, and evaluate skeletal maturity by looking at the Risser's lines at the crest of the pelvis (ossification of the iliac apophysis, occurs from lateral to medial)
- Magnetic resonance imaging (MRI) indicated in a child with <10 years of age, with suspected intraspinal anomaly, or in cases of congenital scoliosis for the same reason
- Patients with neurological abnormalities also require an MRI
- A relative indication for MRI is in patients with left thoracic curve looking for associated pathology

Pitfalls

- Not suspecting curves that are balanced
- Missing rapidly progressive curves
- Not looking for associated pathology
- Attributing pain to the scoliosis

Red Flags

- Night pain
- Fever
- History of trauma

Treatment

Medical

- Nonsurgical treatment depends on the age of the patient, skeletal maturity, and the degree of the curve
- Curves that measure <7° do not need orthopedic referral, only regular follow-up by primary physician
- Curves <10° need follow-up during the period of growth, especially at peak velocity of adolescent spinal development, which starts earlier in girls (around 10–12 years of age)
- Curves <25° in immature patients and those between 25° and 40° in adolescents who have not stopped growing require bracing
- After growth cessation, patients usually are not braced; they are followed for curve progression beyond 45° to 50°, and then are treated with surgical methods. An exception would be a rapidly progressive curve beyond 35° in a growing child
- Bracing is also utilized in an immature child in whom curve progression must be controlled until more spinal length has been attained prior to fusion
- Bracing will not correct the curve, it will only limit progression. Patient compliance most critical factor for effectiveness
- Commonly used braces include the Milwaukee cervical-thoracic-lumbar-sacral orthosis (CTLSO), or lower profile thoraco-lumbo-sacral orthoses such as the Boston brace
- Braces can be used at nighttime, daytime, or full time. There are some evidences for effectiveness of nighttime bracing using orthosis such as the Charleston, and this may be an attractive option for patients with lower thoracic, or lumbar curves

- Bracing carries the risk of lowering self-esteem in young patients, and prolonged use is uncomfortable

Exercises
- Hip, hamstring, and spine flexibility training
- Back and core muscle strengthening, endurance training (no evidence that they halt progression of the curve)
- Aerobic exercises, aquatic rehabilitation

Modalities
- Cryotherapy to reduce pain and muscle "spasm"
- Superficial heat for symptomatic relief of pain
- Electrical stimulation of muscle (no evidence that it alters progression of the curve)

Injection
- Not indicated

Surgical
- Reserved for curves that are either progressive in nature, or curves that cannot be contained with bracing during the growth period
- Those that have reached 45° to 50° and are also out of balance
- Posterior spinal fusion, instrumentation and autologous bone graft is state-of-the-art surgical treatment and the current gold standard to which other procedures have to be compared
- Types of instrumentation include hybrids, rods, hooks, and screws. Usually no bracing is required postsurgery with newer types of instrumentation
- Recovery time is around 6 months for a solid fusion and around 1 year to return to regular daily activities and sports

Consults
- Orthopedic/spine surgery

Complications/side effects
- Short-term complications
  - Blood loss
  - Infection
  - Loss of correction
  - Pseudoarthrosis
  - Neurological deficits
  - Gastric outlet syndrome
  - Cholecystitis
  - Pancreatitis
  - Pneumothorax
- Long-term complications
  - Straight back
  - Crankshaft deformity in patients <10 years of age (appearance of spiral staircase)
  - Junctional pain and instability

Prognosis
- Variable, depending on the cause
- Good for small curves associated with idiopathic scoliosis; these do not progress after growth cessation
- Large curves in young patients have a high tendency to progress

Helpful Hints
- Young patients with scoliosis need close follow-up during the growth spurt
- Rely on radiological findings and not on chronological age
- Educate patients on the condition
- Pain is usually secondary to other causes

Suggested Readings
Peelle MW, Luhmann SJ. Management of adolescent idiopathic scoliosis. *Neurosurg Clin N Am.* 2007;18(4):575–583.

Silva FE, Lenke LG. Adult degenerative scoliosis evaluation and management. *Neurosurg Focus.* 2010;28(3):E1.

Shoulder Dislocation

Marc Safran MD

Description

A shoulder dislocation is an injury to the shoulder joint where the humeral head (upper arm) is displaced from its normal position in the center of the socket (glenoid) and the joint surfaces no longer touch each other. Subluxation of the shoulder is common and is where the ball of the humerus does not stay centered in the socket with shoulder motion and feels like it wants to slip out of place.

Etiology/Types

- Anterior dislocation more common, posterior dislocation unusual
- Some patients can be voluntary dislocators
- Subluxation with repetitive throwing motion or swimming
- Congenital abnormality of socket

Epidemiology

- The shoulder is the most commonly dislocated large joint in the body
- Posterior dislocation may be associated with seizures
- More common in younger individuals, particularly in contact sporting activities or from falls

Pathogenesis

- The shoulder has great mobility at the expense of stability
- The glenoid is a shallow dish for the humeral head to rotate upon
- The ligaments are lax in midranges of motion; dynamic stability depends on the muscles
- The ligaments are important at the extreme ranges of motion, the inferior glenohumeral ligament (IGHL) is important in stability with the shoulder in abduction and external rotation
- Scapular dysfunction may lead to changes in the congruency of the glenoid with the humeral head
- The muscles of the rotator cuff are the most important stabilizers of the shoulder in the mid ranges of motion, pulling the humeral head toward the center of the glenoid
- Most individuals require significant traumatic force to dislocate their shoulders the first time

- To dislocate anteriorly, the arm is usually in a throwing type position (abducted and externally rotated)
- To dislocate the shoulder posteriorly, the arm is usually in front of the person during a fall, or due to significant muscular contraction, such as may occur with a seizure or electrocution

Risk Factors

- Genetically inherited loose joints
- Contact sports (football, wrestling, and basketball)
- Sports that involve repetitive overhead activity such as baseball, volleyball, swimming
- Sports that require forceful lifting, hitting, or twisting
- Previous shoulder dislocations or sprains
- Shoulder fracture
- Poor physical conditioning (strength/flexibility)
- Congenital abnormality, such as a shallow or malformed joint surface or ligament disorder

Clinical Features

- Severe pain in the shoulder at the time of injury
- Loss of shoulder function and severe pain when attempting to move the shoulder
- Feeling like the shoulder wants to slip out of place

Natural History

- Following reduction, healing of ligaments by 6 weeks
- Younger patients (under the age of 20 years) high risk of recurrent dislocation (90%)
- Those over the age of 40 years at the time of their first dislocation have a higher chance of having an associated rotator cuff tear
- There is an increased risk of shoulder arthritis associated with shoulder dislocation (though repeated dislocations do not necessarily increase the risk further)

Diagnosis

Differential diagnosis

- Fracture
- Voluntary dislocation
- Multidirectional instability
- Rotator cuff tear
- Brachial plexus injury

History
- Severe pain in the shoulder at the time of injury
- Loss of shoulder function and severe pain when attempting to move the shoulder
- Feeling like the shoulder wants to slip out of place
- Pain moving the shoulder and pain at night
- Numbness or paralysis in upper arm
- Crepitation with shoulder motion

Exam
- Deformity (fullness in the axilla)
- Tenderness and swelling
- Pain with active or resisted shoulder motion
- Pain/weakness with muscle testing of the shoulder
- Apprehension
- Sensory loss upper arm (test the lateral shoulder for reduce sensation associated with axillary nerve injury)
- Crepitation
- Decreased wrist pulse (rare)
- Decreased external rotation with posterior shoulder dislocation

Testing
- X-rays (anteroposterior [AP] and axillary lateral) demonstrate the shoulder dislocation, bony fracture of the glenoid rim, and/or greater tuberosity
- Magnetic resonance imaging (MRI) can identify the Bankart lesion (avulsion of the anterior-inferior labrum for anterior dislocation), strain or tear of the rotator cuff, and a Hill-Sachs lesion (impression fracture of the humeral head on the edge of the glenoid fossa)

Pitfalls
- Overinterpretation of imaging studies
- Not obtaining an axillary radiographs of the shoulder (may miss a dislocation on the AP view)

Red Flags
- Infection
- Fracture
- Neoplasm
- Neurological dysfunction
- Weakness in patients over 40 years

Treatment
Medical
- Reduction (usually performed closed with medications to relax the patient)
- Sling or brace for 3 to 6 weeks for anterior dislocation, 6 to 8 weeks after posterior dislocation (shorter time of immobilization for older patients to avoid adhesive capsulitis)
- Nonsteroidal anti-inflammatory medications
- Analgesics

Exercises
- Strengthen the rotator cuff and scapular stabilizers
- Increase range of motion, initially avoiding the abduction-external rotation position (for anterior dislocators) or the adduction-internal rotation-flexion position (for posterior dislocators) for at least 6 weeks
- The success of rehabilitation in preventing recurrent dislocation is 20% in younger patients, 80% in older patients, and 70% to 90% following posterior dislocation
- The success of a rehabilitation program for atraumatic multidirectional shoulder stability is about 80%

Modalities
- Heat
- Ice
- Transcutaneous electrical nerve stimulation
- Ultrasound

Injection
- Intra-articular injection may provide some pain relief when reducing the shoulder

Surgical
- Reserved for people who have recurrent shoulder dislocations or subluxation that affects activities of daily living and/or sports activities despite 3 to 6 months of rehabilitation
- Occasionally recommended for young patients or throwers after the first dislocation (controversial)
- May also be performed in a patient who has had a prior operation for shoulder instability
- Arthroscopic stabilization to reattach the labrum and tighten the capsule
- Open surgery for stabilization to reattach labrum and tighten capsule
- Open surgery to internally fix fractured glenoid rim
- Open surgery to transfer bone block (coracoid) if significant bone loss from the glenoid or engaging Hill-Sachs Lesion
- Tendon transfer can be considered for posterior shoulder dislocation

Consults
- Orthopedic surgery

Complications/side effects

- Damage to the axillary nerve and less commonly, the suprascapular nerve
- Fracture or joint cartilage injury
- Rotator cuff tear when first dislocate
- Repeated shoulder dislocations
- Unstable or arthritic shoulder
- Adhesive capsulitis (especially in older patients)

Prognosis

- Good
- High risk of recurrence with surgery for those with multidirectional shoulder instability

Helpful Hints

- For young patients with traumatic anterior shoulder dislocation, reduction, sling, and physical therapy should be attempted, but counsel the patient about the risk of recurrence of dislocation
- For patients over 40 years of age, evaluate with MRI to rule out associated rotator cuff tear
- Always perform a neurological examination of a patient with shoulder dislocation before and after performing shoulder reduction (axillary patch over the deltoid for sensation of the axillary nerve)

Suggested Readings

Dodson CC, Cordasco FA. Anterior glenohumeral joint dislocations. *Orthop Clin North Am.* 2008;39(4):507–518.

Kowalsky MS, Levine WN. Traumatic posterior glenohumeral dislocation: classification, pathoanatomy, diagnosis, and treatment. *Orthop Clin North Am.* 2008;39(4):519–533.

Safran MR, Dorey FJ, Hodge D. How should you treat an athlete with a first time dislocation of the shoulder. In: MacAuley D, Best T, eds. *Evidence Based Sports Medicine.* 2nd ed. Malden: Massachusetts; 2007:361–290.

Shoulder Instability, Atraumatic

Phillip T. Henning DO ▆ Jay Smith MD

Description

Spontaneous subluxation/dislocation of the glenohumeral joint, often found bilaterally but usually asymmetrically symptomatic

Etiology/Types

- Classified by direction and voluntary/involuntary nature
- Direction: anterior, posterior, or multidirectional. Most have multidirectional laxity, but may have instability symptoms in only one direction (eg, anterior or posterior)
- Voluntary vs involuntary. Voluntary types may be associated with psychiatric illness
- Regardless of type, poor or abnormal neuromuscular control of the shoulder girdle thought to be pathoetiological in symptoms

Epidemiology

- Often seen in association with generalized ligamentous laxity and connective tissue disorders

Pathogenesis

- Redundant joint capsule
- Laxity of glenohumeral ligaments
- Flat concavity of glenoid
- Increased retroversion of glenoid
- Small or degenerated labrum
- Incompetent scapulothoracic and glenohumeral stabilizing musculature

Risk Factors

- Genetics
- Younger age
- High or repetitive mechanical loading
- Generalized ligamentous laxity
- Connective tissue disorders (Ehler-Danlos syndrome)

Clinical Features

- Laxity of the glenohumeral joint: either unidirectional or multidirectional
- Hyperextension of other joints: for example, elbow, fingers, wrists, or patellofemoral joint subluxation

Natural History

- Not well defined
- Often spontaneous resolution with increasing age

Diagnosis

Differential diagnosis

- Rotator cuff tear/tendinopathy—often secondary to instability of joint, which stresses the cuff
- Acromioclavicular or sternoclavicular joint laxity
- Bankart lesion/Hill-Sachs lesion/posterior labral tear (seen in traumatic shoulder dislocations)
- Superior labral anterior and posterior (SLAP) lesion
- Subacromial bursitis
- Cervical spinal cord syrinx, radiculopathy (C5-C6), brachial plexopathy, peripheral neuropathy (suprascapular or axillary nerves)—neurological reasons for dysfunctional neuromuscular control

History

- Pain with overhead activities
- Sense of instability or frank dislocation without traumatic force
- Transient paresthesias or "dead arm"
- Sense of weakness of poor arm control

Exam

- Reproduction of pain with anterior and/or posterior apprehension tests
- Laxity with anterior and posterior load and shift
- Positive sulcus sign
- Evidence of rotator cuff injury
- Scapular dyskinesis
- Tight posterior capsule or other soft tissue asymmetries

Testing

- Plain radiography usually normal; used to assess for bony humeral or glenoid lesions that can lead to instability
- Sonography examines extra-articular pathology as well as the extent of rotator cuff involvement
- No specific magnetic resonance imaging (MRI) findings; can be useful to assess for other pathology that is amenable to surgical correction
- Electromyography as indicated to rule out contributing and/or concurrent diagnoses

Pitfalls
- Missing surgically correctible lesions
- Failure to assess for and correct abnormal scapulothoracic mechanics
- Failure to identify voluntary subluxators/dislocators who may require psychological intervention

Red Flags
- Unresolving shoulder pain associated with overhead activity may be due to undiagnosed instability
- Night pain

Treatment

Medical
- Analgesics
- Nonsteroidal anti-inflammatory medications

Exercises
- Scapulothoracic and rotator cuff strengthening
- Manual resistance training, rhythmic stabilization exercises
- Kinetic chain strength and conditioning program
- Selected soft tissue stretching to remove imbalances

Modalities
- Ice
- Electromyography (EMG) biofeedback

Injection
- Injections used selectively to treat associated disorders such as synovitis, tendinitis, or bursitis

Surgical
- Inferior capsular shift
- Labral repair or other surgery directed at treating identifiable contributing cause

Consults
- Orthopedic surgery

Complications/side effects
- Progressive pain and dysfunction
- Recurrent dislocations
- Neurovascular injury
- Hill-Sachs (fracture of the humeral head), or Bankart lesion (avulsion injury of the glenoid labrum, with or without fracture)

Prognosis
- Often responds to initial rehabilitation within 3 months
- Usually resolves with increasing age

Helpful Hints
- Assessment of entire kinetic chain for biomechanical abnormalities can make rehabilitation more successful
- Establish maintenance rehabilitation program to reduce reoccurrence of pain

Suggested Readings
Eisenhart-Rothe R, Matsen F, Eckstein F, et al. Pathomechanics in atraumatic shoulder instability. *Clin Orthop.* 2005;433:82–89.
Paxinos A, Walton J, Tzannes A, et al. Advances in the management of traumatic anterior and atraumatic multidirectional shoulder instability. *Sports Med.* 2001;31(11):819–828.
Tzannes A, Murrell G. Clinical examination of the unstable shoulder. *Sports Med.* 2002;32(7):447–457.

Sinding-Larsen-Johannson Syndrome

Mimi D. Johnson MD

Description
Sinding-Larsen-Johannson syndrome is a traction apophysitis of the inferior pole of the patella.

Etiology
- Repetitive traction exerted by the patellar tendon pulling on the inferior patellar apophysis

Epidemiology
- Occurs with greatest prevalence in boys, ages 10 to 13 years
- Typically occurs in active/athletic preadolescents

Pathogenesis
- Repetitive traction of the apophysis at the proximal insertion of the patellar tendon
- Often seen in running and jumping athletes
- Pain is usually of gradual onset, but can be acute
- It can be unilateral or bilateral
- The severity of pain can range from mild to severe
- The duration of symptoms can range from 3 to 18 months

Risk Factors
- Involvement in running and jumping activities
- Pre- to early adolescence
- Inflexibility of hamstrings and quadriceps

Clinical Features
- Pain with jumping, running, squatting/kneeling, stair climbing
- Point tenderness at the inferior pole of the patella
- Mild, localized soft tissue swelling

Natural History
- During early adolescence, jumping and running activities cause a typically gradual, but sometimes acute, onset of pain at the inferior pole of the patella
- Pain often waxes and wanes with activity, and rest results in decreased pain
- It typically resolves within 12 to 18 months

Diagnosis

Differential diagnosis
- Avulsion or sleeve fracture of the patella
- Bipartite patella
- Patellar tendinitis/jumper's knee

History
- Typically, gradual onset of pain with running, jumping, squatting, kneeling, and stair climbing
- Pain may be of acute onset
- Pain intensity is variable, though when severe, there can be pain with walking
- Occasional soft tissue swelling

Exam
- Point tenderness at the inferior pole of the patella
- Soft tissue swelling at the inferior pole of the patella
- Occasional palpable lump at the inferior pole of the patella
- Pain with resisted knee extension
- Range of motion may be painful on full flexion
- No gap is palpable at the inferior pole of the patella

Testing
- X-ray may be normal or with varying degrees of irregular calcification at the inferior pole of the patella
- With growth, the irregular ossifications eventually coalesce and incorporate into the patella
- Infrequently, an ossification can remain as a separate ossicle
- Pitfalls
- Erroneously treating this as a fracture

Red Flags
- In case of acute onset of pain with an abrupt quadriceps contraction suspect an avulsion fracture
- Palpable gap at the inferior pole of the patella, as seen in avulsion fracture

Treatment

Medical
- Rest from aggravating activities (ie, running, jumping, climbing)
- Patellar tendon strap or knee sleeve with infrapatellar buttress may be helpful during activities
- Nonsteroidal anti-inflammatory drugs (NSAIDs)

Exercises
- Flexibility exercises for the hamstrings, quadriceps, and iliotibial band can decrease tension on the patellar tendon
- Strengthening exercises focusing on the core, hip abductors, and quadriceps may be helpful

Modalities
- Cryotherapy
- Superficial heat
- Electrical stimulation

Injection
- Inappropriate, due to risk of tendon rupture

Surgical
- Rarely required

Consults
- Orthopedic
- Physical medicine and rehabilitation
- Sports medicine

Complications/side effects
- Acute avulsion fracture at the inferior patellar apophysis
- Limited tolerance to sports activity

Prognosis
- Good

Helpful Hints
- Sinding-Larsen-Johannson syndrome is a benign and self-limiting disorder
- Anticipatory guidance for patient and parents as to time course until resolution can be helpful
- Presentation and treatment is much like Osgood-Schlatter disease
- Once pain has subsided, a gradual resumption of activity can take place

Suggested Readings
Medlar RC, Lyne ED. Sinding-Larsen-Johansson disease. Its etiology and natural history. *J Bone Joint Surg Am.* 1978;60:1113–1116.
Outerbridge AR, Micheli LJ. Overuse injuries in the young athlete. *Clin Sports Med.* 1995;14(3):503–516.

Spondylolisthesis

Christopher J. Standaert MD

Description

Spondylolisthesis refers to the anterior displacement of one vertebral body on the one subjacent to it.

Etiology/Types

- Classification system for spondylolysis and spondylolisthesis:
  - Type I—dysplastic
  - Type II—isthmic
  - Type III—degenerative
  - Type IV—traumatic
  - Type V—pathological
- Spondylolisthesis is further categorized by the degree of slip, expressed either by quartiles or as a percentage of the anteroposterior diameter of the superior aspect of the subjacent vertebral body
  - Grade I: <25%
  - Grade II: 25% to 50%
  - Grade III: 50% to 75%
  - Grade IV: >75%
  - Spondyloptosis: 100%

Epidemiology

- Isthmic spondylolisthesis (associated with a pars defect [spondylolysis]) usually develops during childhood or adolescence, most commonly at L5/S1
  - Two percent to 3% of the adult population
  - Thirty percent to 50% of those with spondylolysis
- Degenerative spondylolisthesis occurs in about 2% to 3% of males and 9% of females, most commonly at L4/5 and in those over 50 years old

Pathogenesis

- May be associated with hereditary factors, seen in patients with spina bifida occulta
- Extension and rotation forces applied with the lumbar spine
- Instability of the lumbar spine associated with degenerative disc disease, and zygoapophyseal joint arthritis

Risk Factors

- Starting participation at a young age in sports that place high loads in the lumbar spine
- Bilateral spondylolysis
- Degenerative disc disease

Clinical Features

- Spondylolisthesis by itself is rarely symptomatic
- Symptoms may be associated with instability or neural involvement
- Postural abnormalities may be noted with high-grade slips

Natural History

- Progression of low-grade isthmic spondylolisthesis is uncommon
  - Most often seen during the adolescent growth spurt
  - More frequently occurs with initial slips of >20% to 30%
  - Slip progression is generally asymptomatic
  - For low-grade slips, risk not increased by sports participation
- Progression may be more common with other forms of spondylolisthesis
- No substantial increase in problems with low back pain for adults with spondylolisthesis when compared with the general population

Diagnosis

Differential diagnosis

- Lumbar disc herniation
- Lumbar facet syndrome
- Congenital spinal stenosis
- Sacroiliac joint disorders

History

- Axial back pain with activity
- Younger athletes and individuals who exercise
- Leg pain with standing or walking in patients with root compression
- Older individuals with previous diagnosis of disc problems

Exam

- Pain with back motion, particularly extension, which may cause leg radiation
- Step-off defect noted in the lumbar spine in high-level slips (defect usually felt to palpation at L4-L5, or L5-S1 levels)

- Increased lumbar lordosis
- Tight hamstrings and hip muscles
- Neurological examination usually normal at rest, may have deficits in sensation, strength, and muscle stretch reflexes associated with root injury

Testing

- Can generally be seen on plain radiographs
- Standing flexion/extension views may be helpful to document instability
- Computed tomography (CT) may help clarify the etiology of the slip
- Periodic radiographs should be taken during the adolescent growth spurt to monitor for slip progression

Pitfalls

- Overtreating patients who have minimal symptoms or are asymptomatic
- Missing progression of slips in young patients during the growth spurt

Red Flags

- Progressive pain despite treatment
- Neurological deficits
- Night pain (may be associated with infection or tumor)

Treatment

Medical

- Generally no specific treatment required for a low-grade spondylolisthesis that is nonprogressive and asymptomatic
- Analgesics, and anti-inflammatory medications for pain exacerbations
- Consider adjuvant analgesics for patients with neurogenic claudication

Exercises

- Lumbar stabilization exercises may be effective for LBP when a spondylolisthesis is present
- Back flexion exercises in patients who have worsened pain with extension
- Core strengthening
- Low-level aerobic exercise program during periods of exacerbation, cycling may be an alternative

Modalities

- Cryotherapy
- Superficial heat
- Transcutaneous electrical nerve stimulation, electrical stimulation

Injection

- Blocks may be used for patients with radicular symptoms or facet joint pain, particularly older patients with nonprogressive slips

Surgical

- Surgical evaluation for patients with slips over 50%, neurological symptoms, or symptomatic instability
- Fusion, fusion plus instrumentation, and bone grafting are alternatives

Consults

- Orthopedic/spine surgery
- Neurological/spine surgery
- Physical medicine and rehabilitation
- Pain medicine

Complications/side effects

- Progressive pain that limits activity
- Infection, hardware failure, limited back motion following surgery

Prognosis

- Good for the majority of patients
- Low-grade slips rarely progress

Helpful Hints

- Many patients with spondylolisthesis do well with conservative treatment, this should be communicated to patients early
- Try to identify muscle imbalances, weakness, and biomechanical problems, which may be the real cause of pain

Suggested Readings

Herman MJ, Pizzutillo PD, Cavalier R. Spondylolysis and spondylolisthesis in the child and adolescent athlete. *Orthop Clin N Am.* 2003;34:461–467.

Kalichman L, Hunter DJ. Diagnosis and conservative management of degenerative lumbar spondylolisthesis. *Eur Spine J.* 2008;17:327–335.

Muschik M, Hahnel H, Robinson PN, et al. Competitive sports and the progression of spondylolisthesis. *J Pediatr Orthop.* 1996;16:364–369.

Spondylolysis

Christopher J. Standaert MD

Description

Spondylolysis refers to a defect in the pars interarticularis of the neural arch of a vertebra. Isthmic spondylolysis is the classification for the overwhelming majority of painful pars lesions occurring in adolescent athletes.

Etiology/Types

- Congenital/hereditary: associated with spina bifida occulta, and other congenital anatomical variants
- Isthmic: associated with sports such as gymnastics in which stress is applied to the lumbar spine

Epidemiology

- Present in 4.4% of the general population by age of 6 years and 5% to 6% by age of 18 years
- Present in 8% to 15% of high-level adolescent athletes
- Most common cause of persisting low back pain (LBP) in adolescent athletes
- Thirty percent to 50% of those with spondylolysis will develop a spondylolisthesis

Pathogenesis

- Isthmic spondylolysis is felt to represent a fatigue fracture of the bone
- Associated with repeated hyperextension and rotation of the spine

Risk Factors

- Hereditary predisposition
- Spina bifida occulta
- Extensive participation in sports involving spinal extension and rotation

Clinical Features

- A clinical problem restricted to older children, adolescents, and young adults
- Axial LBP, central or unilateral, acute or gradual in onset
- Symptoms often worsen with lumbar extension, but can occur with flexion
- Symptoms worsened by activity, relieved by rest

Natural History

- Majority of pars defects identified on radiographs have occurred without pain
- Unilateral "acute" fractures of the pars have bony healing rates of 75% or more
- "Chronic" appearing symptomatic pars fractures do not obtain bony healing

Diagnosis

Differential diagnosis

- Lumbar facet syndrome
- Lumbar ligaments strain
- Annular tears/contained lumbar disc herniations
- Sacroilitis/spondyloarthropathies

History

- Acute back pain following sports participation
- Gradual onset of axial back pain in young athletes
- Worsens with back extension activities (gymnastics), trunk rotation (tennis), loading and forceful motion of the spine (football linemen)
- Results in limitation of activity

Exam

- Pain with back extension, limited trunk flexion
- Tight hamstrings and hip flexor muscles
- Weak abdominal and trunk muscles
- No neurological deficits
- May present with positive one leg hyperextension test, which reproduces the pain (sensitivity and specificity being debated)

Testing

- Plain radiographs of relatively poor sensitivity compared with other modalities
- Oblique views of lumbar spine allow visualization of the pars; negative films do not rule out an acute process; positive films may reveal an old injury
- Nuclear imaging with bone scan/single photon emission computed tomography (SPECT) represents best screening tool but is not highly specific
  - Positive study correlates with painful pars lesion
- Computed tomography (CT) is highly specific in patients with a positive SPECT
  - Can stage the pars fracture for treatment
- Magnetic resonance imaging (MRI) is less sensitive than SPECT/CT
  - Limited data on application of MRI to clinical care

Pitfalls
- Diagnostic studies may be false negative
- Allowing activity too soon after diagnosis may lead to recurrent symptoms

Red Flags
- Radicular symptoms after initial episode of axial pain
- Night pain, or constitutional symptoms such as fever

Treatment

Medical
- Relative rest, including restriction from all sporting activities
  - Three months for acute or subacute ("progressive") pars fractures
  - Until asymptomatic for chronic pars fractures
- Bracing is controversial, provides a means of limiting gross lumbar motion
- Consider bracing if symptoms not resolving after 2 to 3 weeks of rest
- Comprehensive rehabilitation after appropriate rest
- Majority of affected athletes return to play with minimal to no pain after treatment
- Surgery rarely indicated for management of pain

Exercises
- Back flexion and stabilization
- Hamstring and hip flexor stretching
- Core strengthening
- Balance training

Modalities
- Cryotherapy
- Superficial heat
- Transcutaneous electrical nerve stimulation (TENS), electrical stimulation

- Ultrasound followed by stretching of tight muscles (in older adolescents, avoid growth plates in younger athletes)

Injection
- May be used in chronic pars lesions that remain symptomatic (limited literature on its use)

Surgical
- Rarely indicated, surgical fusion advocated for symptomatic patients with chronic lesions
- Unclear role in acute cases

Consults
- Orthopedic/spine surgery
- Neurological/spine surgery
- Physical medicine and rehabilitation

Complications/side effects
- Limitation of sports activity
- Residual pain in chronic lesions

Prognosis
- Good with early diagnosis and appropriate management

Helpful Hints
- Suspect spondylolysis in any young athlete with back pain
- Negative diagnostic studies, particularly x-rays, do not rule out the diagnosis
- Follow the patient clinically for decisions of return to play, the bone/SPECT may remain positive for several months after the patient is clinically improved

Suggested Readings
Standaert CJ. Low back pain in the adolescent athlete. *Phys Med Rehabil Clin N Am.* 2008;19:287–304.

Standaert CJ, Herring SA. Spondylolysis: a critical review. *Br J Sports Med.* 2000;34:415–422.

Stingers and Burners

Trevin Thurman MD ▧ Mark Harrast MD

Description

Stingers, sometimes called burners, are peripheral nerve injuries in sports that occur at variable points from the exiting cervical nerve roots to the brachial plexus causing radiating arm pain, paresthesias, and/or weakness.

Etiology/Types

- Tensile (stretch) injury to the cervical nerve root or brachial plexus
- Compressive injury to the cervical nerve root or brachial plexus

Epidemiology

- Estimated that over 50% of collegiate football players sustain a stinger each year although the precise incidence is unknown

Pathogenesis

- An acute compressive or tensile load to the cervical nerve roots or brachial plexus
- Cervical roots are at higher risk due to:
  - Cervical foramina narrow with extension and rotation
  - Limited epineural and perineural tissue
- The C5 root is particularly vulnerable as it is the shortest cervical nerve root
- The ventral (motor) roots at all levels are more susceptible to injury as the dorsal root ganglion can dampen force through the dorsal root
- Tensile injuries are most common in younger athletes, as their weaker neck and shoulder girdle musculature are unable to dynamically withstand sudden lateral bending loads to the neck
- Cervical root compression is most common in stronger, older athletes, occurring with forceful cervical extension and rotation that narrows the cervical neuroforamen
- Can occur in nonathletes who sustain trauma, such as in rear end motor vehicle accidents

Risk Factors

- Weak neck and shoulder girdle muscles
- Cervical neuroforaminal stenosis

Clinical Features

- Sudden burning pain in one upper limb following trauma
- Player often exits the field holding the affected limb motionless against the abdomen, similar to a shoulder dislocation
- Pain usually lasts seconds to minutes, the first occurrence is often not reported by athletes
- Sensory complaints generally resolve quickly but weakness may persist
- Symptoms usually in a single dermatomal distribution—C5, C6, C7 most common
- C5 myotomal weakness is the most common residual neurological deficit
- Simultaneous bilateral stingers are extremely uncommon and this presentation should be evaluated as a potential spinal cord injury

Natural History

- Generally, symptoms resolve very quickly, from seconds to hours, and less commonly days or longer
- Symptoms often recur if not appropriately treated
- Multiple episodes may lead to permanent neurological injury

Diagnosis

Differential diagnosis

- Transient quadriparesis
- Shoulder dislocation
- Central cord syndrome

History

- Sudden burning pain, paresthesias, or weakness in one upper limb after trauma
- Recurrence often occurs if symptoms not treated initially

Exam

- Cervical range of motion to assess pain provocation and rigidity
- Palpation for body tenderness and/or paraspinal muscle spasm
- Detailed neurological examination focusing on the C5-C7 myotomes
- Serial examinations are necessary until symptoms resolve

Testing

- Cervical magnetic resonance imaging (MRI) or computed tomography (CT) for persistent, severe, or recurrent symptoms
- Electromyography (EMG) if weakness persists beyond 10 to 14 days
- Cervical radiographs including anteroposterior, lateral, flexion, extension, and bilateral oblique views to evaluate for altered cervical alignment, hypermobility, fracture, and foraminal narrowing

Pitfalls

- Unrecognized spinal cord injury in athletes with bilateral symptoms

Red Flags

- Neurological symptoms in both upper limbs or all four limbs

Treatment

Medical

- Nonsteroidal anti-inflammatory medications

Exercise

- Gentle stretching
- Directed strengthening of the cervical paraspinals, upper thoracic and scapular stabilizers, global trunk and core postural stabilizers
- Specific strengthening of focal muscle weakness due to the initial stinger
- Sports- and position-specific exercise

Modalities

- Thermal agents
- Manual traction

Injection

- Cervical epidural steroid injections for persistent symptoms

Surgical

- Surgical decompression of foraminal stenosis if progressive motor loss—rare

Consults

- Physical medicine and rehabilitation or neurology for electrodiagnostic studies (EMG)
- Physical medicine and rehabilitation or anesthesiology for epidural injection
- Neurosurgical or orthopedic-spine if surgical decompression is considered

Complications/side effects

- Persistent weakness in severe or recurrent cases

Prognosis

- Number of previous stingers guides return to play as more severe and persistent motor deficits occur in athletes with recurrent stingers
- Following initial stinger, if full recovery is demonstrated within 15 minutes, then return to competition is allowed
- Following initial stinger, if full recovery occurs within a week after the initial stinger, then return to competition is allowed the next week
- With recurrent stingers, the player is held from competition the number of weeks that correspond to stingers incurred in a given season (eg, 2 weeks for a second stinger)
- If more than three stingers occur in a season, restricting the athlete from play for the remainder of the season must be considered, particularly if there is significant weakness, signs of axonopathy on EMG, and focal cervical disc herniation or significant foraminal stenosis on MRI

Helpful Hints

- Preventive preparticipation-conditioning programs may reduce interplay stingers
- Shoulder pad lifters and cervical rolls to reduce lateral bending and cervical hyperextension
- Comprehensive rehabilitation addressing postural faults and other mechanical factors should be prescribed after sustaining a stinger

Suggested Readings

Harrast MA, Weinstein SM. Cervical spine. In: Kibler WB, ed. *Orthopaedic Knowledge Update: Sports Medicine 4*. Rosemont, IL: AAOS; 2009.

Weinberg J, Rokito S, Silber JS. Etiology, treatment, and prevention of athletic "stingers." *Clin Sports Med.* 2003;22(3):493–500.

Stress Fracture of the Ankle and Foot

John C. Cianca MD

Description
Stress fractures are common in running sports, resulting from repetitive stress due to excessive muscular forces or from fatigue of the structural supports of the bone.

Etiology/Types
- Reaction to repetitive stress
- Low, medium, and high-risk fracture sites (Table 1)

Epidemiology
- Common and rare sites of fractures (Table 2)
- Common in runners, dancers, walkers, jumping sports, military recruits
- Tibia and second metatarsal are most common sites in general

Pathogenesis
- Repetitive loading increases forces at a bone, which increases osteoclastic degradation such that it exceeds osteoblastic repair

Table 1. Stress Fracture Risk Assessment

Low	Medium	High
Fibula	Medial malleolus	Navicular
Lateral malleolus	Proximal fifth	Talus
Calcaneus	metatarsal	Proximal
Cuboid		second
Cuneiforms		metatarsal
Distal and midshaft metatarsals		

Table 2. Stress Fracture Location

Common Stress fractures	Rare stress fractures
Distal tibia	Medial malleolus
Fibula	Cuboid
Calcaneus	Cuneiforms
Second to fifth metatarsals	First metatarsal
Talus	sesamoids
Navicular	

- Periosteal stress reaction, which includes edema and microfractures
- A cortical break occurs if the repetitive loading continues
- Risk factors may cause faster onset and progression

Risk Factors
- Females >> males
- Cavus feet and overpronation of feet
- Metabolic bone disease
- Eating disorders
- Late menarche, irregular menstrual periods, or amenorrhea
- Rapid increase in training

Clinical Features
- Localized sharp pain
- Worsened with initial weight bearing and prolonged weight bearing
- Localized edema and a palpable bump at the site
- Limits ability to run or jump; even walking may be difficult

Natural History
- Initially pain occurs with onset of exercise and is less localized
- Pain intensifies, localizes, and becomes more frequent and limiting
- Responds quickly if repetitive loading is reduced early in the clinical course
- High-risk fractures are at risk for delayed or nonunion

Diagnosis

Differential diagnosis
- Varies with the location of the stress fracture
- Distal tibia: shin splints, compartment syndrome, popliteal artery entrapment
- Ankle: degenerative joint disease (DJD), tendinopathy
- Heel: tarsal tunnel syndrome, plantar fasciitis, fat pad contusion
- Mid foot: anterior tarsal tunnel syndrome, tendinopathy, Lisfranc injury
- Forefoot: DJD, gout, tendinopathy, synovitis

History

- Rapid increase in training duration, frequency, or intensity
- Progressively worsening pain that becomes localized
- Point tenderness
- Progressive disability
- Talar and navicular stress fractures may be more vague and less localized

Exam

- Point tenderness, local induration
- Hop test causes reproduction of pain
- Look for excessive pronation in tibial and tarsal stress fractures
- Hypomobile feet in metatarsal stress fractures
- Tenderness over the proximal dorsal surface of navicular (N spot) for stress fractures

Testing

- X-rays unreliable early in course of a stress fracture. Periosteal reaction may be seen as a fuzzy, gray area
- Bone scan may be very sensitive; may be positive 2 days after onset of symptoms. All three phases are positive in an acute stress fracture
- Magnetic resonance imaging (MRI) often the test of choice, but may pick up clinically asymptomatic areas of "stress" such as the calcaneus
- Diagnostic ultrasound is helpful in bones that are easily visualized

Pitfalls

- Talar and navicular stress fractures are often misdiagnosed due to vague pain
- Consider accessory navicular with navicular pain

Red Flags

- Tarsal coalition is associated with talar stress fractures
- "N" spot pain is very characteristic for navicular stress fractures
- Menstrual irregularity or amenorrhea
- Eating disorders

Treatment

Medical

- Cessation of offending activity
- Pain relievers as needed
- Check shoes and feet
- Low- and medium-risk fractures require protected weight bearing
- High-risk fractures require strict non-weight bearing

Exercises

- Water exercise or reduced weight bearing exercise such as cycling initially
- Gradual return to activity after pain subsides for 10 to 14 days
- Core strengthening

Modalities

- Acupuncture may reduce pain, speed healing
- Bone stimulators may also promote healing

Injection

- None

Surgical

- Surgical fixation may be needed in middle one-third navicular, and proximal second and fifth metatarsal fractures
- Surgical excision of lateral process of talus is done for some talar stress fractures

Consults

- Podiatry: orthotic fabrication for excessive pronation or other functional deformities
- Endocrinology: metabolic bone disease
- Obstetrics and Gynecology: menstrual disorders
- Nutrition: eating disorders

Complications/side effects

- Delayed or nonunion in high-risk stress fractures

Prognosis

- Excellent with early recognition and activity modification
- Guarded in high-risk fractures or in individuals with intrinsic risk factors

Helpful Hints

- Inquire about menstrual cycle and eating habits
- Do not be fooled by negative x-rays

Suggested Reading

Brukner P, Bennell K, Matheson G. Stress fractures of the foot and ankle. In: Brukner P, Bennel K, Matheson G, eds. *Stress Fractures*. Malden, MA: Blackwell Science; 1999:163–186.

Fredericson M, Fabio J, Beaulieu C, et al. Stress fracture in athletes. *Top Magn Reson Imaging.* 2006;17(5):309–325.

Stress Fracture of the Femur

Michael Fredericson MD FACSM

Description

Accelerated bony remodeling in response to repetitive submaximal stresses. With an increase in physical activity, the osteoclastic activity exceeds the rate of osteoblastic new bone formation and eventually a full cortical break occurs.

Etiology/Types

- Two categories of stress fracture: fatigue fractures (excessive, repetitive stress on normal bone) or insufficiency fractures (normal activity in bone that is deficient in structure or quantity)
- Most common sites: femoral neck and shaft
- Lesser trochanter stress fractures: a subgroup of femoral neck fractures
- Distal femoral stress fractures: rare
- Two types of stress fracture of the femoral neck: the distraction or tension type (typically in older osteoporotic patients) and the compression type (younger athletic patients)

Epidemiology

- Stress fractures: 10% of all injuries seen by sports medicine specialists
- Femoral neck stress fractures: 11% of all stress fractures in athletes
- Femoral shaft stress fractures: 3.5% of all stress fractures in athletes
- Women affected more than men

Pathogenesis

- Repetitive response to stress leads to osteoclastic activity that surpasses the rate of osteoblastic new bone formation, resulting in temporary weakening of bone
- If the physical activity is continued, trabecular microfractures result
- If the osteoclastic activity continues to exceed the rate of osteoblastic new bone formation, a full cortical break occurs
- Stress fractures occur owing to the increased load after fatigue of supporting structures and/or to contractile muscular forces acting across and on the bone

Risk Factors

- Training errors: sudden increase in the intensity or volume of exercise
- Gender: females are at greater risk than males
- Intrinsic factors: lower extremity alignment (leg length inequality, coxa vara), low bone mass, amenorrhea, metabolic disorders (diet or hormonal imbalance)

Clinical Features

- Pain begins after a change in the usual activity regimen or an increase in its intensity
- Localized pain that is not present at the start, but occurs after or toward the end of physical activity
- Vague groin, hip, or anterior thigh pain that worsens with continued weight bearing
- Limited or painful range of motion of the hip
- Local tenderness over the involved bone difficult to elicit in the hip

Natural History

- Untreated stress fractures display pain that progresses during the physical activity
- With continued training, pain will persist into daily ambulation
- The severity of the pain may limit or prohibit activity. Some patients may also experience night pain
- If there is no change in activity, pathological fracture can occur

Diagnosis

Differential diagnosis

- Proximal femur: avascular necrosis, infection, transient osteoporosis, iliopsoas bursitis, synovitis, synovial herniation pit, muscle or tendon injury, and neoplasm
- Femoral shaft pain: quadriceps muscle strain, contusion, infection, or neoplasm
- Distal femoral pain: internal knee derangement, femoral condyle avascular necrosis, infection, tendon and ligament injury, or neoplasm

History

- Change in the training regimen during the preceding 2 to 6 weeks

- Localized pain that progresses during physical activity
- Limitation of activity

Exam
- Palpation over the hip joint may reproduce a patient's symptoms related to stress fractures of the femoral neck
- Pain at the extremes of passive range of motion of the hip
- Hop and fulcrum tests exacerbate pain and may help to localize the site of femoral stress fractures

Testing
- Radiographical findings may not be seen until 2 to 8 weeks after onset of symptoms
- Radionuclide (Tc-99) scanning is a more sensitive but less specific method for imaging bony stress injuries
- Magnetic resonance imaging plays an important role in the diagnosis of femoral stress fractures and the differentiation of femoral stress fractures from other causes of thigh pain. Identification of early marrow edema on fat-suppressed T2-weighted images (initial sign of bone response to stress). T1- and T2-weighted images used to identify areas of femoral stress fracture
- Computed tomography scan is useful in differentiating conditions that mimic stress fractures on bone scan, such as osteoid osteoma, osteomyelitis with Brodie abscess, and various malignancies
- Bone mineral density testing as indicated

Pitfalls
- The most common misdiagnosis of a stress fracture is bone sarcoma because of the periosteal reaction

Red Flags
- Neoplasm
- Delayed diagnosis can result in a complete or displaced fracture that requires more aggressive treatment

Treatment

Medical
- Prevention: education and identification of risk factors
- Period of non-weight bearing: length of time dependent on location, extent of injury, and underlying bone quality
- Pain control: avoid nonsteroidal anti-inflammatory drugs (can impede bone healing); acetaminophen and analgesics if needed
- Nutrition: assess for adequate calcium and vitamin D
- Hormone replacement therapy: consider in amenorrheic females if unable to elicit normal menses

Exercises
- Modified activity program to maintain strength and fitness but to reduce impact loading to the skeleton
- Activities such as swimming, pool running, elliptical exercise, or cycling when pain-free
- Progressive physiotherapy program for closed kinetic chain pelvic and lower extremity stabilization

Modalities
- Cryotherapy (for symptomatic relief)
- Heat
- Electrical stimulation

Injection
- Not indicated

Surgical
- Rarely needed
- Indication for internal fixation: failure of nonoperative management, prophylactic stabilization of a fracture at high risk for displacement, a tension-side femoral neck stress fracture, any displaced femoral stress fracture

Consults
- Sports medicine
- Orthopedic surgery

Complications/side effects
- Displacement of the fracture
- Nonunion, malunion, osteonecrosis, and arthritic changes
- Avascular necrosis after stress fracture of the femoral head with displacement

Prognosis
- Return-to-play and activity based on a combination of radiographical healing and ability to progress pain-free weight-bearing activity

Helpful Hints
- Importance of prevention: education and identification of risk factors

Suggested Readings
DeFranco MJ, Recht M, Schils J, et al. Stress fractures of the femur in athletes. *Clin Sports Med.* 2006;25(1):89–103.

Fredericson M, Jang K, Bergman G, et al. Femoral diaphyseal stress fractures: results of a systematic bone scan and magnetic resonance imaging evaluation in 26 runners. *Phys Ther Sport.* 2004;188–193.

Fredericson M, Jennings F, Beaulieu C, et al. Stress fractures in athletes. *Top Magn Reson Imaging.* 2006;17(5):309–325.

Nguyen JT, Peterson JS, Biswal S, et al. Stress-related injuries around the lesser trochanter in long-distance runners. *Am J Roentgen.* 2008;190(6):1616–1620.

Stress Fracture of the Tibia

Matthew C. Thompson MD ■ Stacy L. Lynch MD ■ Anne Z. Hoch DO

Description

Tibial stress fractures are a common cause of lower leg pain, often resulting from a sudden increase in repetitive activity that results in localized pain that returns with the onset of activity and may progress to pain at rest. Repetitive stress exceeds the bone's native ability to repair itself and results in a microfracture of the tibia.

Etiology/Types

- Compression side fractures occur on anterior-medial aspect of the tibia, with the junction between the middle and distal third being most common
- Tension side fractures usually occur on the anterior edge of the tibial midshaft and usually occur in well-trained athletes whose sport involves repetitive running or jumping

Epidemiology

- Universal, involving both well-trained and casual athletes
- Increased incidence with activities involving repetitive running, jumping, or walking
- Three and a half times higher in females and military recruits
- Two times higher in whites than African Americans

Pathogenesis

- Often seen with increased repetitive activities involving running and jumping
- Due to repetitive loading of tibia, the major weight-bearing bone of the lower leg, leading to microtrauma with deficient bone remodeling

Risk Factors

- Running and jumping activities
- Rapid increase in activity or duration
- Menstrual or hormonal disturbances
- Poor physical condition
- Female gender, military recruits
- Low bone turnover rate
- Reduced bone mineral density (ie, osteopenia/osteoporosis)
- Decreased cortical bone thickness/pathological bone states
- Dietary/nutritional deficiencies
- Body size extremes/composition
- Training on uneven/irregular surfaces
- Poor flexibility
- Inadequate muscle strength
- Inappropriate footwear
- Poor body mechanics/limb and foot alignment (i.e., genu valgum, leg length discrepancy, rigid cavus foot, or excessively pronating foot)
- Smoking

Clinical Features

- Initial presentation may be medial tibial stress syndrome (MTSS), athletes continued to train and pain worsens
- Pain progresses, develops earlier with activity, and progresses to pain at rest

Natural History

- Heal with activity modification
- Anterior tibial fractures may not heal and require surgery

Diagnosis

Differential diagnosis

- MTSS
- Tibial traction periostitis
- Compartment syndrome
- Muscle strain
- Nerve entrapment
- Fascial abnormality
- Popliteal artery entrapment
- Posterior tibial tendinosis

History

- Recent increase in intensity and/or duration of repetitive activity
- Mild pain early, often toward end of activity, which progresses to earlier activity and often at rest
- Night pain frequent

Exam

- Localized pain over fracture site (anterior or anterior-medial most common)

- Edema and/or erythema may be present over fracture site
- Palpable lump or fullness representing new bone formation
- Tuning fork at distal site may elicit pain at fracture site
- Positive hop test (pain with jumping usually in symptomatic leg)
- Fulcrum test (with the patient sitting and the knee and leg extended, the examiner applies downward pressure to the patients knee, while applying upward pressure to the patients leg reproducing symptoms of pain in the tibia)
- Thump tests (with the patient sitting or supine apply pressure "thumping" to the heel and pain may be reproduced)

Testing
- Plain radiographs may reveal dreaded black line, periosteal elevation, bony callous formation (Figure 1)
- Bone scan (triple phase bone scan very sensitive but not specific)
- Magnetic resonance imaging (MRI)
- A four-stage progression of bony injury based on MRI results is used to grade stress fractures
  - Stage I: inflammation of the periosteum (STIR)
  - Stage II: inflammation of the marrow and periostial edema (T2)
  - Stage III: more significant marrow edema (T1)
  - Stage IV: extensive marrow edema with incidence of a visual fracture line

Pitfalls
- Initial radiographs may be negative, taking up to 10 weeks after symptom onset to show fracture

Red Flags
- Reduced bone mineral density
- Amenorrhea or menstrual dysfunction
- Disordered eating
- Repetitive stress fractures

Treatment
Medical
- Physical therapy for strengthening and conditioning
- Activity modification/proper techniques
- Avoid nonsteroidal anti-inflammatory drugs (NSAIDs) and smoking
- For compression side fractures, limit impact loading, no running or jumping for 8 to 12 weeks, and casting/walking boot for limited time, which reduces atrophy and stiffness
- For tension side fracture, immobilization in cast (non-weight bearing for 3 to 6 months due to high nonunion rate)
- Thorough screening and treatment for the female athlete triad or other associated nutritional, metabolic, and biochemical risk factors

Exercises
- Gastrocnemius/soleus stretching
- Ankle muscle strengthening
- Proprioceptive balance training

Modalities
- Ice may provide pain relief
- May benefit from electrical stimulation

Injection
- Not indicated

Surgical
- If nonoperative treatment fails, cortical drilling, bone grafting, or intramedullary nailing is considered

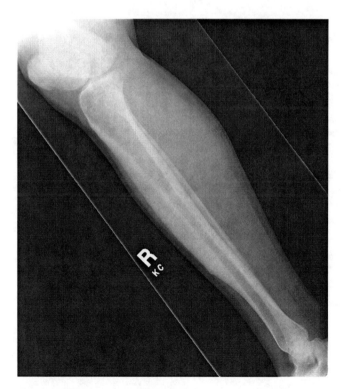

Figure 1. Tibial stress fracture "dreaded black line."

Consults
- Sports medicine
- Orthopedic surgery
- Nutritionist

Complications/side effects
- Nonunion (higher for tension-sided stress fractures)

Prognosis
- Return to previous activity if properly diagnosed and treated
- Healing time is variable and based on severity of injury; may take 2 or 3 weeks up to 6 months, though some athletes may require a year or more for full recovery

Helpful Hints
- Caution with initial negative radiographs
- Slow return to activity after proper treatment
- Screen for the female athlete triad

Suggested Readings

Hoch AZ, Pepper M, Akuthota V. Stress fractures and knee injuries in runners. *Phys Med Rehabil Clin N Am.* 2005;16:749–777.

Raasch WG, Hergan DJ. Treatment of stress fractures: the fundamentals. *Clin Sports Med.* 2006;25:29–36.

Sanderlin BW, Raspa RF. Common stress fractures. *Am Fam Phys.* 2003;68(8):1527–1532.

Suprascapular Neuropathy

William Sullivan MD

Description

Suprascapular neuropathy was first described in the English literature in 1959. Isolated injuries uncommon, but the suprascapular nerve is the most frequently injured brachial plexus peripheral nerve amongst athletes. It is predominantly a motor nerve, sensory to acromioclavicular joint (AC), glenohumeral joint, subacromial bursa, and ligaments. The nerve arises from the upper trunk of the brachial plexus.

Etiology/Types

- Associated with overhead sports
- Entrapment or injury at suprascapular notch may cause pain because of involvement of deep sensory structures, and weakness of the supraspinatus and infraspinatus
- Injury at the spinoglenoid notch causes no sensory symptoms, or pain but results in infraspinatus weakness
- May be associated with neuralgic amyotrophy/brachial plexitis/Parsonage/Turner syndrome

Epidemiology

- Good epidemiological studies lacking
- Up to 45% of volleyball players have infraspinatus involvement, often asymptomatic
- Eight percent of all nerve injuries in athletes
- One percent to 2% of painful shoulder disorders
- Throwing, overhead athletes, weightlifters, and dancers at risk

Pathogenesis

- Suprascapular notch most common site of entrapment
- Distal entrapment at spinoglenoid notch less common
- Nerve immobile at trunk and suprascaplular notch
- Transverse scapular ligament may be ossified
- Shoulder complex is very mobile, which may lead to increase traction or entrapment at ligament sites
- Rare cases of metastatic carcinoma, sarcomas
- Ganglion cysts at spinoglenoid notch, often secondary to labral pathology can cause entrapment
- Iatrogenic injury during surgical procedures: for example, rotator cuff repair and positioning for other conditions (eg, lumbar spine surgery)
- Vascular injury to suprascapular artery, microvascular injury

Risk Factors

- Position dependent in overhead sports, volleyball, baseball, and tennis
- Heavy manual labor
- Viral illness, or immunizations (Parsonage/Turner syndrome)

Clinical Features

- Signs and symptoms depend on location of entrapment
- Many athletes asymptomatic with teres minor assisting with infraspinatus function
- Pain may be deep, worse with shoulder movement

Natural History

- Athlete with infraspinatus involvement may continue to participate in sports
- Unknown, varies based on cause
- Most reports demonstrate resolution with nonoperative care
- Some reports identify asymptomatic lesions, conclude a benign condition without need for further treatment

Diagnosis

Differential diagnosis

- Rotator cuff tendinopathy
- C5-C6 radiculopathy
- Neuralgic amyotrophy
- Thoracic outlet syndrome
- AC joint degeneration
- Glenohumeral instability

History

- Pain with overhead activity
- Weakness and loss of velocity of tennis serve, baseball pitch, and overhead spike in volleyball

Exam

- Protraction of scapula may increase traction on suprascapular nerve
- Tenderness at suprascapular notch
- Infraspinatus atrophy easier to observe due to partial covering by trapezius muscle

- Weakness of shoulder abduction (supraspinatus) and external rotation (infraspinatus), but other muscles also perform these motions

Testing
- Electrodiagnostic testing
  - Document supraspinatus and/or infraspinatus involvement
  - Rule out other conditions
  - Motor nerve conduction studies not specific for suprascapular injury, but useful to identify other conditions
  - Sensory nerve conduction studies not helpful for suprascapular neuropathy, but performed to identify other conditions involving plexus
  - Needle electrode examination most helpful
  - Sample other muscles to exclude cervical radiculopathy or other plexus lesion

Imaging
- X-rays usually nondiagnostic, but may identify callus after scapular/clavicular fracture or calcified transverse scapular ligament
- Magnetic resonance imaging (MRI) helpful to identify rotator cuff tears, other soft tissue pathology, and mass lesions
  - May identify ganglion cysts than compress nerve at spinoglenoid notch
  - Atrophy of rotator cuff may be identified

Treatment

Medical
- Trial of nonoperative care indicated for those cases attributable to repetitive trauma, especially in the absence of a compressive lesion (eg, glenoid cyst)
- Nonsteroidal anti-inflammatory drug (NSAID)

Exercises
- Posterior capsule stretching may decrease traction on suprascapular nerve, theoretically reducing tension on the transverse scapular ligament
- Strengthening of scapular stabilizers and rotator cuff
- Postural retraining, scapular retraction
- Sports-specific training

Modalities
- Cryotherapy

- Superficial heat
- Electrical stimulation

Injections
- Diagnostic injection proposed, but sensitivity studies lacking
- Percutaneous aspiration of ganglion cyst with computed tomography (CT) or ultrasound guidance (ganglion cysts associated with labral tears)
- Fifty percent failure/recurrence after aspiration

Surgical
- Release of transverse scapular ligament, notchplasty
- High-quality data on surgical outcomes lacking: retrospective, small numbers, short follow-up

Consults
- Physical medicine and rehabilitation
- Orthopedic surgery

Complications/side effects
- Chronic residual weakness
- Pain with overhead activity

Prognosis
- Good for function
- May return to overhead sports following rehabilitation (despite residual infraspinatus weakness)

Helpful Hints
- Repetitive nerve compression injuries may result in irreversible muscle atrophy and loss of mobility so early treatment is important
- Awareness of the condition, especially in overhead athletes (volleyball), may increase diagnostics

Suggested Readings

Dumitru D, Zwarts MJ. Brachial plexopathies and proximal mononeuropathies. In: *Electrodiagnostic Medicine*. 2nd ed. Philadelphia: Hanley and Belfus; 2002:805–806.

Preston DC, Shapiro BE. Proximal neuropathies of the shoulder and arm. In: *Electromyography and Neuromuscular Disorders: Clinical-Electrophysiologic Correlations*. 2nd ed. Philadelphia: Elsevier Butterworth-Heinemann; 2005:501–503.

Safran MR. Nerve injury about the shoulder in athletes, part 1: suprascapular nerve and axillary nerve. *Am J Sports Med*. 2004;32:803–810.

Tarsal Tunnel Syndrome

Channarayapatna R. Sridhara MD ■ Thomas Savadove MD MPH

Description

Tarsal tunnel syndrome (TTS) is an uncommon unilateral entrapment neuropathy of the posterior tibial nerve or any of its distal branches as it passes across the ankle (Figure 1).

Etiology/Types

■ Idiopathic causes
- Fibrosis and thickening of the flexor retinaculum
- Hypertrophic abductor hallucis
- Presence of accessory muscles
- Obesity

■ Trauma and posttraumatic changes
- Ankle fractures
- Direct contusion
- Athletics (running, jogging)
- Scar tissue
- Flexion-eversion injuries of the ankle (joint hypermobility)

■ Biomechanical causes related to joint structure or deformity
- Talocalcaneal coalition
- Heel varus or valgus
- Pes planus/overpronation
- Tenosynovitis

■ Systemic diseases
- Diabetes
- Rheumatoid arthritis
- Peripheral vascular disease
- Leprosy
- Endocrine pathologies including acromegaly, hypothyroidism

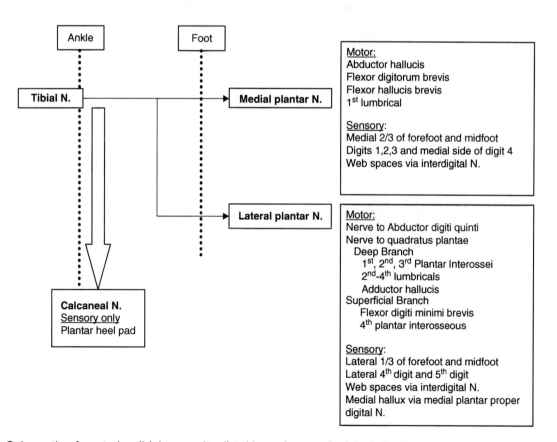

Figure 1. Schematic of posterior tibial nerve, its distal branches, and related structures.

- Space-occupying lesions/structures causing compression
  - Lipoma, schwannoma, neurilemmoma
  - Neurofibrosarcoma
  - Varicosities, hemangioma
  - Ganglion cysts

Epidemiology

- The most common site of tibial mononeuropathy
- Associated with ankle trauma and participation in running and jumping sports
- Seen in individuals with hyperpronation, pes planus, and weak posterior tibial muscles

Pathogenesis

- Difficult to determine the exact pathogenesis of TTS. Associated with compression or traction of the nerve at the level of the tarsal tunnel
- The tarsal tunnel in the medial ankle tunnel is roofed by the flexor retinaculum (lancinate ligament), runs between the medial malleolus and medial calcaneus, and has a bony floor formed by the medial ankle and talus
- With the tibial nerve beneath the retinaculum are the tibial artery and vein, and the tendons of the tibialis posterior, flexor digitorum longus, and flexor hallucis longus in their own compartments
- Within the tunnel, the tibial nerve branches into the medial calcaneal, medial plantar, and lateral plantar nerves, which travel in their own fibrous tunnels along medial edge of abductor hallucis
- The lateral plantar nerve is the smaller of the two terminal branches. The first branch of the lateral plantar nerve is known as the lateral calcaneal nerve (Baxter's nerve) and runs under the quadratus plantae laterally, innervating the abductor digiti quinti; compression of this branch may cause heel pain
- The medial plantar nerve courses distally under the abductor hallucis beneath a fibrous slip that envelops the flexor hallucis longus and flexor digitorum longus tendons and binds to the medial plantar surface of the navicular bone (Master Knot of Henry) and may be an area of entrapment
- The tibial nerve may be compressed:
  - In the distal leg between the lower edge of the gastrocnemius muscle and the posteromedial tibia (high TTS)
  - In the ankle beneath the flexor retinaculum (classic TTS)
  - After it exits from beneath the flexor retinaculum in any of its distal branches (distal TTS)

Risk Factors

- Pes planus
- Underlying ganglion cyst or space-occupying lesion

Clinical Features

- Pain along the medial ankle and foot
- Tingling and burning sensations in the sole of the foot
- Pain occurs at rest and is intensified after standing or walking

Natural History

- Pain and intolerance to activity worsens if not appropriately treated
- May improve with conservative treatment

Diagnosis

Differential diagnosis

- L5 or S1 radiculopathy
- Peripheral neuropathy
- Sciatic neuropathy
- Lumbosacral plexopathy
- Proximal tibial neuropathy
- Interdigital neuropathy (eg, Morton's neuroma)
- Medial plantar proper digital neuropathy (eg, Joplin's neuroma)
- Plantar fasciitis

History

- Patient may present with burning, tingling, and/or numbness in the toes, ball of foot, and heel in the distribution of the branch involved
- Pain may be expressed as throbbing, cramping, or tightness and may radiate to the medial calf
- Prolonged standing or walking exacerbates symptoms, and less commonly may awaken the patient at night with relief of symptoms by rest and removal of footwear

Exam

- Tinel sign at the tarsal tunnel posterior to the medial malleolus is the most helpful physical finding

- Sensory loss tested objectively by pinprick or two-point discrimination with comparison to the unaffected side may reveal loss of sensation in the distribution of the medial plantar, lateral plantar, or calcaneal nerve or in combination
- Weakness of the intrinsic muscles of the foot and abductor hallucis is difficult to detect and is not a common finding but there may be intrinsic muscle wasting or clawing of the second through fifth digits, indicating more severe and longstanding nerve injury
- The dorsiflexion-eversion test: examiner holds the foot in maximal ankle dorsiflexion and eversion while simultaneously maximally dorsiflexing all the metatarsophalangeal joints for 5 to 10 seconds, with reproduction or intensification of symptoms
- Palpable soft tissue mass posterior to the medial malleolus
- Ankle movement and deep tendon reflexes are not affected

Testing
- X-rays to identify bony deformity or fractures
- Ultrasound or magnetic resonance imaging (MRI) may reveal occupying lesion or tendinopathy
- Electrodiagnostic testing
  - The greatest diagnostic yield is found in the sensory or mixed nerve conduction studies (NCS) with slow conduction velocity, small amplitude, or absent response (detection rate of 90% vs 50% for motor NCS alone)
  - Prolonged distal tibial motor onset latency with recording over the abductor hallucis and abductor digiti minimi pedis muscles
  - Electromyography (EMG) findings of positive sharp wave and fibrillations in the abductor digiti minimi pedis, abductor hallucis, and intrinsic (first dorsal interosseous) muscles of the foot with reduced recruitment

Pitfalls
- Missing the diagnosis because of lack of suspicion
- Not addressing the specific etiology

Red Flags
- Severe ankle pain
- Progressive weakness and sensory loss
- Pain at night

Treatment

Medical
- Treatment depends on finding the root cause of the entrapment
- Systemic disease (eg, diabetes, hypothyroidism, acromegaly) should be treated accordingly
- Look for correctable causes (footwear, biomechanics) and adjust accordingly
- Activity modification
- Orthoses (eg, medial heel wedge)
- Anti-inflammatory medications
- Adjuvant analgesic such as gabapentin, tramadol, and pregabalin
- Lidocaine patches

Exercises
- Achilles tendon stretching
- Anterior tibial, posterior tibial, peroneal, and foot intrinsic muscle strengthening
- Cross training/aquatic rehabilitation

Modalities
- Cryotherapy
- Superficial heat
- Transcutaneous electrical nerve stimulation (TENS)

Injection
- Local injection with corticosteroids may be effective in combination with a rehabilitation program

Surgical
- Surgical release of the flexor retinaculum and associated nerve tunnels accompanied by excision of space-occupying lesions and varicosities
- Patients undergoing surgical release of only the flexor retinaculum, or with a history of prior surgery on the foot, may not show substantial benefit from decompression
- Immediate mobilization with a protective, soft dressing to encourage the formation of a gliding bed in the surgical plane prevents adherence to the tissue and discourages scarification and fibrosis of the nerve

Consults
- Orthopedics/foot and ankle surgery
- Podiatry
- Physical medicine and rehabilitation

Complications/side effects
- Chronic ankle and foot pain

- Infection
- Intolerance to activity

Prognosis
- Variable
- Improves with early diagnosis and correction of biomechanical and structural abnormalities
- Results may not be as good in patients following fracture with severe ankle deformity

Helpful Hints
- Identify treatable causes early to help with treatment success

Suggested Readings

Bashir WA, Connell DA. Imaging of entrapment and compressive neuropathies. *Semin Musculoskelet Radiol.* 2008;12(2):170–181.

Dellon AL. The four medial ankle tunnels: a critical review of perceptions of tarsal tunnel syndrome and neuropathy. *Neurosurg Clin N Am.* 2008;19:629–648.

Mullick T, Dellon AL. Results of decompression of four medial ankle tunnels in the treatment of tarsal tunnel syndrome. *J Reconstr Microsurg.* 2008;24(2):119–126.

Patel AT, Gaines K, Malamut R, et al. Usefulness of electrodiagnostic techniques in the evaluation of suspected tarsal tunnel syndrome: an evidence-based review. AANEM practice topic. *Muscle Nerve.* 2005;32:236–240.

Triangular Fibrocartilage Complex Injuries

David A. Soto-Quijano MD FAAPMR

Description

The triangular fibrocartilage complex (TFCC) contains the ligamentous and cartilaginous structures that form the ulnar aspect of the wrist. It is composed of an articular disc, dorsal and volar radioulnar ligaments, a meniscus homolog, the ulnar collateral, ulnolunate, and ulnotriquetral ligaments and the sheath of the extensor carpi ulnaris (ECU).

The TFCC is the main stabilizer of distal radioulnar joint (DRUJ), contributes to ulnocarpal stability; helps in the distribution of axial loading, increases the gliding surface of the carpus, and supports the proximal carpal row.

Etiology/Types

Palmer classification for TFCC injuries
- Class 1: Traumatic
  - A: central perforation—most common
  - B: ulnar avulsion with or without distal ulnar fracture
  - C: distal avulsion—ulnolunate and ulnotriquetral ligaments
  - D: radial avulsion with or without sigmoid notch fracture
- Class 2: Degenerative
  - A: TFCC wear
  - B: TFCC wear with lunate and/or ulnar chondromalacia
  - C: TFCC perforation with lunate and/or ulnar chondromalacia
  - D: TFCC perforation with lunate and/or ulnar chondromalacia and lunotriquetral (LT) ligament perforation
  - E: TFCC perforation with lunate and/or ulnar chondromalacia, LT ligament perforation, and ulnocarpal arthritis

Epidemiology

- Ulnar-sided pain is one of the most common problems of the wrist—the "low back pain" of the joint

- No studies on the specific prevalence or incidence of TFCC

Pathogenesis

- Degenerative tears are caused by excessive wrist joint loading
- With normal axial loading, approximately 20% of the force is transmitted through the ulna and 80% is transmitted through the radius
- Changes in ulnar variance—the relative length of the ulna with respect to the radius—will affect the distribution of axial loading and promote TFCC injuries
- Distal radius fracture that affects radial length can also change the load distribution
- Can be associated with bone fractures, especially of the distal radius

Risk Factors

- Sports that require upper extremity loading—that is, gymnastics
- Occupational activities with high or repetitive mechanical loading of hands

Clinical Features

- Ulnar-sided wrist pain, frequently accompanied with clicking on pronation/supination that improves with rest and worsens with activity
- Traumatic injuries may be associated with falls onto a pronated and hyperextended wrist, the use of power tools, and distraction force applied to the volar forearm or wrist

Natural History

- Symptomatic traumatic tears with neutral ulnar variance do not worsen over time; one-third of patients are asymptomatic at 9.5 years of follow-up
- Symptomatic traumatic tears with ulnar positive variance worsen over time in two-third of patients

- TFCC degeneration begins in the third decade of life and progressively increases in frequency and severity with time
- TFCC defects are present in 53% of cadaveric asymptomatic elderly wrists
- TFCC was perforated in 46% of wrists in elderly cadavers (mean 76.6 years)

Diagnosis

Differential diagnosis
- LT instability
- LT ligament injuries
- Midcarpal instability
- ECU tendinopathy/subluxation
- Flexor carpi ulnaris (FCU) tendinopathy
- DRUJ arthritis
- Pisotriquetral joint arthritis
- Hook of hamate fracture
- Pisiform fracture
- Hypothenar hammer syndrome
- Essex-Lopresti lesion—proximal radial fracture, disruption of the interosseous membrane, and the DRUJ
- Cervical radiculopathy

History
- Ulnar-sided wrist pain
- Pain with forced forearm pronation and supination
- Pain with gripping and ulnar deviation
- Clicking on pronation/supination
- Pain improves with rest and worsens with activity
- Fall onto a pronated, outstretched extremity
- Axial load of wrist
- Rotational injury of forearm
- No neurological deficits

Exam
- Tenderness to palpation between ECU and FCU, distal to the styloid, and proximal to the pisiform
- Painful grinding or clicking with wrist range of motion (ROM)
- TFC load test—axial load applied on an ulnarly deviated wrist
- Ulnar grind test—extension of wrist, axial load, and ulnar deviation
- Piano key sign (for radioulnar joint instability)—examiner tries to force the radius manually in dorsal and palmar directions vs the ulna, compares with contralateral side; excessive mobility suggests a complete peripheral tear of the TFCC

Testing
- X-rays—neutral forearm rotation, posterior-anterior (PA) and lateral
- Magnetic resonance imaging (MRI)—useful for diagnosis, variable findings in clinical studies depending on MRI machine parameters and radiologist expertise
- MR arthrography (may improve diagnostic yield)
- Wrist arthrograms, triple injection (radiocarpal, midcarpal, and distal radioulnar joint)—not specific, positive in 27% of asymptomatic adults, not frequently used
- Computed tomography (CT) arthrography
- Wrist arthroscopy—more accurate; diagnostic or therapeutic tool used in patients who fail conservative treatment
- Diagnostic injection—may localize pain source

Pitfalls
- Lack of suspicion may lead to missed diagnosis
- Not identifying cause (poor technique in tennis stroke, overload associated with floor exercises in gymnastics)

Red Flags
- Worsening symptoms with activity
- Pain at rest

Treatment

Medical
- Eight to 12 weeks of conservative therapy before considering surgery
- Nonsteroidal anti-inflammatory drugs (NSAIDs)
- Immobilization in slight flexion and ulnar deviation
- Long-arm casting for 4 to 6 weeks for traumatic tears
- Short-arm casting 3 to 4 weeks for degenerative tears

Exercises
- ROM
- Wrist ROM: flexion, extension, ulnar and radial deviation
- Forearm ROM: pronation, supination
- Stretching exercises when sharp pain goes away
- Wrist stretching: flexion, extension
- Strengthening exercises when stretching is nearly painless
- Wrist strengthening: flexion and extension
- Grip strengthening

Modalities
- Heat—paraffin
- Cryotherapy
- Transcutaneous electrical nerve stimulation
- Ultrasound

Injection
- Corticosteroid joint injections—no research studies

Surgical
- Open vs arthroscopic repair; trend toward arthroscopy
- Open reduction needed if DRUJ is unstable

Consults
- Orthopedic surgery
- Physical medicine and rehabilitation

Complications/side effects
- Continued pain with activity
- Inability to participate in sports
- Loss of grip strength

Prognosis
- Usually good

Helpful Hints
- Suspect TFCC injury in athletes with dorsal ulnar wrist pain
- Look for positive ulnar variance in x-rays

Suggested Readings
Ahn AK, Chang D, Plate AM. Triangular fibrocartilage complex tears: a review. *Bull Hosp Jt Dis.* 2006;64(3–4):114–118.

Henry MH. Management of acute triangular fibrocartilage complex injury of the wrist. *J Am Acad Orthop Surg.* 2008;16(6):320–329.

Loftus JB, Palmer AK. Disorders of the distal radioulnar joint and triangular fibrocartilage complex: an overview. In: Lichtman DM, Alexander AH, eds. *The Wrists and its Disorders.* 2nd ed. Philadelphia, PA: WB Saunders Company; 1997:385–414.

Wright PE. Wrist disorders. In: Canale ST, Beaty JH, eds. *Campbell's Operative Orthopaedics.* 11th ed. Philadelphia, PA: Mosby Elsevier; 2008:4044–4102.

Thoracic Disc Herniation

Joshua A. Thomas DO MBA ■ Larry H. Chou MD

Description
Thoracic disc herniation (TDH) is the displacement of the nucleus pulposus through a tear in the annulus fibrosis in the thoracic spine (rib-bearing vertebrae).

Etiology/Types
- The thoracic spine is an uncommon site of disc herniation due to the stabilizing effect of the rib cage
- The lower thoracic spine is most frequently involved
- Degenerative changes are the most common cause, although trauma may contribute:
  - Mild when the anterior epidural fat is preserved
  - Moderate when the epidural fat is obliterated, and the thecal sac is displaced
  - Severe when the cord is effaced or the nerve root is displaced
- Thoracic intervertebral discs can herniate vertically through the vertebral endplate and are called Schmorl's or cartilaginous nodes
- TDH classification
  - Central (70% of cases)
  - Centrolateral
  - Lateral
  - Intradural (<10% of cases)

Epidemiology
- TDH least common type of symptomatic intervertebral disc herniations (0.15%–1.8%)
- Up to 73% of asymptomatic individuals have abnormal thoracic disc findings such as bulges, herniations, annular tears, endplate deformation, or spinal cord compression
- At least 37% of asymptomatic individuals have at least one TDH, half of whom have multiple protrusions, many with deformation of the spinal cord
- Neurological findings due to TDH are estimated to be one in 1 million annually

Pathogenesis
- The discs are susceptible to injury with torsional and axial loads
- The kyphosis of the thoracic spine places the cord closer to the posterior longitudinal ligament (PLL),

vertebral bodies, and discs making the cord more susceptible to compression
- The thoracic spine houses a small spinal canal with narrow epidural space; small disc herniations may produce spinal cord compression
- Axial pain may be due to the nerves innervating the annulus fibrosis or PLL
- Radicular pain may be due to impingement or inflammation of the nerve root by the disc or due to stretching of the nerve root

Risk Factors
- Aging leads to decreased disc hydration, disc height, and increased axial load on the spine. This can lead to disc herniation
- Scheuermann's kyphosis can marginally increase the risk of thoracic herniations
- Any sport or activity that involves axial rotational of the spine

Clinical Features
- Pain is the most common symptom in 60% of patients
- Bladder and/or bowel symptoms are the presenting symptoms in only 2% of patients
- Cord compression is found in 70% of patients at the time at diagnosis
- Symptoms are often vague and poorly defined
- Patients with thoracic nerve root compromise may present with radicular pain and sensory disturbances. Weakness in the trunk or hands (with high TDH at T1-T2) may rarely occur
- TDH may present like an upper acute lumbar radiculopathy due to compression of the low thoracic nerve roots
- Central protrusions may cause spinal cord compression, and patients may present with myelopathic symptoms
- Schmorl's nodes usually do not cause symptoms and are rarely painful

Natural History
- TDH may be completely asymptomatic

- Preexisting thoracic herniations remain relatively unchanged, approximately 27% improve over a 3-year period
- In a series of patients with TDH, 27% required surgery due to progressive neurological decline or intractable pain

Diagnosis

Differential diagnosis

- DDD, stenosis, fracture, infection, Arteriovenous malformation (AVM), syrinx, and neoplasm should be considered
- Cardiovascular, pulmonary, renal, or gastrointestinal disorders may have similar symptoms
- Postherpetic neuralgia
- Intercostal neuralgia

History

- Weakness, paresthesias, radicular pain, and bowel and bladder dysfunction associated with myelopathy
- TDH most commonly has an insidious presentation without history of a significant antecedent trauma
- The initial symptom is pain followed by neurological deficits

Exam

- Examination may be normal
- It may reveal motor and sensory deficits, upper motor neuron signs (clonus, Babinski sign, spasticity, hyper-reflexia in the lower limbs), or rarely lower motor neuron signs (flaccidity, atrophy)
- If a sensory level is established, myelopathy should be strongly considered
- Maneuvers that stress the cervical and lumbar nerve roots should be performed to help rule out cervical and lumbosacral pathology

Testing

- X-ray findings include disc space narrowing, osteophyte formation, calcification, and kyphosis; but not diagnostic of TDH
- Disc calcification can be seen on plain radiograph not diagnostic of TDH
- Magnetic resonance imaging (MRI) can detect TDH, cord compression, disc degeneration, and nerve root impingement
- Electromyography may reveal findings suggestive of radiculopathy but it is difficult to establish a level in the thoracic spine
- Plain radiographs, MRI, and computed tomography (CT) alone or in combination can help rule out

other diagnostic possibilities such as compression fractures, rheumatological diseases, infection, and malignancies

Pitfalls

- Overinterpretation of imaging studies; improperly labeling a structural radiological abnormality as the pain generator

Red Flags

- Infection, fracture, neoplasm, and neurological dysfunction must be ruled out

Treatment

Medical

- Nonsteroidal anti-inflammatory medications, steroids, analgesics, muscle relaxants, and adjuvant analgesics

Exercises

- Goals are to improve posture, maintain flexibility, strengthen muscles, and prevent deconditioning
- Specific muscles to train are the rhomboids, trapezius, latissmus dorsi, spinal extensors, and deep abdominal musculature
- Training in posture and body mechanics
- Limit activities that increase intradiscal pressure such as twisting with an axial load, lifting, straining, sitting, and bending

Modalities

- Heat
- Ice
- Transcutaneous electrical nerve stimulation
- Ultrasound

Injection

- Epidural steroid injections may be used, but efficacy not clearly documented

Surgical

- Indications for surgical intervention include myelopathy or progressive neurological deficit
- Decompression is the mainstay of treatment and fusion is rarely required for TDH
- Anterior or lateral decompression via a thoracotomy with or without fusion is preferred unless the disc is easily accessible posteriorly

Consults

- Neurosurgeon
- Orthopedic/Spine surgeon
- Physical medicine and rehabilitation

Complications/side effects
- Progressive pain, weakness, and myelopathy are possible complications

Prognosis
- This is highly variable
- Return to previous activity occurs in 80% of patients who have no evidence of myelopathy

Helpful Hints
- High level of suspicion required to make early diagnosis

Suggested Readings

Are M, Burton AW. Thoracic spinal pain. In: Slipman CW, Derby R, Simeone FA, Mayer TG, eds. *Interventional Spine: An Algorithmic Approach*. Philadelphia, PA: WB Saunders Company; 2008:777–784.

Sheikh H, Samartzis D, Perez-Cruet MJ. Techniques for the operative management of thoracic disc herniation: minimally invasive thoracic microdiscectomy. *Orthop Clin North Am*. 2007;38(3):351–361.

Tokuhashi Y, Matsuzaki H, Uematsu Y, et al. Symptoms of thoracolumbar junction disc herniation. *Spine*. 2001;26(22):512–518.

Thoracic Outlet Syndrome

David J. Kennedy MD ■ Joel Press MD

Description

Any acquired, functional, or congenital anatomical change in the architecture of the cervicoaxillary canal that compromises the subclavian vessels or brachial plexus

Etiology/Types

- Arterial compression: <5%
- Venous compression: <5%
- True neurogenic: <5%
- Symptomatic: vast majority >90%. May represent mild or early form of vascular or neurogenic

Epidemiology

- Due to the lack of no objective tests, there is disagreement in regards to incidence, ranging from 3 to 80 cases per 1000 people
- Onset usually occurs between 20 and 50 years of age with 3:1 female-to-male ratio
- Most common groups that develop thoracic outlet syndrome (TOS) are post motor vehicle collision and nonergonomic computer users

Pathogenesis

- Compression of the lower trunk of the brachial plexus and/or subclavian vessels as they course through three narrow passageways from the base of the neck toward the axilla and the proximal arm
- The most common sites of compression are the costoclavicular space between clavicle and first rib (costoclavicular syndrome), the triangle between anterior scalene muscle and upper border of first rib (anterior scalene syndrome), and between the coracoid process and the pectoralis minor insertion (hyperabduction or pectoralis minor syndrome)
- Poor posture with protracted scapula and depressed shoulders can decrease diameter of cervicoaxillary canal
- Congenital abnormalities (including complete cervical rib, incomplete cervical rib with fibrous bands, fibrous bands from transverse process of C-7, and clavicular abnormalities) can compress the neurovascular bundle
- Traumatic fracture of clavicle with subsequent malunion, exuberant callus formation, or crush injury of upper thorax can also lead to neurovascular compromise

Risk Factors

- Poor posture with depressed shoulders and protracted scapula
- Repetitive overhead work or improper workstation ergonomics including assembly line workers, painters, plasterers, slaughterhouse workers, cash register operators, and welders
- Motor vehicle collision
- Overhead athletes (such as swimmers, volleyball players, and baseball pitchers), musicians, hikers, and weightlifters

Clinical Features

- Neck, shoulder, and arm pain; numbness, or impaired circulation to the upper extremities (causing discoloration, parathesias, aching, or heaviness)
- Arterial compression: coldness, weakness, intermittent blanching, easy fatigability of arm, and diffuse pain
- Venous compression: edema, cyanosis, increased circumference of upper extremity, distension of superficial veins of upper limb and shoulders
- Often nonspecific arm and hand numbness

Natural History

- Usually nonprogressive

Diagnosis

Differential diagnosis

- Cervical spondylosis and/or herniated cervical disc with radiculopathy
- Entrapment neuropathies such as carpal tunnel syndrome and ulnar nerve lesions at elbow

- Shoulder disorders such as impingement syndrome, rotator cuff injury, labral injuries; and shoulder instability
- Myofascial pain, or fibromyalgia
- Tendonitis or epicondylitis
- Complex regional pain syndrome
- Acute coronary syndrome
- Multiple sclerosis
- Vasculitis
- Pancoast tumor
- Neurofibroma
- Syringomyelia

History
- Gradual onset of upper extremity pain, parathesias, aching, or heaviness that is worse with overhead activities or sleeping with arm over head

Exam
- Physical examination to rule out other cervical or shoulder pathology
- Provocative maneuvers place the arm in a position to decrease the thoracic outlet diameter reproducing symptoms or decreasing radial pulse. Individually, they have high false positive and negative rates with poor sensitivity and specificity
- Costoclavicular and hyperabduction maneuvers
- Adson maneuver (performed with the patient sitting with hands on the thighs. The examiner palpates both radial pulses as the patient takes a deep breath and holds it while extending the neck and turning the head toward the affected side. If the radial pulse on the affected side is significantly diminished or there is numbness or tingling in the hand, the result is regarded as positive
- Wright test (hyperabduction of the arm with palpation of the radial pulse, reduction of pulse is considered a positive test)
- Roos stress test (ask the patient to abduct the shoulder to 90°, flex the elbow 90°, closed and open the hands for 1 to 3 minutes, reproduction of symptoms constitute a positive test)

Testing
- Chest, cervical, and shoulder x-rays
- Cervical radiography to evaluate for sources of referred pain
- Arterial and venous Doppler duplex scanning
- Somatosensor (SSEP) and electromyography with nerve conduction studies, and F-waves to may be useful to rule out other pathology

Pitfalls
- Failure to recognize symptoms or rule out other potential causes

Red Flags
- Signs of acute denervation on electromyography (EMG)
- Loss of strength
- Vascular findings on physical examination including discoloration, edema, or blanching

Treatment
Medical
- Usually no medications needed
- Nonsteroidal anti-inflammatory drugs (NSAIDs) or acetaminophen for symptomatic relief

Exercises
- Mainstay of treatment for all forms of TOS
- Focuses on "opening up" thoracic outlet by correcting abnormal posture
- Initially correct protracted and depressed shoulders with aggressive pectoralis and scalene stretching combined with correction of any scapulothoracic dysfunction
- Manual medicine to focus on: soft tissue mobilization, mobility of first rib, and resorting motion to sternoclavicular and acromioclavicular joints
- Side bending and cervical retraction can correct head forward posture by stretching soft tissues of lateral cervical spine
- Thoracic extension and brachial plexus stretching as tolerated
- Weight loss, stress reduction, and aerobic fitness have been shown to be beneficial

Modalities
- Typically none indicated
- Treatment of venous compression is often conservative with strict arm elevation, compression wraps, and possibly anticoagulants

Injections
- Trigger point injections controversial with limited studies evaluating their efficacy
- Injection of short-acting anesthetic into the anterior scalene, subclavius, or pectoralis minor muscles can assist in the diagnosis of TOS. This is referred to as a "scalene block"
- Botulinum toxin into the scalene muscles may be considered for patients with a positive diagnostic

scalene block, although there are limited data on the efficacy of this treatment

Surgical

- Cervical rib resection for patients with vascular compromise caused by complete cervical rib
- Neurogenic TOS that does not respond to aggressive upper limb and shoulder girdle therapy with identifiable anatomic correlate may need a surgical referral

Consults

- Physical medicine and rehabilitation
- Physical and occupational therapy
- Pain medicine for chronic TOS

Complications/side effects

- Deep vein thrombosis with venous constriction

Prognosis

- Symptomatic TOS usually responsive to conservative measures
- Vascular and true neurogenic are less likely to resolve completely with conservative measures and often require surgery to relieve pressure on the affected vessel or nerve

Helpful Hints

- Symptomatic TOS is a diagnosis of exclusion
- Think of TOS with any vague upper extremity symptoms

Suggested Reading

Sanders RJ, Hammond SL, Rao NM. Diagnosis of thoracic outlet syndrome. *J Vasc Surg.* 2007;46(3):601–604.

Trigger Finger

Gregory M. Worsowicz MD MBA

Description
Trigger finger or stenosing tenosynovitis of the hand results in difficulty with finger flexion to the point that the finger snaps or triggers into flexion and is difficult to extend. Progression can lead to locking of the digit in a flexed position.

Etiology/Types
- Inflammatory changes in the retinacular sheath and peritendinous tissue lead to involvement of the flexor tendon sheaths
- Overuse/repeated hand activity

Epidemiology
- Found in up to 2% to 3% of the general population
- Two peaks occur: under the age of 8 years and more commonly in the fifth and sixth decade
- Reported up to 10% in individuals with diabetes mellitus
- Female incidence greater than male
- Children less common, but thumb is affected in 90% of cases in this population

Pathogenesis
- Results from a discrepancy in the diameter of the flexor tendon and its sheath at the level of the metacarpal head
- High pressures occur at the proximal edge of the A_1 pulley on maximal flexion and tight grip; this is the most common site of pathology
- Inflammation of the A_1 pulley results in "pinching" of the flexor tendon that may lead to thickening and a nodule formation
- This discrepancy between the size of the flexor tendon sheath and the size of the tendon results in "triggering," which cannot be overcome by the finger extensors, hence finger is stuck in flexion
- Triggering of the digits results in further enlargement of the tendon and pulley with continued inflammation and degenerative changes

Risk Factors
- Repetitive finger movements or compressive forces on A_1 pulley
- Repetitive local trauma

- Diabetes mellitus
- Rheumatoid arthritis
- Hypothyroidism
- Osteoarthritis
- Gout
- Amylodosis
- Tendonitis of the upper extremity
- Carpal tunnel syndrome
- deQuervain tenosynovitis

Clinical Features
- Pain at level of distal palmar crease or metacarpophalangeal (MCP) joint
- Painful click as patient flexes finger
- Triggering or snapping with flexion
- Digit locked in a flexed position and difficulty with extension
- Pain with stretching finger into extension
- Palpable swelling or nodule
- Often occurs during sleep

Diagnosis

Differential diagnosis
- Dupuytren's contracture
- MCP sprain
- Fracture

History
- Discomfort in the palm with movement of involved digits
- Painful click with flexion and extension of involved digit
- Finger catching or locking

Exam
- Pain with forceful flexion (gripping)
- Pain on passive extension
- Demonstration of triggering
- Palpable nodule on palmar aspect of tendon at the MCP joint

Testing
- Imaging often not necessary or helpful
- Ultrasound may reveal thickening of the A_1 pulley, including during sleep

Treatment

Medical

- Nonsteroidal anti-inflammatory drugs
- Splinting: flexion blocking (decrease excursion around A_1 pulley), including during sleep
- Ergonomic grip change
- Activity modification

Modalities

- Cryotherapy
- Superficial heat/paraffin
- Ultrasound
- Iontophoresis

Injection

- Corticosteroid injection into the region of the A1 pulley

Surgical

- Percutaneous trigger release (A_1 pulley)
- Open surgical release (A_1 pulley)

Consults

- Hand surgery
- Physical medicine and rehabilitation

Complications/side effects

- Limited hand motion
- Pain/hand weakness affecting hand function
- Infection
- Complex regional pain syndrome

Prognosis

- Treatment with steroid injection leads to resolution of systems in up to 60% to 90% of cases
- Surgery indicated for longstanding or refractory cases
- Patients with diabetes mellitus have decreased response to steroids

Helpful Hints

- In patients with Type 1 diabetes mellitus, surgical release is often the treatment of choice
- Repeat steroid injections have a diminished response in patients who have had multiple injections or have long-standing symptoms
- Success rates of physical therapy and splinting are higher in younger children; decrease as they age

Suggested Readings

Akhtar S, Bradley J, Quinton D, et al. Management and referral for trigger finger/thumb. *Brit Med J.* 2005;331(7507):30–33.

Nimigan A, Ross DC, Gan BS. Steroid injections in the management of trigger fingers. *Am J Phys Med Rehabil.* 2006;85(1):36–43.

Rozenthal TD, Zurakowski D, Blazar PE. Trigger finger: prognostic indicators of recurrence following corticosteroid injection. *J Bone Joint Surg.* 2008;90(8):1665–1672.

Trochanteric Pain Syndrome (Bursitis)/Hip Abductor Tendinopathy

Steve Geringer MD

Description

In the past, *trochanteric bursitis* was used to describe nearly any musculoskeletal condition causing pain at the lateral hip. It now seems clear that many conditions that cause trochanteric pain syndrome are not bursitis. Hip abductor tendinopathy is the most common other diagnosis leading to this regional pain syndrome.

Etiology/Types

- Overuse, that is repetitive physical activities
- Abnormal pelvic or gait mechanics, for example with obesity, Trendelenburg gait from any cause, hip degenerative joint disease (DJD), lumbar spine conditions, and so on

Epidemiology

- For the activity-related causes, a young adult population is more widely represented
- For the remaining causes, a middle-age-to-older population prevails

Pathogenesis

- In cases of bursitis, the sac is irritated and inflamed
- With tendinopathy, microtears often occur, as confirmed by magnetic resonance imaging (MRI)

Risk Factors

- Overly aggressive or overly rapid physical activity, that is overuse
- Iliotibial band tightness
- Obesity
- Abnormal lumbar, pelvic, or hip mechanics from any cause

Clinical Features

- Pain in the lateral hip just superior, posterior to, and/or over the greater trochanter
- Pain may refer distally through the lateral thigh toward the knee
- Symptoms worse with physical activity, relieved with rest

Natural History

- Insidious onset most common
- Can arise from a single bout of strenuous activity, especially with a predisposing cause present

Diagnosis

Differential diagnosis

- Iliotibial band syndrome
- Osteoarthritis of the hip
- Lateral femoral cutaneous neuropathy (meralgia paresthetica)
- Femoral head avascular necrosis (AVN)
- Femoral head or neck fracture
- Mid-lumbar radiculopathy
- Lumbar plexopathy

History

- Pain, mostly isolated to the lateral hip
- Recent increase in training regimen, either in frequency or intensity of exercise
- Recent introduction of new dance technique or maneuver
- Suboptimal stretching routine

Examination: bursitis

- Focal tenderness over and superior to greater trochanter
- Pain with Ober's maneuver (patient lies on the uninvolved hip, the symptomatic hip is abducted, extended, and subsequently adducted to the examination table, reproduction of pain may considered a positive test)
- Positive Patrick's test (pain lateral hip, with flexion abduction and external rotation "FABERE")
- Possible predisposing factors: leg length discrepancy, pelvic asymmetry, Trendelenburg gait, and so on

Examination: gluteal tendinitis

- Local tenderness at superior aspect of trochanter
- In some cases, tenderness over origin of gluteus medius at the lateral iliac crest
- Pain with Ober maneuver
- Pain with resisted hip abduction

Testing

- No testing typically needed at first diagnosis
- X-ray if needed to confirm hip DJD
- MRI is indicated with any concern of AVN
- MRI can detect microtears of the hip abductor group, but is rarely needed for that reason

Pitfalls

- It is critical to never miss an unexpected cause of lateral hip pain, for example a fracture or AVN
- Therefore, while diagnostic testing is rarely needed with initial diagnosis, and in particular with "routine" cases, imaging should be done if symptoms persist, especially if they are atypical

Red Flags

- Pain that is not localized directly over the trochanter or just adjacent to it
- Pain that is felt deep within the area, not superficially
- Pain with maneuvers that stress the hip joint

Treatment

Medical

- Weight loss if obesity is a factor
- Correction of mechanical problems, for example leg length discrepancy or abnormal lumbar mechanics
- When overuse is causative, modify training schedule—revert to 80% of prior pain-free level, then advance more gradually

Exercises

- Hip rotator stretching
- Hip and gluteal muscle strengthening

Modalities

- Cryotherapy
- Superficial heat
- Electrical stimulation
- Ultrasound (followed by stretching)

Injection

- Inject down to bursa or insertion of gluteal tendons at superior aspect of trochanter

- Use typical fan-shaped pattern to distribute injectate adequately
- Diagnostic and/or therapeutic injection using anesthetic with or without corticosteroid

Surgical

- Rarely needed; consider for refractory cases in high-level athletes, including dancers
- Iliotibial lengthening/release, debridement of gluteal tendons and bursa

Consults

- Physical medicine and rehabilitation
- Orthopedic surgery if no response to conservative treatment

Complications/side effects

- Usual (rare) complications from injection, especially infection
- Any potential surgical complication

Prognosis

- Usually very good, if the predisposing or causative factor can be successfully addressed
- Guarded with a recalcitrant predisposing factor, for example obesity

Helpful Hints

- Although commonly described as a bursitis, symptoms are associated with insertional tendinopathy
- Management should include muscle strengthening
- In patients who do not improve or have leg pain, consider underlying radiculopathy

Suggested Readings

Alvarez-Nemegyei J, Canoso JJ. Evidence-based soft tissue rheumatology: III: trochanteric bursitis. *J Clin Rheumatol.* 2004;10(3):123–124.

Silva F, Adams T, Feinstein J, Arroyo RA. Trochanteric bursitis: refuting the myth of inflammation. *J Clin Rheumatol.* 2008;14(2):82–86.

Turf Toe

Tiffany C.K. Forman MD ■ Andrew W. Nichols MD

Description

Turf toe is an injury of the capsuloligamentous complex located on the plantar aspect of the first metatarsophalangeal (MTP) joint. The capsuloligamentous complex consists of the sesamoid phalangeal (SP) ligaments, metatarsosesamoid ligaments, intersesamoid ligaments, joint capsule, plantar plate, and collateral ligaments.

Etiology/Types

- Turf toe is classified based upon the severity of injury
- Grade 1 injury: stretch of the capsuloligamentous complex without gross disruption
- Grade 2 injury: partial tear of the capsuloligamentous complex
- Grade 3 injury: complete tear of the capsuloligamentous complex and may also include articular cartilage injury, subchondral bone injury, sesamoid fracture, separation of a bipartite sesamoid, and dislocation of the first MTP joint with spontaneous reduction

Epidemiology

- The incidence of turf toe has increased in parallel with higher exposures to artificial turf surfaces and the usage of lighter, more flexible, and less protective athletic footwear. Fifty-seven percent of US football players report having experienced turf toe injury, and 84% recall that their initial injuries occurred while playing on artificial turf surfaces

Pathogenesis

- Turf toe injury typically results from a first MTP joint hyperdorsiflexion force
- A common mechanism is foot is planted, toes dorsiflexed, while the foot sustains a concomitant axial force to the heel
- The plantar capsuloligamentous structures are stretched with resultant tears that may involve the joint capsule and collateral ligaments, and fractures that may affect the proximal dorsal phalanx, metatarsal head, and sesamoids
- Varus and valgus injuries are also possible

Risk Factors

- Cutting and pivoting running sports
- Excessively light and flexible athletic footwear
- Artificial turf surfaces

Clinical Features

- Pain along the plantar aspect of the first MTP joint with localized swelling and tenderness
- Pain with active and passive motion of the first MTP joint
- Pain with ambulation

Natural History

- May present as an acute injury, chronic injury as a result of repetitive joint stress, and finally osteoarthritis

Diagnosis

Differential diagnosis

- Sesamoid dysfunction/sesamoiditis
- Sesamoid stress fracture
- Bipartite sesamoid diastasis
- Metatarsal or phalangeal fracture
- Flexor hallucis longus/brevis strain or tendinopathy
- Gout
- Osteoarthritis

History

- Significant pain and swelling at the first MTP joint due to a hyperdorsiflexion injury mechanism
- Difficulty pushing off the injured foot and great toe

Exam

- Grade 1: mild edema, no visible ecchymosis, little reduction in joint range of motion (ROM), able to bear weight
- Grade 2: edema and ecchymosis over the first MTP joint, restricted ROM, pain causes limp, partial weight bearing
- Grade 3: marked edema and ecchymosis over the first MTP joint, severe pain and tenderness, markedly restricted ROM, avoidance of weight bearing due to severe pain
- Dorsoplantar translation test is useful to assess joint and capsuloligament complex stability by comparing with the contralateral toe

Testing

- Plain radiographs (anteriopposterior, lateral, oblique, and sesamoid axial views) to identify capsular avulsion, sesamoid fracture, compression fracture, bipartite sesamoid separation, and proximal sesamoid migration
- Hyperdorsiflexion stress view with comparison to demonstrate ligamentous laxity or disruption
- Follow-up radiographs may demonstrate interval proximal migration of the sesamoids indicating a disruption of the plantar plate or sesamoid fracture with callous formation
- Magnetic resonance imaging (MRI) with special imaging protocols should be considered in the presence of x-ray abnormalities, Grades 2 and 3 sprains, and to identify soft tissue injury

Pitfalls

- Sesamoid abnormalities may go undetected if contralateral comparison views and/or follow-up x-rays are not obtained
- Allowing premature return to play
- If not identified and treated promptly, turf toe may lead to significant morbidity, a prolonged recovery, and chronic symptoms

Red Flags

- Worse pain with return to activity
- Continued swelling and limitation of motion

Treatment

Medical

- Initial nonoperative treatment including rest, ice, compression, and elevation
- Nonsteroidal anti-inflammatory drug (NSAID) medications may reduce pain and inflammation
- Restrict first MTP joint dorsiflexion by use of taping, rigid insole, or casting/walking boot
- Grade 3 injuries require immobilization and long-term protective weight bearing

Exercises

- Rest until pain-free full ROM returns
- Begin light stretching and functional rehabilitation once symptoms allow

Modalities

- Ice

- Electrical stimulation
- Pulsed or direct ultrasound
- Iontophoresis

Injection

- Injection with corticosteroids is not recommended as this may inhibit healing

Surgical

- Often indicated in the presence of fractures, osteochondral avulsions, and nonreduced joint dislocations
- Occasionally for sequelae including hallux valgus, claw toe, osteochondral nonunions, sesamoid nonunions, hallux rigidus, and osteoarthritis

Consults

- Orthopedic surgery for Grade 3 and some Grade 2 injuries

Complications/side effects

- Osteoarthritis (hallux rigidus) and instability of the first MTP joint
- Persistent symptoms
- Loss of push-off strength

Prognosis

- Athletes with Grade 1 or 2 injury can usually return to play within 2 to 4 weeks as symptoms resolve
- Athletes with Grade 3 injury require prolonged rest with return to play at 6 to 8 weeks if the joint regains stability

Helpful Hints

- Pain and joint motion most important guideline for determining progression of rehabilitation and activity
- MRI may be useful in determining the severity of injury and guide operative vs nonoperative treatment courses

Suggested Readings

Crain JM, Phancao JP, Stidham K. MR imaging of turf toe. *Magn Reson Imaging Clin N Am.* 2008;16:93–103.

Maskill JD, Bohay DR, Anderson JG. First ray injuries. *Foot Ankle Clin.* 2006;11:143–163.

Mullen JE, O'Malley MJ. Sprains-residual instability of subtalar, Lisfranc joints, and turf toe. *Clin Sports Med.* 2004; 23:97–121.

Ulnar Collateral Ligament Injury of the Elbow

Marc Safran MD

Description

The ulnar collateral ligament (UCL) is a structure that maintains the normal alignment of the humerus and the ulna. This ligament is injured in throwing types of sports or after elbow dislocation or surgery. Damage may occur as a sudden tear or gradually stretch over time with repetitive injury. When torn, this ligament usually does not heal or it may heal in a lengthened position.

Etiology/Types

- Overuse injury associated with throwing sports and repeated overhead activity
- It may occur as a result of a fall on an outstretched hand, with or without an elbow dislocation
- It may occur as a result of surgery
- Ligament sprains are classified into three grades
  - Grade I: lengthened, but is painful
  - Grade II: stretched but still functions
  - Grade III: torn and does not function

Epidemiology

- Increased risk in those involved in throwing sports, such as baseball, javelin, as well as volleyball and tennis
- Increased risk in sports where one may fall on an outstretched hand—wrestling, football, and rugby

Pathogenesis

- Throwing sports may result in repetitive valgus force to the elbow; pitching a baseball has been shown to produce up to 67 Nm of force to the inner elbow, and the UCL has been shown to be able to resist only 32 Nm force
- Repetitive throwing when the UCL is injured may result in overuse of the flexor—pronator muscles of the wrist muscles and ulnar nerve irritation
- Injury and looseness of the UCL may lead to radiocapitellar joint chondromalacia, osteophytes, and loose bodies
- Injury and looseness of the UCL may lead to valgus extension overload, as the olecranon shears and is impacted into the olecranon fossa. This may result in chondromalacia, osteophytes, loose bodies, and loss of elbow motion

Risk Factors

- Throwing and overhead sports
- Poor physical conditioning
- Improper throwing mechanics
- Contact sports

Clinical Features

- Pain and tenderness on the inner side of the elbow, especially when trying to throw
- A pop, tearing, or pulling sensation may be noted at the time of injury
- Swelling and bruising (after 24 hours) at the inner elbow and upper forearm if an acute tear
- Inability to throw at full speed, loss of ball control
- Elbow stiffness, inability to straighten the elbow
- Numbness and/or tingling in the ring and little fingers
- Clumsiness and weakness of hand grip

Natural History

- High level baseball pitchers usually have some looseness of the UCL
- Most people can throw up to 80% of maximum without problems with UCL injury
- The UCL is not needed for day-to-day living but symptoms may be associated with weightlifting
- The UCL usually does not heal sufficiently on its own with nonoperative treatment
- To return to throwing, surgery is often necessary

Diagnosis

Differential diagnosis

- Medial epicondylitis
- Valgus extension overload
- Ulnar neuritis

History

- A pop, tearing, or pulling sensation of the inner elbow may be noted at the time of injury
- Swelling and bruising (after 24 hours) if an acute tear
- Inability to throw at full speed, loss of ball control

- Locking or catching of the elbow
- Inability to fully straighten the elbow
- Pain with gripping

Exam
- Pain and tenderness on the inner side of the elbow, especially when trying to throw
- Elbow stiffness and extension deficits
- Pain and/or laxity with stress testing
- Numbness and/or tingling in the ring and little fingers
- Clumsiness and weakness of hand grip

Testing
- X-rays are usually normal, but may show avulsion fractures (uncommon) or calcification within the ligament
- Stress radiographs showing >2 mm increased widening as compared with the normal side is consistent with UCL
- Magnetic resonance imaging (MRI) may show torn UCL
- MRI arthrogram is more sensitive at detecting UCL tear and coexistent pathology
- MRI arthrograms or computed tomography (CT) arthrogram may show partial tears of the UCL (dye tracking distally, under the ligament at the ulna)
- There is a very high incidence (>80%) of abnormal changes on MRI within the UCL in asymptomatic professional baseball pitchers
- Ultrasound has also been shown to be effective

Pitfalls
- Overinterpretation of imaging studies
- Under diagnosis, laxity is not great and thus the diagnosis is often missed, misdiagnosed, or the severity is underappreciated

Red Flags
- Neuropathic symptoms
- Fracture
- Progressive pain
- Loose bodies

Treatment

Medical
- Nonsteroidal anti-inflammatory medications
- Analgesics
- Splinting acutely

- Bracing

Exercises
- Elbow range of motion
- Elbow and wrist flexion strengthening
- Throwing program for gradual return to throwing
- Throwing mechanics evaluation

Modalities
- Heat
- Transcutaneous electrical nerve stimulation
- Ultrasound

Injection
- Consider for persistent medial epicondylitis symptoms

Surgical
- Reconstruction of ligament

Consults
- Orthopedic surgery

Complications
- Frequent recurrence of symptoms
- Inability to throw at full speed or distance, pain with throwing, loss of ball control
- Injury to cartilage of the outer elbow, loose body formation, injury to the ulnar nerve, and muscles that originate at the medial epicondyle
- Elbow arthritis
- Elbow stiffness

Prognosis
- Complete rupture in nonthrowers is usually well-tolerated
- Some throwers (up to 42%) have chronic injury to the UCL and may continue to throw effectively without surgery. Some may have repeated bouts of intermittent elbow pain
- Complete rupture or attenuation in throwers often requires UCL reconstruction

Helpful Hints
- Suspect UCL injury in any thrower with medial elbow pain

Suggested Reading
Safran MR, Ahmad C, El Attrache N. Ulnar collateral ligament injuries of the elbow: current concepts. *J Arthrosc Relat Surg.* 2005;21(11):1381–1395.

Ulnar Neuropathy

Steve Gnatz MD

Description
Ulnar neuropathy often results from inflammation or compression of the ulnar nerve, which produces paresthesias and weakness in the forearm and hand.

Etiology/Types
- Compression of nerve segments
- Elbow joint derangement
- Elbow intra-articular loose bodies
- Ganglion cysts
- Direct nerve trauma or transection
- Nerve infarction
- Radiation exposure
- Inflammatory processes of the nerve
- Infectious disorders such as herpes simplex, Epstein-Barr virus, and herpes zoster virus can produce sensory loss and motor dysfunction
- Metabolic problems such as diabetes mellitus or hypothyroidism
- Compression of nerve at other sites such as the wrist

Epidemiology
- Ulnar neuropathy at the elbow (UNE) is the second most common entrapment neuropathy after carpal tunnel syndrome (CTS)
- Patients who repeatedly lean on their elbows are at greater risk

Pathogenesis
- Ulnar neuropathy at the elbow
  - Potential sites of entrapment
  - The ulnar groove just proximal to the medial epicondyle
  - The humeroulnar aponeurotic arcade
  - The exit site from the deep flexor pronator aponeurosis
  - Tardy ulnar palsy is described in patients who experience UNE months to years after elbow trauma has occurred
  - Repeated subluxation of the nerve with elbow flexion over the medial epicondyle may also contribute to UNE
  - The cubital tunnel may be congenitally small, and repeated elbow flexion and extension can produce UNE

- Ulnar neuropathy at the wrist
  - The ulnar nerve travels through Guyon's canal into the wrist. Compression can occur in the canal itself or distally, in the proximal hand

Risk Factors
- Family history of diabetes
- Alcoholism
- Presence of human immunodeficiency virus

Clinical Features
- Sensory loss and paresthesias over digits 4 and 5, and the ulnar aspect of the dorsum of the hand
- Weakness of the interosseous muscles of the hand
- Pain in the region of the elbow
- Weakness in finger and wrist flexion
- Claw hand and the inability of the entire thumb to move to the forefinger in a single motion

Natural History
- If nerve damage has been caused by minor trauma such as putting too much pressure on the elbow or wrist, recovery can be complete

Diagnosis

Differential diagnoses
- C8 radiculopathy
- Lower trunk brachial plexus injury
- Martin-Gruber anastomosis (MGA) and CTS

History
- The patient may complain of worsened grip and clumsiness
- Routinely resting the elbow on a hard surface
- Recent surgery where arm was kept in pronation or flexion for prolonged periods
- Fracture of the elbow

Exam
- Numbness/tingling fourth and fifth digits
- Tinel's sign (pain/tingling with tapping over the nerve) in the region of the elbow (high false positives)
- Froment's sign is demonstrated when the patient is unable to grip a piece of paper between the thumb and first digit

- Loss of elbow range of motion or elbow valgus deformity
- Decreased pinch strength
- Atrophy of the hypothenar eminence and/or hand intrinsic muscles in severe cases
- Confrontational strength testing

Testing
- X-ray to evaluate the bony architecture of the elbow should be performed after trauma
- Ultrasonography to exclude ganglion cysts
- Computed tomography or magnetic resonance imaging for deeper structural lesions
- Nerve conduction studies (NCS) demonstrates a drop in amplitude across the entrapped segment and a slowing of motor nerve conduction (Figure 1)
- "Inching" studies (short segmental electrodiagnostic testing) have been recommended to help localize the lesion
- Sensory NCS of the ulnar nerve at the wrist and dorsal ulnar cutaneous nerve can show reduction of amplitude if the lesion is axonal
- Electromyography (EMG): with ulnar axonal type injury, signs of abnormal muscle membrane irritability, such as positive waves and fibrillations are seen in ulnar innervated muscles

Pitfalls
- MGA may result in the mistaken diagnosis of UNE at the elbow if the cross-over fibers of the MGA are very proximal (shows a drop in compound muscle action potential across the elbow during NCS)

Red Flags
- In progressive weakness of hand intrinsic muscles without sensory loss consider motor neuron disease

Treatment

Medical
- Anti-inflammatory drugs
- Membrane stabilizers (gabapentin, pregabalin)
- Splints and cushions
  - Night splints can prevent prolonged elbow flexion at night by holding the elbow in mild flexion
  - Prescribing a foam elbow pad can decrease external pressure on the ulnar nerve

Exercises
- Hand intrinsic muscle strengthening
- Elbow flexor/pronator muscle stretching

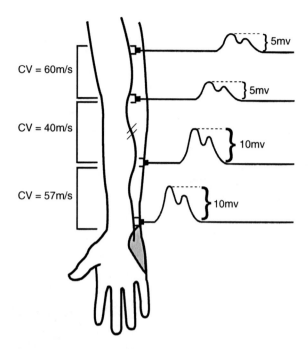

Figure 1. Nerve conduction studies.

Modalities
- Low voltage electrical stimulation can be considered in partial nerve injury

Injection
- Steroid injection, however, local steroids plus splinting may not provide additional relief when compared with splinting alone

Surgical
- Decompression of the nerve under the humerulnar aponeurotic arcade
- Transposition of the nerve anterior to the medial epicondyle
- Medial epicondylectomy
- One study suggested the outcomes of simple decompression and anterior subcutaneous transposition are equivalent; however, simple decompression has a lower complication rate

Consults
- Neurosurgery
- Orthopedic surgery
- Physical medicine and rehabilitation or neurologist for electrodiagnostic studies

Complications/side effects
- Severe injury may result in lasting weakness and muscle atrophy

Prognosis

■ Good if diagnosed early and causative factors are avoided

Helpful Hints

■ Rule out ulnar entrapment in patients with hand numbness and normal median nerve latencies
■ Suspect ulnar entrapment in patients with hand numbness and weakness following surgery

Suggested Readings

Bartels R, Verhagen W, van der Wilt G, et al. Prospective randomized controlled study comparing simple decompression versus anterior subcutaneous transposition for idiopathic neuropathy of the ulnar nerve at the elbow: part 1. *Neurosurgery*. 2005;56(3):522–530.

Gnatz SG. *EMG Basics*. Columbia, MO: Academic Information Systems; 2001:19–25.

Hong CZ, Long HA, Kanakamedala RV, et al. Splinting and local steroid injection for the treatment of ulnar neuropathy at the elbow: clinical and electrophysiological evaluation. *Arch Phys Med Rehabil*. 1996;77:573.

Whiplash

Gerald Malanga MD

Description

Whiplash is an acceleration-deceleration mechanism of energy transfer to the neck that occurs primarily after motor vehicle collisions, although it can occur during other mishaps. This impact may result in bony or soft tissue injuries, which can lead to a variety of clinical manifestations known as whiplash-associated disorders (WAD).

Etiology/Types

- Clinical classification of WAD as per Quebec Task Force on WAD:
  - Grade I—neck complaint of pain, stiffness, or tenderness without physical signs
  - Grade II—neck complaint and musculoskeletal sign(s)
  - Grade III—neck complaint and neurological sign(s)
  - Grade IV—neck complaint and fracture or dislocation

Epidemiology

- Incidence of reported WAD in western countries has increased over the past 30 years
- Annual incidence in North America and western Europe is at least 300 per 100,000 inhabitants

Pathogenesis

- A collision in any direction can cause whiplash, but classically occurs with rear-end impact
- Within 50 to 75 ms after impact, the lower cervical spine is thrust upward and forward. Lower cervical segments are extended while the upper segments are relatively flexed. The net result is an S-shaped cervical spine curve
- By 160 ms postimpact, the head begins to move upward and backward forcing the cervical spine into extension while the trunk is moving anteriorly, pulling the base of the neck moves forward. The net result is extension of the cervical spine
- This results in abnormal separation of anterior elements of the neck and abnormal patterns of compression posteriorly

- Cervical zygapophyseal joints are prone to compressive injuries, including compression fracture, tears of the joint capsule, and hemarthrosis. This may lead to facet-mediated pain
- Muscle strains of posterior muscles
- Fractures of posterior structures including laminae and pedicles can occur
- Injury to the ligamentous structures, including alar ligaments and anterior longitudinal ligament have been documented
- Intervertebral disc pathology is less common than injury to posterior elements
- Fractures of the atlas or axis are possible, but more commonly seen in dramatic events resulting in death or serious neurological injury

Risk Factors

- Inconclusive evidence exists supporting specific risk factors

Clinical Features

- Neck pain
- Headache
- Shoulder, scapular, and/or arm pain
- Dizziness
- Visual disturbances (blurred vision, diploplia)
- Tinnitus
- Low back pain
- Memory and concentration difficulties

Natural History

- Delay in onset of symptoms up to 24 hours is characteristic
- Recovery is extremely variable with reports of 50% to 98% complete recovery within the first year
- Recovery is slower in those with greater initial symptom severity

Diagnosis

Differential diagnosis

- Cervical osteoarthritis
- Cervical radiculopathy
- Cervical myelopathy

- Psychogenic pain disorder
- Polymyalgia rheumatica
- Infection
- Malignancy

History
- Aching pain in posterior cervical region radiating to trapezius ridge, scapula, occiput, and/or down the arms
- Mixed headache pattern
- Blurry vision
- Dizziness or vertigo-type symptoms
- Tinnitus
- Low back pain with or without radicular symptoms

Exam
- Abnormal posture: forward flexed neck, rounded shoulders, asymmetric shoulder heights, neck rotation or tilt
- Local cervical paraspinal point tenderness with muscular tender or trigger points
- Decreased cervical active and passive range of motion (ROM)
- If cervical radiculopathy is present, neurological signs including weakness, decreased sensation, and decreased or absent reflexes

Testing
- No gold standard diagnostic test imaging
- Radiographs indicated for all patients with Grade II or III WAD
- Magnetic resonance imaging (MRI) indicated only if ligamentous or neurological injury suspected
- Electromyography (EMG) if nerve injury suspected

Pitfalls
- Overinterpretation of imaging studies
- Prolonged use of passive treatment and modalities
- Missing concomitant postconcussive symptoms

Red Flags
- Infection
- Fracture
- Neoplasm
- Neurological dysfunction

Treatment

Medical
- Early rehabilitation and resumption of normal activity has the best evidence for recovery and the prevention of chronic symptoms

- The use of passive modalities and treatments should be minimized
- Proper use of analgesics to control pain and inflammation, mitigate deconditioning, and facilitate participation in functional restorative program
- Active physical therapy stressing restoration of motion and improved dynamic muscle strength and head control

Exercises
- Early active therapies with mobilization is imperative
- Multimodal therapy focused on postural conditioning, ROM exercises, proprioceptive retraining, manual treatments, psychological support, and patient education
- Immobilization with/without cervical collar should be avoided

Modalities
- Should be used only as adjuncts to active mobilization
- Transcutaneous electrical nerve stimulation (TENS) in chronic cases after an appropriate trial demonstrates at least a 50% reduction of pain
- Superficial heat in the early phases of pain control and reactivation

Injection
- No strong evidence exists for intra-articular steroid injections or radiofrequency neurotomy for WAD neck pain
- Epidural or selective nerve root injections may provide short-term symptomatic relief
- Trigger point injections with lidocaine or sterile water may be used as an adjunct to active mobilization
- Botox injections remain unproven in this population
- Facet joint injections, medial branch blocks
- Radiofrequency ablation of medial branches that innervates the cervical zygoapophyseal joint

Surgical
- Decompression/fusion for myeloradiculopathy or cervical instability

Consults
- Neurological or orthopedic/spine surgery
- Psychologist or psychiatrist
- Physical medicine and rehabilitation

Complications/side effects
- Persistent pain and dysfunction

- Persistent loss of cervical lordosis
- Altered sleep
- Depression

Prognosis

- Generally very good with 80% fully recovered by 6 months
- Recovery is slower in those with greater initial symptoms severity
- Psychological factors such as postinjury psychological distress and passive types of coping are prognostic of poorer recovery
- Frequent, early utilization of the healthcare system in the first month postinjury is associated with poorer recovery
- Between 14% and 50% of patients may develop chronic neck pain of more than 1 year
- Worse outcomes in patients involved in litigation

Helpful Hints

- Early reactivation and resumption of normal activity has the best evidence for recovery and the prevention of chronic symptoms
- The use of passive modalities and treatments should be minimized
- Physical and psychological issues are interrelated and should be addressed concurrently, particularly in the chronic pain situation

Suggested Readings

Hurwitz EL, Carragee EJ, van der Velde G, et al. Treatment of Neck Pain: Noninvasive interventions: results of the Bone and Joint Decade 2000–2010 Task Force on neck pain and its associated disorders. *Spine.* 2008;33(suppl 4):S123-S152.

Spitzer WO, Skovron ML, Salmi LR, et al. Scientific monograph of the quebec task force on whiplash-associated disorders: redefining "whiplash" and its management. *Spine.* 1995;20(suppl):1S-73S.

Index

Abductor pollicis longus (APL), 67
Acetaminophen
　for adhesive capsulitis, 17
　for ankle sprain, 20
　for calcaneal apophysitis, 37
　for compression fractures, 65
　for epiphyseal injuries, of ankle, 75
　for HOA, 146
　for juvenile OCD, 156
　for lumbar facet syndrome, 117
　for stress fractures, 227
　for thoracic outlet syndrome, 244
Achilles tendinopathy, 6
　footwear modifications, 7
　functional biomechanical deficits, 6
　functional rehabilitation, 7
　heel lift, 7
　jogging, 7
　nonsteroidal anti-inflammatory medications, 7
　overuse injury, 6
Achilles tendon stretching
　for PTTD, 181
　for TTS, 235
Achilles tendon tear, 8
　dynamic strengthening initial exercises, 9
　gradual range of motion of ankle, 9
　nonoperative management, 9
　orthopedic/foot-ankle surgery, 10
　progressive stretching, 9
　static ankle exercises, 9
Acromioclavicular (AC) joint injuries, 11–13
　anti-inflammatory/analgesic treatment, 12
　classification of, 11f
　dynamic strengthening, 12–13
　range of motion exercises, 12
Active assistive ROM (AAROM), for radial head fracture, 191
Active range of motion (ROM), for meniscal tears, 131
Active ROM, for SLL, 204
Activity modification
　biceps tendinopathy, 35
　for calcaneal apophysitis, 37
　for chronic exertional leg compartment syndrome, 59
　for coccygodynia, 61
　for CTS, 39
　for De Quervain's tenosynovitis, 68
　for trigger finger, 247
　for TTS, 235
Acupuncture
　for chest pain, musculoskeletal, 57
　for fibromyalgia, 87

　for lumbar facet syndrome, 117
　for stress fractures, 225
Acute brachial plexus neuropathy. See Neuralgic amyotrophy
Acute calcific tendinitis, of shoulder, 14–15
Adhesive capsulitis, 15
　of shoulder, 16–18
Aerobic exercise
　for arachnoiditis, 31
　for lumbar facet syndrome, 117
　for lumbar myofascial pain, 119
　for meralgia paresthetica, 133
　for MPS, 47
　for scoliosis, 210
　for spondylisthesis, 219
Alcohol avoidance, for osteoporosis, 160
Alendronate (Fosamax), 160
Aluminum splint, for mallet finger, 125
Amitriptyline, for sleep dysfunction
　in fibromyalgia, 86
　for PPS, 168
Anabolic steroids, for quadriceps contusion, 185
Analgesic drugs, for hip adductor strains, 95
Analgesic medications
　for arachnoiditis, 30
　for meniscal tears, 131
Analgesics
　for ACL tear, 26
　for acute calcific tendinitis, 15
　for AVN of hip, 97
　for avulsion injuries, 33
　biceps tendinopathy, 35
　for cervical facet syndrome, 45
　for cervical spinal stenosis, 53
　for CRPS, 63
　for Hamstring strain, 93
　for iliopsoas tendinopathy, 105
　for LLE, 113
　for lumbar myofascial pain, 119
　for MCL injury, 127
　for metatarsalgia, 135
　for MPS, 47
　for neuralgic amyotrophy, 139
　for OA of knee, 151
　for osteitis pubis, 144
　for pain control, in fibromyalgia, 86
　for pes anserine bursitis, 173
　for piriformis syndrome, 174
　for PPS, 168
　for Scheuermann's disease, 207
　for shoulder dislocation, 212

CPSIA information can be obtained
at www.ICGtesting.com
Printed in the USA
LVOW09*1623140317
527186LV00010B/323/P